Canine and Feline Behavior Therapy

Second Edition

Canine and Feline Behavior Therapy

Second Edition

Benjamin L. Hart
Lynette A. Hart
Melissa J. Bain

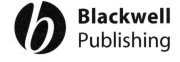
Blackwell Publishing

Blackwell Publishing Professional
2121 State Avenue, Ames, Iowa 50014, USA

Orders: 1-800-862-6657
Office: 1-515-292-0140
Fax: 1-515-292-3348
Web site: www.blackwellprofessional.com

Blackwell Publishing Ltd
9600 Garsington Road, Oxford OX4 2DQ, UK
Tel.: +44 (0)1865 776868

Blackwell Publishing Asia
550 Swanston Street, Carlton, Victoria 3053, Australia
Tel.: +161 (0)3 8359 1011

First edition, 1985
Second edition, 2006

Library of Congress Cataloging-in-Publication Data

Hart, Benjamin L.
  Canine and feline behavior therapy / B.L. Hart, L.A. Hart, M.J. Bain.— 2nd ed.
    p. cm.
  Includes bibliographical references and index.
  ISBN-13: 978-0-683-03912-2 (alk. paper)
  ISBN-10: 0-683-03912-1 (alk. paper)
  1. Dogs—Behavior therapy. 2. Cats—Behavior therapy. I. Hart, Lynette A.
II. Bain, M. J. (Melissa J.) III. Title.

SF433.H36 2006
636.7'089689—dc22

2005028552

The last digit is the print number: 9 8 7 6 5 4 3 2 1

This book is dedicated to our canine and feline companions—past and present—especially Mattie, Thumper, and Monkey, who have so enriched our understanding of companion animal behavior.

Table of Contents

Preface

Behavior medicine is perhaps the most rapidly emerging discipline in animal health care. Increasingly, dog and cat owners are seeking information about the normal behavior of cats and dogs and requesting help in dealing with behavior problems. To some extent, this parallels the increasing sophistication of animal owners concerning the science of animal behavior, an interest stimulated by popular books on dog and cat behavior as well as movies and television specials on animals.

Books on dog and cat behavior frequently refer to behavior problems. In dogs, the most frequent problem is some type of aggressive behavior; in cats, house soiling. Other common problems are those related to fear and anxiety, barking, and destructive activities. Although there are therapeutic approaches to most problem behaviors, clinical research is active and new solutions or improvements are reported on a regular basis. Despite clinical advancements, however, euthanasia is still too frequently the answer to a serious behavior problem. Aside from the unnecessary loss of life of a companion animal, we sometimes have to remind our colleagues in the veterinary medical specialties that to save a pet from the fate of euthanasia by resolving a behavior problem is as meaningful to the pet owner as saving the animal's life by the diligent use of clinical tests or the performance of a skillful surgical operation. Sometimes a behavior problem is the primary disruptive influence in family dynamics, even more so than an illness of the pet.

Despite the image sometimes projected by popular writers, behavior therapy should not be thought of as the art of dealing with overindulged, pampered pets. The concepts and principles of behavior therapy are useful for treating serious problems that occur in relatively normal families.

Behavior therapy is not a highly technical field suitable for only a handful of specialists. Small animal practice is reaching the point where most practitioners are expected to offer their clients help in the behavioral area. Like any discipline in which there are various levels of expertise, different practitioners will find the level at which they feel comfortable. Most of the chapters in this volume offer advice applicable to any small-animal practice. The intended audience is small-animal practitioners, veterinary students, and applied animal behaviorists with an interest in companion-animal problem behavior. Board-certified specialists (diplomates of the American College of Veterinary Behaviorists) will find some parts a convenient update of new research and information on behavior therapy.

Behavior services fall into three categories. One includes treating behavior problems by instructing the client on managing and interacting with the pet differently than before, prescribing a detailed behavior modification program and possibly prescribing a psychotropic drug to facilitate the behavioral and management recommendations. A second category of service is offering advice in identifying causes of specific problems that have occurred, even if the advice applies to the next pet. The advice may help the client prevent a repeat of the problem. Third, we can assist clients in deciding where and when they should obtain a pet and provide information in raising the pet to avoid problems.

This book is a complete revision of *Canine and Feline Behavioral Therapy* published in 1985. The revision reflects not only major advances in the field of clinical animal behavior but also our perception that many readers will also appreciate some introductory comments, where appropriate, on basic canine and feline behavior that relate to problem behaviors. Most serious readers are undoubtedly interested in basic behavior as well as the discipline that focuses on helping owners and caregivers and their companion animals enjoy their relationships more thoroughly.

The authors of the original edition are happy to welcome the full collaboration of Melissa Bain, a diplomate in the American College of Veterinary Behaviorists.

Canine and Feline
Behavior Therapy
Second Edition

Chapter 1

Introduction

Behavior therapy differs from other veterinary and medical specialties in several respects. For one thing, the behavioral history is critical in reaching a diagnosis of the problem, much more so than in internal medicine. Clinical tests, such as hematology and a chemistry panel, although often necessary as a workup for administering psychotropic medications, are not nearly as essential in arriving at a diagnosis as in internal medicine. Pharmaceutical intervention is customary for treatment in internal medicine, but is much less critical for most problems in behavioral medicine. Rather, in behavior therapy the practitioner must astutely assess the client, the companion animal, the problem, and their interactions all in the same setting. Some treatments require an extensive effort by the client at changing the behavior. If the client's commitment appears insufficient for a particular treatment, the clinician must select an option for treating the problem that is more appropriate for the specific client. There are a number of other differences between behavior medicine and internal medicine that have been discussed and elucidated.[1]

A particularly advantageous aspect of behavior therapy is that few situations require immediate attention. Thus, a busy clinician can schedule appointments for slower days. With an appointment at the end of a day, one can even sit down with the client for an hour and discuss a problem. The therapy, whether a great success or just an honest effort on your part, is an effective public relations procedure.

Guiding Principles of Behavior Therapy

Most clinical problems involve behavior that is normal from the animal's standpoint but objectionable to people. We require pets to live in our homes and adapt to our daily schedules where problem behavior may arise from our specific living arrangements. For example, the dog who barks excessively in a tiny apartment because of frequent noises might not bark if housed on a small farm. A cat that urine marks in the home is often just expressing a normal behavior that is adaptive in nature. It is best to reserve the term "abnormal" for behavior patterns that are actually maladaptive to the animal and serve no purpose, even for animals in the wild. Compulsive and stereotypic behaviors, such as flank sucking in dogs and wool chewing in cats, are examples of abnormal behavior. Behavioral changes that are secondary to disease processes in one or more organ systems, such as age-related cognitive impairment, could also be considered abnormal.

The academic areas that contribute to the discipline of clinical behavior include primarily the ethological basis of behavior, the physiological basis of behavior, and learning. The area of ethology follows from the work of biologists and naturalists that have traditionally sought to understand genetically acquired aspects of behavior from the standpoint of the adaptive value for the animal in nature. Since the behavior of dogs and cats includes many behavioral patterns that were vital for survival in their wild ancestors, this field is particularly important.

Many of the innate behavioral patterns inherited from wild ancestors are highly desirable. For example, were it not for an innate tendency to keep their nests or dens clean of eliminative products, dogs and cats would not be popular pets. Watchdog behavior, probably more a reflection of juvenile than adult wolflike behavior, enhanced by selective breeding, is another prized behavior. Understanding the innate aspects of a certain behavior may dictate a certain approach in therapy. We can take advantage of a dog's predisposition to enter into a dominance-subordination relationship rather than fighting. Sometimes problems may be treated or avoided by altering the physiological substrate of an evolved behavior through castration of males, which reduces the likelihood of normal but undesirable male typical behaviors, such as aggression in dogs and urine marking in cats (Chapter 4).

One must also be aware that the innate basis of behavioral patterns seen in evolutionary ancestors may have been "weakened" through our domestic breeding practices, which remove natural selection pressures. Natural selection is overridden when we provide artificial maternal care to young that are neglected by a mother. The young of "poor" mothers are then allowed to survive and may carry on a line of poor mothering. No amount of experience, teaching, punishment, or behavior modification will necessarily transform such animals into good mothers.

Profiling the physiological basis of behavior brings up the fact that problem behavior may be secondary to a disease or abnormality in one or more organ systems, including the brain. Some forms of psychomotor epilepsy involve changes in emotional behavior. Problems with vision have been known to produce otherwise unexplainable occurrences in aggressive behavior. Diseases that are not obvious but cause pain, such as arthritis or prostatic inflammation, may result in irritable aggressive behavior. These examples illustrate the importance of a differential diagnosis in examining the etiology of a problem behavior and the value of a clinical workup.

Some problem behaviors that look as if they have a pathophysiological basis are actually learned behavioral patterns that are attention seeking (Chapter 15). Coughing, lameness, apparent "hallucinations," self-mutilation, and fits have been detected as attention seeking behaviors. A total workup of the problem requires finding no pathophysiological explanations of the problem behavior as well as an understanding of the behavioral interaction between the owner and the animal that may have initiated and that maintains the behavior.

In addition to contributing to the diagnosis of some behavior problems, a physiological approach is involved in the use of psychotropic drugs, especially as an adjuvant to behavior modification procedures (Chapter 3 and 5). The choice of drugs, concerns about drug contraindications, and the monitoring of adverse side effects involve a background in physiology, pathobiology, and medicine.

Learning underlies the development of behavior modification techniques that are so frequently used in the treatment of behavior problems (Chapter 3). We are aware of the learning involved when we teach dogs or cats so-called parlor tricks, but we sometimes fail to realize that our pets are learning all the time. Animals may learn undesirable behavior because there has been some payoff, either in terms of the owner's affection, social interaction, or more tangible rewards such as food. Understanding of the principles of learning is essential in using systematic desensitization, counterconditioning, extinction techniques, and different types of punishment. Keep in mind that there are limitations to the use of behavior modification techniques. Urine spraying in cats may be more easily changed in neutered males by psychotropic medication than by behavior modification, and fighting between male dogs may be more easily altered by castration than by behavior modification.

Finally, one should recognize that there are gaps in our understanding of the behavior of companion animals that reflect human limitations in sensory capacity and orientation to the environment. For example, dogs and cats have olfactory sensitivity that may be 100,000 to 1 million times better than that of humans. This ability is apparent in the performance of dogs for scent tracking and scent matching for search-and-rescue activities and criminal investigations. The degree to which this sensory capacity operates on a day-to-day basis in the home of pet owners is not apparent, but it is safe to assume that dogs and cats are much more aware of what is going on from the standpoint of odors and individual scents than human members of the family.

The Ethological and Illness Models for Behavior Therapy

For some reason there is real temptation, from the standpoint of pet owners and the media, to think about pets as comparable to people with regard to problem behavior and to envision parallels between problem behaviors in dogs and cats and mental illness in humans. This is the illness model, which views behavioral problems in animals as representing a type of maladaptive or abnormal response. The comparison is epitomized perhaps by the analogy sometimes proffered between veterinary behavioral medicine and psychiatry. Because this viewpoint may be superficially appealing does not mean it is correct, and, in fact, this orientation may lead to inappropriate therapeutic approaches including the use of psychotropic drugs. The ethological model, as applied to clinical animal behavior, stems from the concept that, for the most part, problem behaviors in companion animals are not abnormal, but represent normal behavior (at least from the animal's standpoint). The behavior, although normal, may be a major problem for the pet owner. In many respects this contrast is similar to that made by Mills between the medical paradigm and the role of the environment and biology of the species in shaping behavior.[2]

Interestingly, in human psychiatry, the idea that an abnormality in neurotransmitter systems or other types of disorders are responsible for human mental problems has been convincingly challenged by an approach that stems from human ethology.

Nesse, a renowned psychiatrist, shows how a number of psychiatric syndromes such as anxiety, panic disorder, anorexia nervosa, depression, and even child abuse can be viewed as having an adaptive role in human evolutions.[3–5] The mismatch between human biology and ancient behavioral predispositions and the modern environment is viewed as a major cause of behavioral and medical problems.[3] Meanwhile, human-oriented psychotropic drug development races ahead, and our understanding of the functional significance of human behavior problems grows slowly. The lack of basic information about emotions means that there is not the guidance needed on when and where psychotropic drugs should or should not be used.[6]

The ethological model applies to virtually all areas of clinical animal behavior. Examples of common problem behaviors that come to mind are dominance status aggression in dogs, separation anxiety in dogs, and urine marking in cats. The perspective that aggression in dogs toward human family members is normal recognizes the fact that in the wild ancestor of the domestic dog some aspects of aggressiveness (threats, growls, snaps) toward pack members were not uncommon and had an adaptive role in canidae living in nature (Chapter 9).

Applying the ethological model to separation anxiety takes the perspective that in most instances it is normal for dogs, particularly young ones, to become extremely anxious and even to behave in frantic ways if suddenly abandoned by the pack or family (Chapter 10). For a young wolf in nature this would be an appropriate response and may have facilitated reunion with the group. Eventually, young wolves would undoubtedly habituate to the goings and comings of adult pack members and no longer experience separation anxiety.

Urine marking in cats, representing one of the most frequent problem behaviors for which behavior consultation is sought, is also understood by reference to the wild ancestor. Urine marking helps maintain an individual's territory integrity with "advertisement" to other felines passing by that the territory is occupied. In the modern setting the home environment is marked in the same way even though no strange felids may be passing through.

With the ethological model, using a psychotropic drug may be envisioned as elevating a specific neurotransmitter(s), such as serotonin, above normal on a temporary basis to enhance the effectiveness of a behavior modification approach. If successful, such a change allows more variability or gives a client more slack in following prescribed behavioral approaches. After the drug is withdrawn and transmitter levels return to normal, the behavior problem may remain largely resolved. Thus, the psychotropic drugs are viewed as facilitating treatment, not as correcting a transmitter abnormality. In contrast to some viewpoints in both human and veterinary medicine, the fact that an animal improves when treated with a psychotropic drug does not constitute proof that the neurotransmitter was deficient. The track record of reported success of behavior modification techniques, without drug treatment, speaks to the perspective that most problem behaviors in dogs and cats are not due to abnormal neurotransmitter levels or other physiological parameters.

Applying the illness model to problem behavior relies on the assumption that the behavior stems from an imbalance of some neurotransmitter(s), hormones, and other biological factors that influence behavior. This model argues presumably that the behavior in question would be abnormal even in a wild ancestor. Extreme fear-fulness that is never habituated, even with the repeated presentation of the non-harmful stimulus that evokes the response, is an example.

In the illness model, use of a drug is presumed to correct the neurotransmitter imbalance or other physiological abnormality and lead toward normalization of the behavior. This is the model that underlies much of the approach to treating severe-ly mentally disturbed people under the care of a psychiatrist. The illness model would suggest that one would maintain a dog or a cat with a problem behavior on the drug indefinitely because there is a biological abnormality producing the prob-lem behavior.

Perhaps the greatest risk with most behaviors in the illness model is that it is easy for animal owners to have a false sense of security because using drugs may be mindful of treating a medical or physiological condition where there is customarily a much more consistent effect between drug administration and clinical results. Even if effective, there is no guarantee that a drug will continue to control the behavior over time, even if some major changes are initially noted. There are few long-term studies to indicate the degree to which psychotropic drugs will maintain control of the behavior for months or years. One may become lax in administering the drug, or there may be changes in their neurotransmitter receptors making the drug less beneficial. When one looks at the use of psychotropic drugs as only short-term remedies, with a strong emphasis placed on behavior modification and envi-ronmental management, the focus is on phasing the animal off the drug as soon as feasible. An important exception to this principle is the treatment of urine marking in cats, which is a normal behavior but may require long-term treatment with a drug for resolution.

Organization of This Book

This book is organized into four sections. The chapters of Section I provide back-ground information and basis for techniques of behavior therapy, applicable to sev-eral problem behaviors. The principles of behavior modification are discussed as are the indications for hormonal alteration through castration. Two chapters deal with behavioral pharmacology. The section ends with discussion of understanding the behavior of sick animals. This is a useful topic because there is a tendency to consider the behavior of such animals as a reflection of debilitation whereas it is actually an adaptive response to help an animal overcome illness. Section II deals with treating specific problems in dogs and Section III with specific problems of cats. We anticipate that the chapters of Sections I and II will serve as reference sources for clinicians confronted with specific problems. Client relations are increasingly important, not only in dealing with a client's emotions but in effec-tively handling problem behavior. Section IV covers the role of companion dogs and cats in the family, the benefits of pets for human mental and physical health as well as the issues of dealing with difficult or emotional clients, and the difficult area of pet loss.

References

1. Horwitz DF. Differences and similarities between behavioral and internal medicine. Journal of the American Veterinary Medical Association 2000;217:1372–1376.
2. Mills DS. Medical paradigms for the study of problem behaviour: A critical review. Applied Animal Behavior Science 2003;81:265–277.
3. Nesse RM. An evolutionary perspective on psychiatry. Comprehensive Psychiatry 1984;25:575–580.
4. ———. Panic disorder. An evolutionary view. Psychiatry Annals 1988;18:478–483.
5. ———. Is depression an adaptation? Archives of General Psychiatry 2000;57:14–20.
6. Nesse RM, Berridge KC. Psychoactive drug use in evolutionary perspective. Science 1997;278:63–66.

Section I

Basis for Techniques of Behavior Therapy

This section deals with the background for behavior therapy as applied to specific problem behaviors addressed in Sections II and III. Rather than focusing on specific problem behaviors, chapters in this section cover procedures and concepts that generally apply to several specific problems. After a chapter on the medical interview and case assessment, as applied to clinical behavior, subsequent chapters focus on methods of resolving behavior problems through behavior modification, hormonal modification (mostly through gonadectomy), and psychotropic drug administration.

The chapter on behavior modification covers techniques that are employed for almost all problem behaviors. In the chapter on hormones and behavior we are mostly concerned with the therapeutic use of castration and with understanding the behavioral effects of neutering as practiced for pet population control. Behavior therapy will increasingly involve the use of psychotropic drugs that are federally approved for specific problem behaviors or those available from psychiatry and used in an extralabel manner for dogs and cats. To address this expanding area we have included a chapter on general concepts in behavioral pharmacology and a chapter on important groups of psychotropic drugs.

Chapter 2
Medical Interview and Case History Assessment

In general medicine the medical interview and case history assessment are important in developing diagnostic approaches and therapeutic possibilities. These aspects of the case workup are much more important, however, when dealing with behavior problems, because in most instances the medical interview provides the main source of information for the diagnosis of a problem and the recommendations for therapy. Although the approach to behavior consultations in this book is through in-person office appointments, in-home consultations are becoming more common. Certainly the clinician can obtain a more accurate picture of the animal's environment through in-home visits. Some animals are unable to be transported to an office easily for a consultation, and an in-home visit may be the only option. Consultations by telephone, fax, and Internet, although sometimes practiced, do not offer the same level of effectiveness as in-person, hands-on visits, and they may not be consistent with state legal requirements for veterinary care.

During the appointment the clients describe the problem behavior and often attempt to give their evaluation of the problem. As the clinician, you attempt to approach the problem by considering the range of feasible diagnoses that is kept in your mind or shared with the clients. The history may point to a single etiology or set of contributing etiologies, such as a genetic predisposition and early experiences that were cumulative in bringing on the behavior. Part of the diagnostic workup might involve determining whether the behavioral problem is secondary to a disease or abnormality in one or more organ systems, such as the brain, visual system, or endocrine system. Some pathophysiologic diseases that might have secondary behavioral changes are mentioned under the discussion of various problem behaviors in Sections II and III.

The initial appointment may result in a decision to observe the behavior by videotaping the animal at its home with or without the owners present, keeping a journal of the behavior, or, rarely, by hospitalizing the animal for a day or two. Usually there is no particular reason to hospitalize the animal for lengthy observations. Toward the end of the appointment the client is given some instructions verbally. It is strongly recommended that the client be given some form of written instructions, whether a brief review or a more extensive, computer-generated discourse covering history, theoretical approach, and detailed instructions. The ideal approach is at least one follow-up or progress check appointment soon after the initial appointment. Between the initial and follow-up appointments there is time to consult resources regarding further workup and treatment options for specific problems if necessary. This chapter deals with suggestions to get the most out of an appointment in order to evaluate a problem, form a definitive or tentative diagnosis, and consolidate therapeutic approaches. As Internet sources of information about the health and behavior problems of pets become more available,[1] you can expect some clients to be quite conversant about particular problems.

Getting the Most from an Interview

The sections below discuss the importance of instructing the client what to do before the appointment, the client's behavior during the interview concerning the pet's behavioral history, and how the clinician's behavior affects the success of the interview. Several veterinary behaviorists have reviewed essential elements of taking a behavioral history.[2-4] Their perspectives, and others, are incorporated into the discussion below.

Client Preparation for the Appointment

When clients make an appointment, there are some things they can do to help make it most productive. One is to keep a log or journal for a week or so of occurrences of the problem behavior, noting time of day, circumstances, and provoking stimuli. They might also make a videotape of the behavior, both when they are present and not present. It is also helpful if the owners fill out a behavioral questionnaire to be returned before the appointment.

Because the initial interview should be arranged to provide as much information as possible, it is essential for a client to bring in as many other members of the family as possible, including those particularly attached to the pet, those most affected by the pet's behavior, and those least attached to or motivated to work with the pet. The pet, of course, should also be brought into the office. Occasionally, clients ask whether the animal should be brought in, apparently believing that they will simply be discussing the animal in its absence. In addition to having the pet available for physical examination and laboratory tests, by watching the pet interact with one or more family members, you can gain firsthand information about aspects of interactions between family members and the pet that may help in diagnosing some problems. A prime example is observing the degree of affection a dog gets from a client compared with what the client says. If the problem involves fighting between two dogs, both dogs, not just the "culprit," should be brought in. This allows the clinician to watch the interaction between the owners and the dogs to determine the degree to which the owners may be causing the problem. If a dog cannot be in the exam room without endangering staff or clients, a videotape safely made before the appointment may suffice. Having the animal involved at the interview also addresses the legal restrictions necessitating a clinician actually seeing a pet before treatment can be prescribed.

By having more than one member of the family present, you may learn about differences within the family in attitudes toward the pet. Does one family member want to get rid of the pet while another wants to do everything possible to keep it? This usually means that the resolution of the problem will be more difficult because all family members are not pulling together toward a mutually acceptable end result. Even when all family members are in agreement about solving a problem, having several of them present allows the clinician to explain the instructions to all of them.

At the beginning of the interview, or even over a telephone conversation beforehand, it will be useful to mention what to expect at the appointment. For example, they might be told that about 30 minutes will be spent in taking a detailed history, various diagnostic possibilities will be discussed, and the visit will end with a full discussion of the recommended treatment plan. The length of the usual appointment should be mentioned.

Any safety recommendations should be given, such as reminding the owners of dogs to have them on a leash or waiting in the car during check-in if the dog is very aggressive. Any medical records and laboratory tests performed at another veterinary clinic should be brought to the appointment.

Some behavior specialists have a client complete a history questionnaire prior to the appointment, and this is referred to during the visit. One advantage of this exercise is that it gives the clinician an opportunity to at least briefly review the case before the appointment and gets the client thinking about relevant aspects of the problem behavior prior to the visit.

The Client's Behavior

The main contact with clients is through the exam room interview. By definition, an interview is a conversation with a purpose. When interviews lose this orientation, the clinician's time is not used effectively. Despite this purposeful orientation, the clinician must also be prepared to accommodate emotional situations. Clients are often distressed when they see a clinician about a behavior problem, and you must be sensitive to this distress. Although lack of skill or ignorance on the part of the client may have contributed to the behavior problem, it is important that we not convey a value judgment about the client's behavior. Making a judgment is a sure way to cause clients to not provide the most helpful history, or follow through with treatment plans. Most clients respond to compliments such as, "Well, you certainly are taking care of your dog," or, "It was smart of you to come in when you did."

The Clinician's Behavior

Although the interview is all-important in providing information for evaluating and resolving problem behavior, it must be conducted under the constraints of a busy schedule. The pace of the interview is set by the duration of the appointment, and the duration should be reviewed with the client by the clinician.

It is important to be aware of interviewing skills and techniques that play a role in efficiently conducting a medical interview. For one thing, our own behavior should not interfere with the information-seeking goal. The clinician who seems preoccupied or distant (even for reasons not related to the client) will not be maximally effective at obtaining the information needed and will make a poor impression on the client.

Some forms of body language can give clients an impression about the clinician's feelings. For example, arms and legs tightly folded suggest a closed, withdrawn attitude. Leaning back with hands on the head might suggest a supercilious or superior attitude; this may prevent the client from opening up. Leaning slightly forward with arms and legs relaxed is the most advantageous posture to invite the client to speak. Eye contact is also important, but with the pet in the examination room, it is easy to focus the most attention on the pet while talking to the client. Remember you are interviewing the client, not the pet.

Because it is a two-way conversation, the clinician should be aware of the body language of the client. This is especially true in determining whether the client is accepting and buying into the recommendations during the closing phases when treatment plans are outlined. Clients who seem to withdraw, divert eye contact, and/or fold their arms are confused or concerned, and those who maintain eye contact, nod, and move slightly forward (to hear better) are likely to understand and comprehend the specific recommendations. If you see some of the signals that indicate clients are withdrawing, take action to determine the source of their concerns and address them. In addition to being aware of the client's body language—and the body language of all members of the family that are present—you should take into account the interactions of client family members with each other and with the pet or pets in attendance. These important elements of body language and client-patient interactions are one of the reasons that telephone, e-mail, or fax consultations are not nearly as successful as in-person consultations.

Most successful practitioners treat clients and their pet as though they are very special, although they may have seen many such patients. The dog that misbehaves or is unruly in the exam room may be a frequent and irritating behavioral problem, but you will get further by giving the client and dog particular attention rather than by emphasizing that the problem is common.

You can physically arrange the examination room to facilitate eye contact and conversation with the client. Putting the examination table or a desk to the side of the room, rather than between you and the client where it represents a barrier, helps facilitate eye contact. Placing chairs for the client close by, so that you, as clinician, are almost forced to look at the client, may also be helpful. The seating should be as comfortable as possible, because the appointments are often lengthy. Placing stuffed toys on a shelf in the examining room can help provide a diversion for young children so that the children do not disrupt your contact with the client.

It is best to occasionally paraphrase what the client has told you about the pet. In this way you allow the client to check your understanding of the problem, and the client knows that you are listening. When talking to a client, the use of occasional comments such as, "That is interesting," or even, "Yes," generally facilitates the interview. If a client was neglectful or in error in the treatment of a pet, do not criticize. Even a question such as, "Why did you do that?" implies criticism. Most owners will have tried a treatment on the recommendation of someone else.

The style of questions has a role in the success of an interview. Open as opposed to closed questions allow the client some latitude and may reveal information a clinician might not have considered. For example, to ask "When does this occur?" rather than "Did this occur yesterday?" leaves room for the client to give more information than you might otherwise obtain. With a progress check visit, an open-ended question relating to a previously recommended procedure such as, "How are things going with the desensitization?" is more open-ended than "Are things improving with the desensitization?" Of course, closed questions are also needed, especially to obtain specific information, such as when asking how an animal responds to many different stimuli. The problem areas can then be addressed more in depth later. These questions usually follow the open-ended approach. Resolution of most problems will usually require addressing such information as where and when a problem behavior occurs, as well as the frequency and intensity of the problem.

The use of indirect rather than direct comments is useful in sensitive areas. You may, for example, like to recommend castration of a pet but feel the client may be sensitive to this operation. An indirect approach such as, "I was wondering about castration," leaves you more room to assess the client's emotional response than the direct approach of "How about castrating Skippy?" It may be useful to explore a client's reason for being opposed to castration in that it gives you an opportunity to explain some unsupported myths.

Stages of the Medical Interview

Whether the appointment lasts 30 minutes or 3 hours, or is an initial appointment or a progress check, it is best to approach the interview in identifiable stages. Stages are the (1) opening, (2) development and exploration, (3) closing. This orientation focuses the clinician's attention on the necessity of efficiently progressing through the information-gathering process so that in closing there is adequate time to give instructions to the client.

Before beginning an interview, some brief preparation may be necessary. As mentioned, the physical setting of the furniture should be such as to encourage eye contact and comfortable conversation with the client. Before going into the examination room, you should clear your mind, take a deep breath, relax, and be prepared to give full attention to the client. If you schedule appointments of 30 minutes to an hour or more at the end of a day, the stage is set for a more relaxed session. The client should be informed of the plan, which will include an explanation of detailed history, a discussion of diagnostic possibilities, and treatment options. The interview will conclude with some specific recommendations.

The Opening

In addition to exchanging pleasantries and greeting the dog or cat, the opening is when the presenting complaint and much of the history is discussed. Assuming the problem appears to be solvable, and the client seems likely to follow conscientiously the suggestions you make, your next task is to define the problem, or problems, as precisely as you can.

In this stage and throughout the interview, you can evaluate the type of attachment the client has to the pet. Is it a strong emotional attachment, or one in which the client's interest is primarily economic, as in instances where a prized show dog is involved? The client may want to breed the dog, but not if the dog's problem behavior seems incurable or genetically linked. Some clients are on the verge of disposing of their pets and are more or less giving the pet one more chance. A client, in fact, may be hoping that you will tell them the problem is unsolvable; in essence, they may want your permission to have the pet euthanized. Even this process could easily take a 60-minute interview.

Finally, at the end of this phase it may be useful to determine what the client's goals are. You may find it useful to ask, "In the ideal outcome, how would you like your dog to act?" For a dog that is aggressive toward children, the most desirable outcome would, for example, be for the dog to "like" children. Although this goal may not actually be attainable, thinking about and emphasizing it helps to focus attention on the types of information needed and the types of behavior modification indicated. Owners will often complain about more than one behavioral problem. In these instances it is usually best to focus on one problem at a time, unless all the complaints seem to be related to a single causal factor. Explain to the client that improvement in one problem area is often accompanied by improvement in other problem areas as well.

Development and Exploration

This stage of the interview covers additional relevant history, provides the material for the diagnosis, and points the way to treatment options. This is also the stage where the duration of the interview can get out of hand, forcing too much curtailment of the closing stage. A major problem can be extensive pet storytelling or rambling by the pet owner about a behavior that goes beyond that needed for evaluation purposes. The clinician must remain in control of the conversation. You can control such distractions by leaning back and diverting eye contact to suggest tactfully that the interview must move on. Alternatively, you can simply mention the need to move on.

Within the context of controlling the conversation, several issues must be considered, depending on the nature of the problem and the pet's household. With the specific behavior problem (or problems) identified, it will be necessary to determine the context of the problem behavior. What specific stimuli or situations, such as the time of day or location, seem to be related to the occurrence of the behavior? Attempt to determine whether any rewarding contingencies are maintaining the behavior. Does the behavior seem to be primarily learned, or is it partially a reflection of the animal's individual genetic makeup or breed membership? Although some breeds are more predisposed to excessive barking than others (Chapter 11), excessive barking may occur because the dog gets a frequent payoff, such as being let into the house. Such barking may also be due to the natural alarm tendencies of dogs in response to noises and movements outside the home.

Although most interviews center around the problem behaviors, during the development stage is the time to learn when the pet is behaving appropriately. This is just as important as identifying when an animal is misbehaving. This information gives you an idea of what conditions might be explored to help solve the problem. Is the pet good at certain times of the day or with certain family members but not others?

The issue of a genetic predisposition may arise. Questions regarding behavior of the dam, sire, and siblings may clarify the degree to which a genetic predisposition is present. It is important to consider the behavior of several related animals rather than just the dam, and it may be necessary for the client to contact owners of the sire and littermates later.

If there are indications of mistreatment of a pet, such as excessive punishment, teasing when the animal was a kitten or puppy, or leaving it alone for extensive periods, avoid expressing an accusing tone while asking the owner about these adverse experiences. If expressed, your negative feelings, however justified, might evoke answers that are more defensive than informative. Learning about the background of a pet is also useful. Dogs and cats obtained from animal shelters, pet shops, or large breeding operations may not have been properly socialized. Clients that obtain a pet with an unknown prior history may try to blame its problems on previous abuse, whereas the problem may not be due to abuse. If the prior history is truly unknown, speculation on this aspect is not very helpful. However, the owner's reasoning should be taken into consideration in determining the approach to the treatment. Be sure to ask what the clients did to attempt to resolve the problem and the animal's reaction to their attempts. If the clients' approach was somewhat successful, you might consider building on the aspects of their approach that *were* successful.

Seasoned behaviorists learn a lot by watching interactions between the clients and their pets. This is most evident with dogs, but a cat should be allowed out of the transport crate if it wishes. On rare occasions you may wish to hospitalize the animal in an attempt to observe a highly unusual behavioral pattern. If the behavior never occurs when the animal is unaware that anyone is watching, but occurs when the owner or hospital staff is present, this may be an indication that the behavior is maintained through an audience effect. Much more useful would be to have the owner videotape the behavior in the home setting.

A physical examination is conducted at this stage in the interview, especially if you are seeing a client as a referral and are unsure of the degree of a medical workup that has been performed in the recent past. This is also the time when, if indicated, blood may be drawn or urine taken for analysis.

The diagnostic possibilities and a tentative or definitive diagnosis are reached during the end of the development and exploration stage. In the initial approach to diagnosis you would have ruled out (or ruled in) the possibility that the behavior reflects an underlying pathophysiological process in one or more organ systems. Clients sometimes expect that a behavioral problem is due to a brain tumor or other brain abnormality, but this is relatively uncommon. Brain tumors usually have to involve suppression of bilateral areas to produce behavioral signs. Thus, most brain tumors with behavioral signs are on the midline and in the hypothalamic region where deficits in vision, appetite, water consumption, and function controlled by the pituitary gland might also be evident. Examples of abnormal behavior related to such brain dysfunction are the changes in emotionality and aggressiveness associated with psychomotor epilepsy. An extremely painful condition may cause an animal to threaten or bite if the tender area is handled. Acute inflammation of the prostate gland is an example of a painful disorder that may not be immediately obvious. A dog may tolerate handling by one owner, but it may act irritable if handled by others. Sometimes aggressiveness initially induced by a painful inflammation persists even after the inflammation has been completely resolved.

The Closing

This is the most difficult and important part of the interview. The first part of the closing is to present a general evaluation, which includes a single diagnosis or multiple diagnoses, assessment of causes of the problem, and an overview of treatment possibilities to be followed by a discussion of specific instructions. Topics that are of concern during the closing are discussed in the following sections.

Diagnosis or diagnoses

Even if tentative, your diagnosis or diagnoses should be shared with the client. Having a named diagnosis, even if as vague as "excessive anxiety" or "fear of children" can be expected to instill the client's confidence in you. A more scientific-sounding label, such as "territorial aggression complicated by dominance-related aggression," is more impressive. The important thing is to let the client know you have made progress in narrowing down the problem and its causes. Do not rush through this stage of the interview. It is better to cut off the development stage or save some of your closing comments for the next visit than to be caught short of time and risk having instructions misunderstood or forgotten.

Relationship of family to the pet

During the closing is the time to consider the relationship of the pet with various family members. Is it disliked by some and loved by others? Are the pet and its problem keeping family members from addressing important difficulties in their family relationship? Sometimes therapeutic suggestions can go in the direction of helping reduce divisiveness in a family. At other times advice can inadvertently add to the divisiveness, as when taking sides with a husband or wife in solving a problem about which the couple have a disagreement. An example is that of a dog that is aggressive to a couple's newborn baby. One person may not comprehend the seriousness of the problem and want to keep the dog, while the other is extremely frightened of the situation. Clients should be asked whether their whole family can follow through with a treatment plan.

In choosing the right treatment, the interactions between a client and pet, as observed during the interview, may affect the choice of treatment. Family composition and the family schedule also play a role. For example, it could be clear that the easiest solution to a mild problem of aggressive dominance in a young, small dog is a verbal reprimand for occasional aggressive acts. However, most dog owners are unable, either emotionally or physically, to discipline a dog appropriately, so it probably is not an appropriate treatment recommendation. One study evaluating client compliance for the treatment of separation anxiety revealed that clients that were given more than five instructions at the appointment were significantly less likely to follow the treatment regimen than if they were given five or fewer instructions.

Environmental management

Keep in mind that there may be possibilities for the client to avoid or reduce a problem by environmental management rather than change the animal's behavior through a specific behavior modification technique or drug intervention. You might suggest confining the pet to a certain location during some parts of the day for certain misbehaviors. Problems of urine marking or inappropriate elimination in a dog may be lessened if the pet is allowed access to the outdoors when the owners are not home. If separation anxiety does not seem to occur inside the house but only when the dog is left alone outside, a solution might be to leave the dog inside or install a dog door.

Seeking additional information

There are times when it is difficult to devise a therapeutic approach. You might mention that you would like to consult other clinicians. You might ask the client to collect more useful information, such as looking into the occurrence of the behavior in the dam or siblings, or determining the degree to which the behavior occurs in the client's absence. They could then return to the office in a week for further discussion of treatment.

Exam room demonstrations

In most behavior cases, the challenge is to lead the client toward a new pattern of interaction with the pet. This type of client education is best learned with practice demonstrations by the clinician or an assistant. Encourage the client to practice the new procedure briefly in the examination room and offer additional advice. Clients may feel silly rehearsing a conditioning approach in the office, but it will enable them to feel more confident when the training sessions begin at home. This is also the time to fit a dog with a head halter and go over its basic use. A knowledgeable technician may work with the client in these circumstances. If a family with two dogs is to transfer the role of the "favored" and "privileged" dog to the other dog to resolve a problem of fighting (Chapter 9), the shift may come more easily after the family members have actually practiced interacting with the dogs in your exam room. If you recommend affection control for dominance-related aggression directed toward a family member, go through a few practice attempts in the examination room. This is a good time to work out the specific variables for desensitization and counterconditioning programs such as duration and number of trials (Chapter 2).

Experimenting with a therapeutic program

Often clients find it difficult to follow suggestions that run counter to their previous interactions with the animals, such as affection control for dominance-related aggression. In such cases, you can suggest that they give the full behavior treatment in a very consistent manner for one full week and come back for a follow-up appointment.

The question of euthanasia

During some behavioral consultations the question of euthanasia may surface. This may come up after hearing of the time commitment needed to attempt to resolve a serious problem with a questionable prognosis and with no guarantees. Although euthanasia for a behavior problem is not uncommon, keep in mind that it is likely to be more emotionally upsetting for a pet owner to accept euthanasia when it is performed because of some behavior problem in a physically healthy pet than when it is performed to end the suffering of a pet with a terminal illness. Owners have a strong tendency to feel guilty or inadequate for possibly having caused a problem behavior. It may be necessary to emphasize the parallel between some types of behavior problems and terminal or incurable disease, emphasizing that the client is not really at fault. Risk of injury to people should be pointed out as a justifiable reason for euthanasia. A client that feels guilty about the euthanasia of a pet may not get another pet and thereby deprive themselves of the enjoyment and benefits that pets offer. Therefore, time spent in dealing with this issue is worthwhile.

Delaying a euthanasia decision by offering the client the behavior modification program, even one that has a low probability of succeeding, is sometimes worthwhile. After making a further effort to correct the pet's behavior, the client knows he or she has tried everything and feels less conflict in making the choice for euthanasia. It may help to mention to the client that, no matter what decision they make regarding euthanasia, family members may be upset with their decision. The performance of euthanasia brings up the prospect of dealing with the grief reactions of clients, which is handled in Section IV (Chapter 29).

Facilitating client compliance

Virtually all behaviorists believe that the success of a behavioral outcome depends on a client's compliance with instructions. Although outcome is not necessarily always correlate with compliance,[5] it is essential to take reasonable steps to facilitate compliance. One step involves helping clients remember instructions. Keep in mind that clients tend to forget instructions, rather than the history or diagnosis. Limited research reveals that a list of fewer instructions, especially those that are simpler and less time consuming, brings about the best compliance and the most improvement; at least this is what was found in evaluations of outcomes for treatment of separation anxiety.[6]

Here are three suggestions for instructions:

1. Give the client a written summary of instructions. At a minimum, you could use hospital letterhead for handwritten instructions with a copy for hospital files. More beneficial would be instructions written on computer with a printed copy for the client. The main thing is that there should be little delay in getting these instructions to the client. Instructions should be as specific as possible. It is too much to expect a client to work from a general theory to a particular situation—that is the clinician's job. The more concrete and specific the instructions are, the less the client will forget and the more compliant the client will be with instructions. Some behavior specialists use handouts or computer templates to supplement the specific instructions for a client. As mentioned, fewer instructions and those that are the most simple and least time consuming are likely to produce the best results.
2. Schedule one or two additional follow-up appointments at intervals ranging from a week or two to a month, depending on the problem. This not only allows the clinician the ability to reduce the number of instructions required per visit, but provides the opportunity to review and make adjustments in the instructions. It is important during these visits to reinforce the efforts of the client verbally in addressing the problem, even if the progress is only minimal.[7]
3. Telephone the client, or have a technician familiar with the problem call, to see how things are progressing between office visits. The time for such calls should be arranged during the first visit. Again, the client should be verbally reinforced for even small increments in progress; this will encourage further progress and let the clients know you are aware of their efforts.

References

1. Bergman L, Hart BL, Bain MJ. Evaluation of urine marking by cats as a model for veterinary diagnostic and treatment approaches and client attitudes. Journal of the American Veterinary Medical Association 2002;221:1282–1286.
2. Crowell-Davis SL, Houpt KA. Techniques for taking a behavioral history. Veterinary Clinics of North America: Equine Practice 1986;2:507–518.
3. Hunthausen W. Collecting the history of a pet with a behavior problem. Veterinary Medicine 1994;(Oct)954–959.
4. O'Farrell V. Owner attitudes and dog behaviour problems. Applied Animal Behaviour Science 1997;52:205–213.
5. Lane J. Client compliance and outcome of behavior cases. Paper presented at the World Veterinary Congress, Minneapolis 2005.
6. Takeuchi Y, Houpt KA, Scarlett JM. Evaluation of treatments for separation anxiety in dogs. Journal of the American Veterinary Medical Association 2000;217:342–345.
7. Lane J. Understanding and improving client compliance. Veterinary Technician 2003:850–853.

Chapter 3
Principles of Behavior Modification

Behavior modification procedures provide the most important tool in solving behavior problems. Throughout Sections II and III, which discuss the treatment of specific problem behaviors of dogs and cats, references will be made to a number of conditioning or modification procedures. The purpose of this chapter is to discuss these procedures in a unified way, with a theoretical basis for their use. The term *behavior modification* implies the intentional or structured use of conditioning or learning procedures to modify behavior (the term *conditioning* is used interchangeably with *learning*). There are, of course, other approaches for solving specific behavior problems. One of these is environmental or household management, such as making an outdoor-indoor cat an indoor-only cat, keeping a dog inside when human family members are gone, restricting an animal's exposure to other animals outside or inside the house, and removing odors from inappropriately soiled areas. Two other approaches to problem behavior are hormonal alteration through castration (Chapter 4) and the use of psychotropic drugs (Chapter 5). When environmental management, hormonal alteration, and pharmaceutical approaches are employed, the concurrent use of behavior modification procedures is usually still indicated. In fact, drugs should be viewed as facilitating a behavior modification program.

The time available for an office consultation to discuss behavior modification procedures with a client can vary widely. Some of the procedures require a considerable time commitment from the client with daily practice sessions. Before spending the time needed to discuss the details of such a program, it may be desirable to determine the extent to which the client is able to stay with the demands.

When confronted with a behavior problem, it will be necessary for the clinician to select the appropriate procedure and then determine how this procedure can be customized for the specific case. This involves a diagnosis and an understanding of the cause, or causes, of the problem. Sometimes the diagnosis will automatically suggest a specific therapeutic approach. For example, the diagnosis of attention-seeking behavior automatically suggests a program to extinguish the learned behavior by removal of reinforcing attention.

A useful tip to keep in mind is that clients will usually have tried some sort of punishment or other behavior modification before seeking your advice. Because your advice is being sought, their attempts have not resolved the problem. Therefore, think along the lines of trying something that is different from what the client has tried. If the client has tried interactive punishment, for example, think of using social or remote punishment and/or counterconditioning techniques. Sometimes the client has seen progress with some approaches and your task may be to use the principles of behavior modification to extend the improvement to more complete resolution.

An oversimplified first-level approach to dealing with some behavior problems is to think of two possibilities. One is rewarding desirable behavior and the second is discouraging behavior that is undesirable. This requires an investigation into the circumstances in which an animal is behaving appropriately, as well as determining the circumstances in which its behavior is undesirable. If a dog is being destructive around the house, for example, it is important to also know when it is being good around the house.

The conditioning techniques that can be used to accomplish therapeutic goals are systematic desensitization, typically used to eliminate learned or innate fears and anxieties; counterconditioning to establish a new emotional response that is incompatible with the existing undesirable fear or anxiety; operant conditioning of new responses; extinction of an existing learned response; and punishment of some type to reduce the likelihood of the undesirable behavior. With dogs, the use of a head halter (e.g., Gentle Leader), covered at the end of this chapter, can facilitate some desensitization and counterconditioning programs. To set the stage for discussion of therapeutic techniques, several topics dealing with learning processes are discussed first.

Learning Processes

The techniques discussed in this chapter, such as systematic desensitization and counterconditioning, are best understood if they are related to some of the basic concepts involved in learning, namely habituation, classical conditioning, and operant conditioning. The clinically useful techniques are derived from these learning processes. A few examples are mentioned to illustrate both the conditioning procedures and the therapeutic techniques, but specific details for the employment of these techniques are covered under the specific behavior problems in Sections II and III.

Habituation

Every animal has a set of behavioral patterns that are innate and that serve to protect it in nature against predators, aggressive conspecifics, and other dangerous situations. These include startle responses to sudden unfamiliar stimuli, fear or anxiety from exposure to strange objects or strange conspecifics, and anxiety from being abandoned or left alone. These responses are genetically programmed and have been shaped by natural selection and selective breeding. On the other hand, every environment produces strange and startling but harmless stimuli, and animals have the ability to habituate to such stimuli that are repeated over and over again without adverse consequences. In nature this allows young animals to adapt quickly to potential startle- or fear-evoking, but harmless, stimuli typical of its specific environment. Habituation saves an animal from being continuously and needlessly startled or frightened all day by harmless stimuli. When the animal habituates to a stimulus, it is to that specific stimulus and not to everything that might cause a startle response. An animal that habituates to the loud screech of birds overhead may not have habituated to the sound of a heavy object falling on the ground.

Both in nature and with domestic animals, young animals habituate more readily than do adult animals. Hence, it is suggested that situations that evoke fear or anxiety in dogs and cats, such as being taken in an automobile, handled by children, walked through heavy traffic or loaded into an airline shipping crate, be performed in a safe and positive manner when animals are very young. Hunting dogs are usually habituated to gunshots when they are puppies by being exposed to the firing of a starter pistol. Habituating a dog to gunshots when it is an adult is a more laborious and lengthy process. Cats have a natural fear response to close interactions with dogs, but kittens may even be habituated to rough-and-tumble playful interactions with puppies at a very young age. It is almost impossible to habituate an adult cat to this degree of interaction with dogs.

The paradigm for habituation may be given as follows:

Unconditioned stimulus (gunshot) → Emotional activation

Unconditioned stimulus (gunshot)—Repetitive presentations → Weak emotional activation

Unconditioned stimulus (gunshot)—Repetitive presentations → No emotional activation

An intentional or structured habituation program is referred to as *desensitization*. When the stimulus or stimuli are presented repetitively at full strength the desensitization process is referred to as *flooding*. As mentioned, this type of habituation works well with young animals. Generally pet dogs and cats are habituated, by virtue of unintentional flooding, to the ordinary stimuli that are in the urban environment, such as automobile rides, machinery noises, sounds of a vacuum cleaner, power tool noises, wearing a collar, and the like. Dogs and cats that grow up in areas where there are frequent thunderstorms usually habituate to these sounds.

Habituation is an active process, and for animals to continue to be habituated they must be periodically exposed to the stimuli. A puppy that has been habituated to gunshots may regain the innate startle and emotional fear of this type of loud sound if it does not hear any gunshots for a couple of years. In other words, habituation is a learning process that requires maintenance.

In the clinical setting you are confronted with adult animals that have unhabituated fear or anxiety reactions. Such fears may occur because the animal was never habituated to the stimulus that causes the reaction, or perhaps the potentially fear-inducing stimulus was not continued on a long-term basis and the animal lost the habituation. In adult animals, unhabituated fear reactions are often much more intense or severe than in young animals. Dogs may throw themselves through sliding glass doors at the crack of a thunderbolt or upon hearing firecrackers, if they are not habituated to the stimuli. Usually the animal attempts to be where the caregiver is, and if the caregiver is outside and the dog inside, the animal will do anything it can to get outside and vice versa.

Unhabituated anxiety or fear reactions in adult animals can be enhanced through experiencing these stimuli if the stimuli are actually associated with unpleasant or painful consequences. A dog that gets hurt when it reacts violently to the sound of a thunderstorm may be basically proving to itself that thunderstorms are harmful, and this enhances the fear reaction the next time. Sometimes just the visceral turmoil associated with a fear-inducing sound enhances the fear reaction.

Unhabituated fears may also be enhanced when the caregiver understandably attempts to comfort the animal when it shows signs of fear. This comforting can be rewarding to the animal, so it learns that the fear which comes naturally also pays off in terms of extra comfort and affection. In dealing with unhabituated fear and anxiety reactions in adult animals, one usually has to examine the possibility of reinforcement that may have intensified the reaction.

The usual therapeutic approach to unhabituated fear and anxiety reactions in adult animals is gradual habituation, which is referred to as *systematic desensitization*. If one presents the stimulus that evokes the reaction at full force repeatedly (flooding), as one might with a puppy, the emotional state produced may be so intense and aversive that it enhances the fear reaction. This can prevent the animal from being desensitized. However, if one presents the stimulus that produced the fear reaction repeatedly in a very mild fashion, the fear or anxiety can be habituated at that mild level. After this is accomplished, one can increase the intensity of the stimulus slightly and again repeatedly present the stimulus at this new level, accomplishing habituation at the new level. Over a series of systematic stages the stimulus intensity is gradually increased until the animal is habituated to the stimulus at full strength, or at least somewhat near full strength.

The technique of systematic desensitization is used with unhabituated fears and with fears or phobias that may be acquired by virtue of classical conditioning (see next section). The manner in which a stimulus is initially presented in a mild form, and later gradually increased, depends on the nature of the stimulus. For loud sounds the gradient is usually volume intensity; for separation anxiety the gradient is duration of time the animal is left alone; and for fear of strangers the gradient may be the distance to the stranger.

Classical Conditioning

The two ways by which animals may acquire new responses are through classical conditioning and operant conditioning. Classical conditioning involves responses that are basically involuntary or reflexlike associated with the contraction of smooth muscles and secretion of endocrine glands, rather than the contraction of skeletal muscle. Operant conditioning, covered in the next section, involves responses mediated by skeletal muscles and typically considered voluntary movements. Classical conditioning occurs when a stimulus that was previously neutral to the animal takes on the power to elicit a reflexlike response. The responses that can be conditioned to a neutral stimulus are limited to those that have already been preprogrammed into an animal's central nervous system. Two categories of responses that are important clinically are those categorized as pleasant or appetitive and those that are unpleasant or aversive; these two types of responses are discussed next.

Conditioning of pleasant or appetitive emotional reactions

Most people are familiar with the paradigm for classical conditioning associated with salivation in dogs. This type of learning was made famous through the classical work of Ivan Pavlov around the turn of the century when he studied the conditioning of salivation as a model for learning. Salivation is, of course, simply an external manifestation of a variety of internal, generally pleasant or appetitive, responses associated with food. The term *classical conditioning* refers to the work of Pavlov as being classical in the field.

   Classical conditioning involves the occurrence of a neutral stimulus immediately prior to the unconditioned stimulus that evokes an internal or visceral response. After usually several pairings, depending on the type of response being conditioned, the neutral stimulus will eventually evoke the visceral response alone. The following is a paradigm for classical conditioning of an internal appetitive (positive) response to a clicker which represents a neutral stimulus:

Unconditioned stimulus (food) → Internal appetitive emotion
Conditioned stimulus (clicker) → Unconditioned stimulus (food) → Internal
   appetitive emotion
Conditioned stimulus (clicker) → Internal appetitive emotion

   In the Pavlovian tradition the unconditioned stimulus would be meat powder, the conditioned stimulus would be a bell, and the response would be salivation. Conditioning is most efficient when the neutral stimulus precedes the unconditioned stimulus by an interval of only a few seconds. As mentioned, this type of conditioning involves responses normally under an animal's "involuntary" control. For example, without the use of some suitable food to activate food-related visceral responses innately, it would be impossible to train a dog to salivate and have food-related positive internal feelings on command. When a dog is salivating for food or tail-wagging with facial expressions that owners recognize as happy, the internal emotional state, which cannot be observed, is assumed to be pleasurable or appetitive to the animal.

Conditioning of unpleasant, aversive emotional reactions

A clinically important group of classically conditioned responses produces an aversive internal state innately brought on by a painful or fear- or anxiety-evoking stimuli. Such aversive states can be conditioned to the sight of a person or an environment associated with the administration of pain. Painful stimulation in an animal usually causes an increase in blood pressure, slowing of intestinal motility, and a variety of other visceral reactions that stem from the release of hormones from the adrenal medulla (epinephrine) and the adrenal cortex (corticosteroids). Responses usually associated with fear or anxiety produce internal emotional states that are aversive or unpleasant. The paradigm for this type of conditioning is as follows:

Unconditioned stimulus (pain) → Aversive emotional reaction
Conditioned stimulus (sight of syringe) → Unconditioned stimulus (pain) →
   Aversive emotional reaction
Conditioned stimulus (sight of syringe) → Aversive emotional reaction

Although pain will innately evoke an aversive emotional reaction, some other stimuli will also. These include abandonment, some types of restraint, a sudden change in stimulus intensity such as falling, and intense physical stimuli such as loud noises. Thus, the sound of car keys can be classically conditioned to the aversive emotional reaction seen in separation anxiety (abandonment). Slapping a puppy with a folded newspaper probably produces an aversive emotional reaction because of the swift hitting movement and intense auditory stimulus, not because it is painful. Neutral stimuli that accompany or slightly precede a stimulus that innately evokes an aversive emotional reaction may be conditioned by only one or two pairings. A dog that is in an automobile accident may thereafter refuse to go in the automobile. The automobile, which was previously a neutral or even a pleasant stimulus, was paired with a painful stimulus that evoked a very aversive emotional reaction in just one trial. The adaptive value of such one-trial learning with regard to what might be life-threatening situations is obvious. This is in contrast to the slower acquisition of classically conditioned appetitive responses.

When some stimuli or situations evoke aversive emotional reactions, an animal may try to attenuate the reactions by escaping from or driving away the conditioned stimulus that evokes the reaction. Hence, fear-biting behavior in dogs is maintained and enhanced if the behavior has paid off by driving away the fear-inducing stimulus. Being handled on a part of the body may be classically conditioned to the pain of an inflammatory process in that body part. With inflammation in the hips of a dog with hip dysplasia, the animal may respond with signs of defensive aggression when it is touched or handled in the rear quarters. After the inflammation has been decreased by medical treatment, the conditioned response to handling the rear quarters may remain, and the animal may still react with conditioned fear and show signs of defensive behavior.

A conditioned response that has received considerable attention is the aversive emotional reaction associated with the gastrointestinal upset and nausea caused by food poisoning from bacterial endotoxins. An animal may reject a food based on the taste or smell of the food causing the poisoning, even if the gastrointestinal upset occurred hours or a day later.[1] This conditioning to the food may persist long after the toxin is removed from the implicated food. This response, often referred to as a *conditioned food aversion,* protects animals in nature from future poisoning. The response has been used by sheep ranchers to produce aversion in coyotes to sheep by exposing them to a bait of lamb skin containing lamb meat laced with the illness-inducing toxin, lithium chloride.[2] Although a variant of this technique has been suggested as a possible remedy for coprophagy in dogs or killing chickens or sheep by dogs, for various reasons these applications have not worked out.

Other responses

A variety of visceral responses that are difficult to categorize as appetitive or aversive can also be classically conditioned. These include milk ejection, which is commonly conditioned to stimuli associated with the nursing of newborn; secretion of insulin, which is normally elicited by ingestion of sugar but can be conditioned to the taste of sweet food; and asthmatic reactions, which are normally caused by foreign proteins, but can be conditioned to the environment in which the foreign protein is administered.

Extinction of classically conditioned responses

Reduction or elimination of classically conditioned responses, referred to as *extinction,* occurs when the neutral stimulus is presented repeatedly without being followed by the stimulus that innately evokes the response. This is easily seen regarding an appetitive emotional reaction evoked by a neutral stimulus associated with food. If presentation of the conditioned stimulus, such as the box that contains dog treats, is no longer followed by giving the dog treats from the box, the connection is extinguished and the box no longer evokes an appetitive emotional reaction. The extinction of classically conditioned fear or anxiety responses is much more difficult, which is perhaps a reflection of the survival value in nature of a fear response to a stimulus related in the past to dangers.

When a therapeutic approach calls for reduction or elimination of an acquired fear response, such as a fear of men, it can be almost impossible to extinguish the fear reaction when the full-blown, fear-evoking stimulus is presented. However, the process of presenting the conditioned fear-inducing stimulus at very low intensities, which evokes only a mild fear reaction, can lead to extinction. In the case of fear of men, for example, a mild stimulus might be the sight of a man at a distance. After the fear response is extinguished at the mild level, the intensity may be increased by presenting the sight of a man at a closer distance. This process is continued until the fear-evoking stimulus can be presented at full strength.

The process of presenting fear-evoking or anxiety-evoking stimuli in gradually increasing intensities to extinguish classically conditioned fear responses is also referred to as *systematic desensitization*; this is virtually the same process that is used for gradually desensitizing unhabituated innate fear reactions. Sometimes it is not even necessary to diagnose whether fear reactions are unhabituated responses, classically conditioned responses, or a combination, because the treatment, systematic desensitization, is the same for each.

Operant Conditioning

The concept of operant conditioning is quite simple. Operant conditioning concerns voluntary responses involving skeletal muscles. In this respect it differs from classical conditioning, which involves the smooth muscles and glands that are normally associated with involuntary responses. If a response is followed by a reward, usually called a *reinforcer,* the probability of the response occurring again increases. For example, when begging behavior by a dog occurs at the table and is followed by a reinforcement, such as a piece of cheese, begging behavior tends to be repeated. Operant conditioning is responsible for a number of unwanted behaviors in pets, including jumping up on people, barking to get inside, digging holes in a flower bed, waking up owners at 3:00 a.m. to be fed, and engaging in a variety of attention-seeking behaviors that may resemble medical problems. Operant conditioning is also used to train animals in a number of useful and desirable behavioral patterns.

Most circus performing animals are currently trained on the basis of operant conditioning.

Positive reinforcement

It should always be remembered that reinforcement increases the probability of an animal repeating the behavior in the future. Reinforcements for operant conditioning may be positive or negative. We usually think of reinforcement as positive. Reinforcers such as food, water, social contact, and exploratory behavior are positive, which means that their presentation, or addition, will result in learning. With most positive reinforcers, such as food, it may be more motivating that an animal be at least modestly deprived before it can be reinforced. Sleep is reinforcing only to a sleep-deprived animal. Finding an appropriate place to urinate is reinforcing to an animal with a full urinary bladder. Some positive reinforcers require hardly any deprivation. This may be true of highly favored foods, such as hamburger or cheese, even to a satiated dog. Social contact and petting are also examples of reinforcers that require little or no deprivation. An example of the paradigm for positive reinforcement is

Stimulus (command to "sit") → Response (sitting position) → Reinforcement
   (food or petting)

Because there often is a delay between the response and delivery of the reinforcement, a bridging stimulus, like a clicker or whistle, can be used to signal that reinforcement is coming. If the bridging stimulus is paired with reinforcing food treats whenever they are given, the bridging stimulus takes on the properties of the reinforcing treat by virtue of classical conditioning; at this time the bridging stimulus is referred to as a *secondary reinforcer*. A bridging stimulus in the form of a clicker was introduced as a practical way of facilitating teaching animals tricks by B. F. Skinner[3] and is the basis for so-called *clicker training*.[4] Actually most dog and cat owners use the words "good boy," "good girl" and "good kitty" as bridging stimuli in training.

Negative reinforcement

Reinforcers that are negative are aversive stimuli which, when removed, increase the probability of the response. Termination of pain or the reduction of fear are negative reinforcers. Animals learn tasks, including escaping or growling, if such behavior results in the fear-inducing stimulus going away. One can see the process of negative reinforcement at work when an animal is approached by someone who evokes fear. The animal, by threatening or snapping, drives away the person, which leads to a reduction of the fear. Hence, the threatening behavior tends to be repeated in the face of the fear-inducing stimulus. An example of the paradigm for negative reinforcement is

Stimulus (person and onset of fear) → Response (growl) → Reinforcement
   (termination of fear)

Negative reinforcement is easily confused with punishment. Punishment, discussed below, is the presentation of an aversive stimulus or removal of a pleasurable stimulus after an undesirable behavior has occurred. When punishment is delivered it tends to stop the behavior and reduces the likelihood of the behavior occurring in the future.

Successive proximation

Operant conditioning techniques work well to enhance a behavioral pattern that is already in an animal's repertoire. Scratching at a door, for example, occurs every once in a while without any conditioning. This is what is called the operant level of the response. When the door-scratching is reinforced by allowing the dog inside, the probability of door-scratching increases.

Successive approximation is the process by which "parlor tricks"—such as rolling over or jumping through a hoop, which are not normally in an animal's repertoire—are conditioned. In teaching such tricks a behavioral goal is derived, and a gradient from the starting point to the goal is determined. For example, in teaching a cat to jump through a hoop, one could initially place the hoop on the floor and stand on the side of the hoop opposite to the cat, with food that the cat can see and smell, and say "jump" when the cat walks through the hoop. It is then given the food treat. This is repeated until the cat readily walks through the hoop when "jump" is said and food offered. This is a starting point. The process of successive approximation is then used when the hoop is raised an inch from the floor. The cat is asked to "jump" through the hoop and given a food treat every time it steps over the raised hoop. After a few trials at this level, the hoop is raised a bit more and the cat is again reinforced every time it jumps or steps over the hoop. Over a series of many trials the hoop is very gradually raised until it is a foot or two off the floor. The word "jump" is also gradually dissociated with showing the cat the food treat.

The key to the use of successive approximation is to determine a beginning point and define a goal as specifically as possible. One must devise a gradient along which the criterion is gradually raised for reinforcing an animal's performance. In using successive approximation to shape behavior, the animal should be reinforced with praise, affection, and favored food treats each time it behaves appropriately. Use of a clicker or other bridging stimulus will greatly facilitate training the new operant through successive approximation, because responses in the direction of the goal can be reinforced in less than a second and the exact response can be rewarded immediately. After the desired behavior is learned one may reinforce the behavior on an intermittent schedule.

An animal may learn complex tasks without intentional training through successive approximations. Learning to open a closed gate latch may have been the last step along a gradient that started with someone leaving a gate latch partially closed so it was easily pushed open by a dog randomly moving about.

Extinction of operant responses

After a conditioned operant response has been learned, it is generally maintained as long as reinforcement is at least occasionally presented. If the reinforcement is withheld permanently, an animal will make fewer and fewer responses until the behavior drops to the previous operant level. As noted before, this process is called *extinction*. Note that extinction is an active process, requiring behavioral responses to be made.

Extinction should be distinguished from forgetting, which is a passive process representing the decrement of response strength through the passage of time. A learned, feigned lameness, which is maintained because it evokes attention from the dog's owner, would eventually be extinguished if the owner decided to withhold all attention from the dog whenever the behavior was exhibited. Extinction will work with many of the common unwanted behavioral patterns that dogs show, such as scratching on screen doors and begging for food, if the behavior is never again reinforced.

Sometimes extinction is impossible because the reinforcing aspects of the behavior cannot feasibly be removed from the behavioral acts. For example, when dogs jump up on people the reinforcement is built into the response; by jumping, the dog gets close to the face of people, which is reinforcing, and people tend to contact the dog by pushing away with their hands. Other behaviors that have a built-in reinforcement are digging holes in the backyard to create a cool bed and being destructive in the house as a manifestation of reinforcing escape from boredom. These behavior patterns are solvable by other means, namely punishment and counterconditioning.

Schedules of reinforcement

Successfully teaching animals new operants, as well as resolving objectionable acquired behavioral patterns through the process of extinction, requires an understanding of the consequences of intermittent versus continuous schedules of reinforcement. In teaching an animal a simple trick, one usually attempts to reinforce each response with food or praise. This is referred to as *continuous reinforcement*. After an animal learns something, however, it is not necessary that it be rewarded each time; intermittent reward can usually maintain the behavior. A major difference between behavior that has been maintained by continuous and intermittent reinforcement is that the latter is much more resistant to extinction.

Consider the typical behavior of a dog scratching a door to be let in. The animal is obviously putting out many scratches, perhaps 100, before it is allowed in; that is, reinforcement is intermittent. If one wanted to extinguish door scratching, the behavior could be eliminated by permanently withholding all reinforcement. Undoubtedly, thousands of responses would be made by the dog before its behavior would be extinguished. The extinction would be much easier if the dog had been allowed in the house almost every time it scratched at all. What usually happens, however, is that not only has reinforcement been intermittent, but the milder forms of door scratching have been extinguished because they never paid off. Only the more intense and frequent forms of scratching actually led to reinforcement.

There are two types of intermittent reward schedules. One of these is a ratio schedule. If an animal must make an exact number of responses before it is reinforced one time, then it is on a fixed ratio schedule. If the number of responses per reinforcement is variable, the animal is being reinforced on a variable ratio schedule. In practice, most reinforcement is given on a variable ratio rather than a fixed ratio schedule. On both fixed and variable ratio schedules, operants are emitted rapidly because the sooner the required number of responses are made, the sooner reinforcement is attained.

The other type of intermittent reinforcement is the interval of time, which may be either relatively fixed or variable. Interval schedules are commonly seen in animals that engage in waiting behavior. In a fixed interval schedule an animal is not reinforced until a specific amount of time has elapsed since the preceding reinforcement. The dog that waits at the door each evening before it is taken out on its routine 8 o'clock walk is being reinforced on a relatively fixed interval reinforcement schedule. If an animal is reinforced on a variable interval schedule, it means that the duration of time elapsed since the preceding reinforcement varies, but still may be represented by an average interval duration. Animals that are reinforced on this type of schedule are likely to display waiting behavior for a longer period that is still related to the predicted time to return. Some dog owners may feel that their dogs "know" when they are coming home when, in fact, they are showing a learned waiting behavior maintained on an interval reinforcement schedule.

Therapeutic Techniques

Therapeutic techniques are derived from conditioning processes and are designed for specific problem behaviors. These techniques include systematic desensitization, counterconditioning, operant conditioning, extinction of operant conditioning, and various types of punishment.

Systematic Desensitization

Systematic desensitization is usually applied to anxiety or fear reactions and allows the habituation of innate fears and anxieties or the extinction of classically conditioned fears or anxieties to occur gradually. The physiological reactions that generally accompany fear and anxiety are in themselves aversive. Even fear-evoking stimuli that are not accompanied by external pain are difficult to habituate or extinguish. However, if such stimuli are presented at lower intensities, the fear-evoking stimuli produce little or no aversive emotional reaction, and desensitization occurs to the low-level stimuli. The stimulus intensity may then be increased slightly without evoking noticeable emotional responses while the desensitization continues at this new level. If this procedure is continued, eventually a stimulus may be presented at full strength and the animal is no longer fearful, as the fear reaction is entirely desensitized.

This technique is referred to as *desensitization* because the intense emotional response to the stimulus is desensitized, much as one might desensitize an animal to an allergen or antigen. The term *systematic* is used because the stimulus is presented at gradually increasing degrees of intensity on a systematic and orderly basis. Systematic desensitization is useful in treating the various fear and anxiety reactions, which include innate and acquired fears of sounds or strange people, fear aggression, and separation anxiety.

It is important to be aware of the types of gradients that are used in systematic desensitization. When designing a program of training sessions, it is critical to build in a gradient with increments that gradually increase the stimulus intensity for the animal in some measurable or logical fashion. At the beginning of the gradient, the animal should experience at a low level the same stimulus that, which if presented in full strength, would be sufficient to evoke the fear and related aversive emotional reaction. One usually first presents the stimulus close to full intensity to make certain that the stimulus does in fact evoke the fear or anxiety. For example, in using a commercial recording of fireworks to desensitize a dog to fireworks, one should play the firework recording at full strength to make certain the stimulus is adequate to evoke the fear response. After performing this first critical test one should next find a starting point along the sound volume gradient just short of where a visible anxiety reaction is seen. One then structures ways of measuring points of increased volume in a systematic way. By talking with the owners, the clinician can help outline a stimulus gradient. Figure 3-1 schematically illustrates the desensitization paradigm.

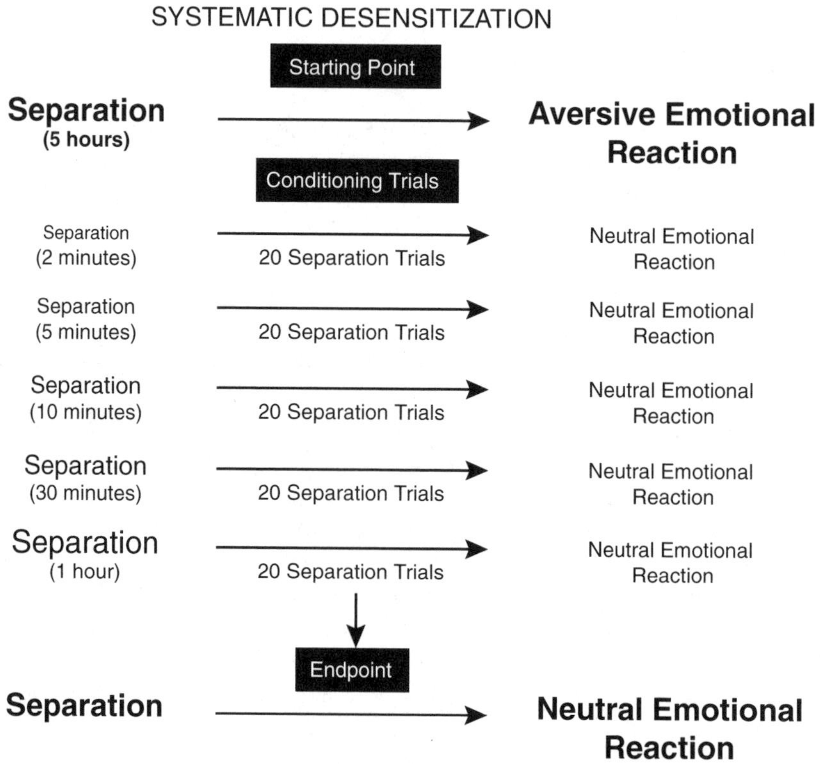

SYSTEMATIC DESENSITIZATION

	Starting Point	
Separation **(5 hours)**	⟶	**Aversive Emotional Reaction**

	Conditioning Trials	
Separation (2 minutes)	⟶ 20 Separation Trials	Neutral Emotional Reaction
Separation (5 minutes)	⟶ 20 Separation Trials	Neutral Emotional Reaction
Separation (10 minutes)	⟶ 20 Separation Trials	Neutral Emotional Reaction
Separation (30 minutes)	⟶ 20 Separation Trials	Neutral Emotional Reaction
Separation (1 hour)	⟶ 20 Separation Trials	Neutral Emotional Reaction

	Endpoint	
Separation	⟶	**Neutral Emotional Reaction**

Figure 3-1 Use of systematic desensitization to treat separation anxiety in a dog. In this example, the initial problem is an aversive emotional reaction, manifested by extreme anxiety, when the dog is left alone for more than 15 minutes. The starting point of treatment is short departures (2 minutes), representing a weak separation stimulus. The weak separation stimulus should evoke a neutral emotional reaction, and with multiple separations the dog will become desensitized to short separations. The dog is continuously desensitized to longer periods of separation.

When the owners plan their sessions, they should keep a journal of the stimuli, the gradients, and the animal's reactions. They should ideally plan to hold multiple sessions per day for the quickest resolution, with each session lasting only a few minutes. The clinician should brainstorm with the clients on how the clients can most efficiently do this within the context of their other daily responsibilities.

The first published account of the use of systematic desensitization to treat problem behaviors in dogs applied this technique to an Old English Sheepdog that had acquired an intense fear of thunderstorms.[5] At the first indication of an impending storm, the dog would begin accelerating its aimless pacing and exhibit profuse salivation and marked panting. These responses were climaxed by the dog throwing his body against doors in an attempt to escape. A thunderstorm recording was used to desensitize the dog.

Systematic desensitization of fear reactions to certain people, such as strange men, can also be approached using distance as a gradient. Training sessions can be planned in which a man who normally evokes a fear response enters a room at a distance far enough from the animal that the man is seen but the fear reaction is not evoked. The man makes an appearance at a given distance, say 10 times in a row, and this constitutes a training session. Over subsequent sessions the man moves slightly closer each time. As mentioned the gradient being used here is distance.

Although systematic desensitization refers to the clinical use of desensitization to resolve problem behavior, desensitization is occurring regularly in the lives of animals and people. When one moves to a home next to the railroad tracks, the people, dogs, and cats all become desensitized to the roar of trains in the middle of the night. One might refer to such desensitization as *autonomous* to help differentiate it from that which is intentionally arranged. Of course, the stimuli involved generally occur at full strength, so such desensitization is basically flooding.

SYSTEMATIC DESENSITIZATION

- Identify anxiety-provoking stimulus.
- Do not force the animal to experience stimulus.
- Test the conditioning stimulus for its effectiveness.
- Gradually increase intensity of stimulus during planned trials.
- Use a gradient starting with a "safe" distance or intensity.
- Do not expose to full stimulus until program reaches that stage.
- Combine with counterconditioning for best response.

Counterconditioning

Although this technique is used along with systematic desensitization, the emphasis in counterconditioning is on establishing a new emotional response that is generally incompatible with the aversive emotional response underlying the undesirable behavior. That is, an aversive emotional reaction associated with an outside manifestation of fear may be reduced when a positive or appetitive emotional response is classically conditioned to the same stimulus that evokes the fear. By pairing a stimulus, such as a food treat, that produces an appetitive emotional reaction with a very mild form of the fear- or anxiety-evoking stimulus, the pleasant emotional reaction replaces the aversive reaction. As the animal is successively desensitized to higher and higher levels of the fear-evoking stimulus, the animal is counterconditioned to successively more intensive forms of the same stimulus (Fig. 3-2).

Both counterconditioning and systematic desensitization are generally conducted simultaneously. As an illustration, consider a dog that is very fearful of the sound of fireworks. One can arrange training sessions to expose the dog to the sound of fireworks using a cap gun and working up to using a starter pistol, available through sporting catalogs or retail stores. A pistol fires .22 caliber blank cartridges so it sounds and smells like firecrackers. The sound can be muffled by several layers of boxes and blankets (Fig. 3-3). If the shots are sufficiently muffled, the dog can be told to "sit" and focus on the owner and the emotional disturbance will be mild or nonexistent. One can then start the counterconditioning by giving the dog a bit of favored food after each muffled shot of the starter pistol, but only if the dog is calm and not anxious. It is convenient for a training session to consist of a full cylinder of blank shots. The food will create an internal appetitive emotional reaction that is classically conditioned to the sound (and smell) of muffled gunshots. After a few

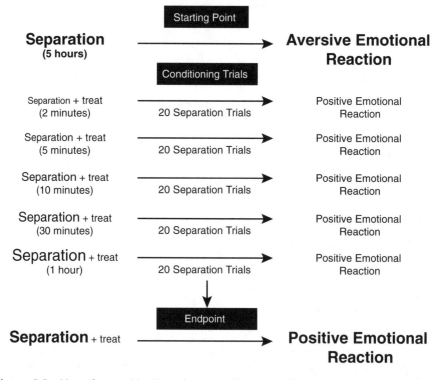

Figure 3-2 Use of a combination of systematic desensitization and counterconditioning to treat separation anxiety in a dog. The systematic desensitization aspect is the same as in Figure 3-1 except that by adding counterconditioning with a food treat paired with the departure, a positive emotional reaction is associated with separation.

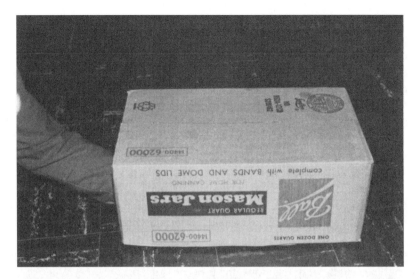

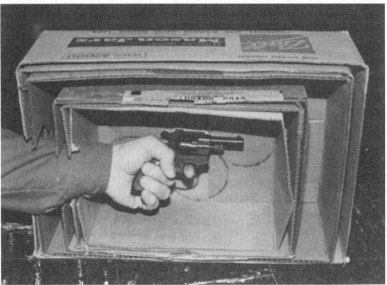

Figure 3-3 Nested cardboard boxes muffle the sound produced by a .22 caliber starter pistol to desensitize a dog to firecrackers. The boxes are placed with the open ends on a floor. Systematic desensitization proceeds as the nested boxes are uncovered, one at a time, over a series of training sessions. Blankets may be used instead of boxes.

training sessions the muffled shot may come to produce this desirable emotional reaction. This reaction is incompatible with the aversive emotional state and fear response previously evoked by fireworks.

As mentioned, in the training sessions the fear response should not be apparent because the gunshot sound is so muffled. As the muffling blankets are removed, layer after layer, the gunshot sound becomes louder, but the degree of aversive emotional reaction remains weak. This is because, with each session, the animal's fear and aversive emotional responses are desensitized, and an appetitive emotional response is conditioned to the sound. With an ideal outcome, the pistol eventually can be fired with no muffling and, instead of evoking the fear reaction, an appetitive emotional reaction is produced. More often one would expect the dog to show only mild disturbance to a gunshot. In outlining this process to clients it may be useful to explain that the goal is to condition the dog eventually to "love" to hear gunshots.

There are other options available for the desensitization process. The owners can start sessions with a recording of fireworks played at a low volume and progressively increase the volume. First one should play the recording at full volume once to determine whether the dog reacts to it, because if the recording does not accurately portray the real thing, the desensitization and counterconditioning sessions will probably not affect any change.

Although it is common to think of counterconditioning as useful primarily for resolving fear and anxiety reactions, the process is useful for other types of behavior therapy. The establishment of a positive emotional reaction through counterconditioning may be used to create a favorable disposition in a dog toward people, a process referred to as affection control in the treatment of dominance-related aggression (Chapter 8).

Consider, for example, a dog that had been strongly attached to an unmarried man. After the owner marries, the dog frequently threatens and even occasionally bites the wife. The dog may have been punished by the husband for this aggressiveness with no influence on the problem. Counterconditioning was employed when the husband was instructed to withdraw all affection and attention from the dog for a 2-week period. The dog was to obtain social interaction, praise, affection, and favored food treats only from the woman. When the dog approached the man he was simply to turn away. A positive association toward the wife was thus counterconditioned. The problem was further resolved when the woman was instructed to take advantage of the opportunities to gain the upper hand in control of the dog by requiring the dog to respond to some commands, such as "sit down," before giving the dog rewards.

Counterconditioning is also routinely used to deal with separation anxiety. Because of the fear and anxiety produced by being left alone, some dogs engage in a variety of misbehaviors, including defecating and urinating in unacceptable places, vocalizing excessively, and being destructive. This problem behavior is dealt with in detail in Chapter 10. One aspect of solving the problem involves staging short departures that result in no perceivable anxiety. After a history of short departures where the dog comes to anticipate being left alone only a short time, one gives the dog a long-lasting treat, such as a food stuffed toy or a knucklebone upon leaving. The dog will associate being left for brief periods with the reinforcing properties of the treat. The treats paired with departures should lead to the departures being counterconditioned to the appetitive emotional reaction induced by the food treats; this may be strong enough to overcome the mild anxiety that follows a short departure. As training sessions progress, the dog is gradually desensitized and counterconditioned to departures of longer and longer durations.

COUNTERCONDITIONING
• Use with systematic desensitization. • Pair treats with gradients of stimulus.

Drug-Facilitated Desensitization

It is becoming increasingly common to administer an anti-anxiety medication on a chronic basis to facilitate desensitization, especially when it is difficult to establish a graded stimulus presentation due to the owner's schedule, or because of an extreme reaction by the animal, or the inability to avoid the stimulus. Reducing the emotional reaction by administration of antianxiety medication allows more flexibility with the starting point and presumably more slack in the exposure to the fear-evoking stimulus. Sometimes autonomous desensitization occurs and the medication can be gradually phased out while systematic desensitization is employed, as necessary, to more completely resolve the problem. It is conceivable that for a fear reaction that is reduced pharmacologically, an intentional systematic desensitization schedule may not be necessary, but in most instances one can expect less-than-complete resolution. Figure 3-4 illustrates the concept of drug-facilitated desensitization; combining the use of anti-anxiety drugs as adjuvants in desensitization is discussed

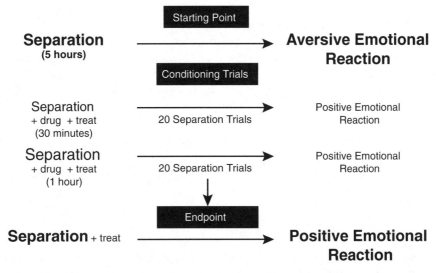

Figure 3-4 Use of a psychotropic drug to facilitate desensitization and counterconditioning to treat separation anxiety in a dog. The drug eliminates or weakens the aversive emotional reaction to separation anxiety and induces a positive emotional reaction evoked by a food treat that is associated with the departure stimuli. After several weeks, the drug dosage is gradually reduced, and the end point is the same as that when systematic desensitization and counterconditioning are used without a drug. The theoretical advantage of the drug facilitation is to allow departures to be longer and more flexible.

in Chapter 5. Separation anxiety, one of the most common anxiety-related problems for dogs, is commonly treated with anti-anxiety medication, which helps allow for some desensitization to departures without the rigid adherence to a departure training schedule. It is recommended that some form of planned desensitization and counterconditioning be used along with antianxiety medication for the best resolution of anxiety- or fear-related problem behaviors, including separation anxiety. The use of counterconditioning potentiates the desensitization process.

Therapeutic Use of Operant Conditioning

A process similar to counterconditioning but which does not focus on emotional responses is to condition an operant that is incompatible with an undesirable operant response. If a dog is digging holes, for example, and the digging behavior does not stem from anxiety, one might solve the digging problem by training the dog to dig in a spot that is acceptable.

The use of operant conditioning techniques to solve some problems often involves shaping a desirable response through the process of successive approximation. In such instances it is necessary to define the behavioral goal in precise terms, determine a beginning point for conditioning, and devise a gradient from the beginning point to the behavioral goal. Teaching a dog to stay around the backyard to solve a roaming problem illustrates this principle. Initially, one could go out into the backyard every 5 or 10 minutes and reinforce a dog for being there with a food treat. The behavior being rewarded is simply hanging around and may take different forms such as sleeping, playing, and watching people. The average time between reinforcements is gradually increased and the intervals are varied (variable interval schedule). One can also make the yard more exciting by placing food treats around the yard so that the dog is rewarded for exploring.

Another example of using successive approximation of operant conditioning to solve misbehavior is teaching a dog to ring a bell rather than scratch on the door to get human family members to open the door to allow it to come in. A bell, mounted on a bracket, can be placed close to the spot where the animal is scratching so that it cannot help but hit the bell when scratching the door. All scratching behavior is ignored and the owner simply waits for the animal to hit the bell before letting it in. After a few days most dogs will be hitting the bell rather than scratching at the door. Over a period of the next few days the bell can be gradually moved to a final desirable location.

Extinction of an Operant Response

An operant response may be eliminated by permanently withholding any further reinforcement, resulting in extinction of the response, and, as mentioned, extinction is easier with responses that have been reinforced on a continuous rather than an intermittent basis. One of the best uses of the extinction technique is in dealing with attention-seeking behaviors, even ones such as feigned lameness, snapping at imaginary flies, or tail chasing. By simply walking away whenever the animal shows the attention-seeking behavior, the behavior is eventually extinguished. An example of such an approach is illustrated in a case in which a client complained that his cat was biting its tail as though it were irritated and itching. No dermatologic problem, peripheral neuritis, or other medical cause could be found. Nevertheless, the cat continued to chew on its tail, which became so mutilated that it had to be amputated so the cat could no longer reach it. Still the cat attempted to grab at its phantom tail. Careful questioning of the owner revealed that the cat chased its tail only in the owner's presence, and when it did so, the owner invariably picked up and comforted the cat. The client was instructed to no longer reinforce the tail-chasing behavior with comforting and to walk away from the cat whenever the behavior occurred. For the first few days, when the client walked away from the cat, the animal would sometimes follow him into the next room and begin his little act again. The owner continued simply to walk away and over about 2 weeks the tail chasing behavior completely disappeared.

Extinction is almost impossible to use for cases in which reinforcement is closely linked to the behavior and cannot easily be separated. For example, this would be true for a dog jumping up on people. The reinforcement is built in because as soon as the dog jumps up, it receives interaction with a person. The interaction can be positive or negative, for even yelling at a dog is a form of interaction and attention. For undesirable operants in which extinction is not feasible, the best approach is to condition alternative behaviors that are acceptable.

One of the interesting aspects of extinction is that in the initial part of the extinction process, an animal may engage in the behavior more frequently and intensely before it tapers off, as if to try harder before giving up; this is referred to as an *extinction burst*. In giving clients advice in using extinction, it should be emphasized that for a period of time after the reinforcement is withheld, the behavior may get somewhat worse before it gets better.

Another point to emphasize when recommending the extinction approach is that when a pet owner decides to start extinguishing a behavior, the withdrawal of the reinforcement must be complete. One must not give in, even occasionally, to relieve the more objectionable extremes of behavior. If one gives in, the behavior then becomes reinforced on an intermittent schedule and at the same time the more objectionable parts of the behavior are shaped. By giving in even once, one makes the whole extinction process much more lengthy. Extinction is an active process and one is simply waiting for a number of responses to be emitted before elimination of the behavior finally takes place.

Punishment

Punishment is a complex process that involves elements of an animal's innate behavioral predispositions, classical conditioning, and operant conditioning. Punishment is defined as the application of an aversive stimulus (positive punishment) or removal of a rewarding (reinforcing) stimulus (negative punishment), contingent upon the performance of a particular behavior, that decreases the probability of that behavior occurring in the future. One uses punishment with the intention that the effects will endure and that the animal's behavior will change as a result of the experience. When this happens there is usually some sort of conditioning process involved. Punishment is not the same as negative reinforcement. Negative reinforcement is the removal of an aversive stimulus to increase the probability of behavior.

In this section three forms of punishment are discussed: interactive punishment, remote punishment, and social punishment. In all instances, one goal is to stop the ongoing undesirable behavior and another is to discourage the animal from engaging in that behavior in the future. Often several applications of punishment may be needed to have a lasting effect on behavior. This is due to the enduring aspects of punishment requiring some sort of learning, either by classical conditioning, operant conditioning, or extinction of an operant. It is important to distinguish between the different types of punishment because the particular punishing technique that is recommended should be clearly designed for the problem one is trying to resolve.

Interactive Punishment

When a person hits an animal with his or her hand or with an instrument such as a rolled-up newspaper, or shouts at it in a threatening way, this is interactive punishment. A hallmark of interactive punishment is that the animal associates the unpleasant stimulus with the person. Interactive punishment is not recommended clinically for resolving problem behavior. When used for misbehavior, interactive punishment may stop the ongoing behavior, but it has little enduring value. Clearly it is fruitless to administer interactive punishment hours, or even minutes, after an act of misbehavior.

The disadvantages of interactive punishment aside, many people who successfully raise and interact with their dogs have, at one time or another, exerted this type of punishment when their pet showed signs of aggressiveness, barked and frightened people, or were at risk of running into a situation where they were at danger. Almost without thinking one may use this type of punishment to stop an ongoing unwanted behavior in dogs such as jumping up onto people, getting into the cat litter box, or chasing a cat. When used in such special situations and infrequently, mild interactive punishment often accomplishes the immediate goal and does no harm.

A common difficulty with the use of interactive punishment is inconsistency on the part of the owner. Jumping up on people may be allowed on weekends when the owners are in old clothes, but the behavior may be verbally admonished on weekdays when the owners are dressed for work. Because punishment and reward are administered on an intermittent basis, the behavior continues. The primary disadvantage of interactive punishment is that with harsh or frequent use, the person

---

INTERACTIVE PUNISHMENT

- Involves discipline, such as hitting, yelling, grabbing
- Not recommended as a therapeutic measure
- Contraindicated for fear-related problems
- May evoke aggression from cats

delivering the punishment can evoke classically conditioned fear and aversive emotional reactions in the animal. The use of harsh, interactive punishment may lead to the situation of fear of certain classes of people resembling the person who delivered the punishment.

Another disadvantage of using interactive punishment is that the animal can differentiate between when the owner is present or not. A dog that is punished only by interactive punishment for knocking over the garbage can quickly learn that it cannot knock over the can when the owners are present, but is free to do so when the owners are gone and not around to punish it.

Remote Punishment

The most effective type of punishment for acts of misbehavior is remote punishment. An example is the use of a motion-activated water sprinkler to punish a dog for digging underneath a gate to escape. Except for dogs that love water sprays, this is harmless but still aversive, and the punishment is delivered immediately after the digging begins. This type of punishment is referred to as "remote" because the connection between the punishing stimulus and the person responsible for the punishment is removed. The aversive stimulus not only stops the ongoing undesirable behavior, but an aversive emotional reaction may be classically conditioned to the performance of the behavior, at least in the situation where the behavior occurred. Remote punishment can be successfully used with cats as well as dogs.

Most of the devices marketed for altering pet behavior, such as buried perimeter wires that shock a dog approaching a boundary, electronic mats that mildly shock a dog or cat that jumps on furniture, and loud sirens that are triggered by the motions of a pet approaching, are all examples of remote punishment devices, although the product literature may not use the term "punishment." The use of water sprayers or upside-down plastic carpet runners to discourage cats from walking on countertops is another example, as long as the person is not seen doing the spraying.

There are conventional principles for the successful use of remote punishment for resolving problem behavior that should be reviewed every time punishment is recommended:

1. Punishment techniques should be employed after arrangements are made for the animal to engage in an acceptable alternative to the undesirable behavior. Thus, providing an appropriate digging area should be done before a dog is punished for digging in the unacceptable area.
2. Before punishment is used, an attempt should be made to reduce the animal's motivation to engage in the unacceptable behavior. Thus, one might castrate a male dog before punishing it for urine marking in the house.
3. As much as possible, every act of misbehavior should be punished. Inconsistency in punishment will retard the establishment of a classically conditioned aversion to the circumstances or target of the misbehavior and the punishment is less likely to have lasting effects. Thus, if used for excessive barking, bark-activated collars should punish every barking episode.
4. The undesirable behavior must be punished within seconds. The longer the delay between the misbehavior and the punishment, the less likely there will be

an enduring effect of the punishment. Using a water sprayer on a cat after it has already jumped off the counter is useless. Punishment of a dog for digging an hour or two later is similarly useless.

5.   The requirement for consistency and immediacy of the punishing stimulus may necessitate limiting opportunities for the misbehavior unless punishment can be delivered. To punish a cat for scratching on a chair, for example, it may be necessary to cover the chair with plastic sheeting except when remote punishment can be delivered.

One of the classic examples of remote punishment is the electric shock collar used for misbehavior in dogs. Although the brunt of lots of bad press, the shock collar, when used correctly and for serious problems, often appears to be an effective type of remote punishment for such life-threatening behaviors as chasing bicyclists and cars. The shock collar has been shown to be more effective than drugs in suppressing acral lick dermatitis[6] and can save a dog from the misery of wearing an Elizabethan collar the rest of its life to prevent excessive licking.

The collar designed to deliver a burst of citronella spray when remotely triggered is an alternative to the shock collar. With both the citronella and shock collars the aversive stimulation is associated with the act of misbehavior or with the object to which the behavior is directed. The collar, or a dummy collar, must be worn at non-training times so that the animal does not make an association between the collar weight and the likelihood of punishment. Experience has shown that if the collar is not effective in altering behavior in the first few trials, it will not change the misbehavior with repeated trials. Not only must one follow the principles of remote punishment in using such collars, but it is necessary to use the triggering device out of view of the dog so the aversive stimulus is not associated with the person.

In the bark-activated collar, a sensor in the collar detects vibrations that are produced by barking. The advantage of a bark collar is that one does not have to be present to activate the shock or spray of citronella. A disadvantage is that one cannot judge the dog's reaction to every aversive stimulus occurrence. Some dogs may be so highly motivated to bark that the aversive stimulus may not suppress the bark or the dog may find a way of barking that is too weak to activate the collar. With a citronella collar, a dog may learn that it can empty the collar by barking a certain number of times, thereafter being able to bark without punishment. More work is needed to understand the relative effectiveness of the citronella versus shock collar for suppressing excessive barking. One report on citronella collars found that barking was most effectively reduced when the dogs wore the collar intermittently, a finding inconsistent with one of the principles of punishment outlined above.[7]

REMOTE PUNISHMENT

- Lower motivation for undesirable behavior.
- Reward acceptable behavior.
- Stage punishment sessions if necessary.
- Deliver punishment immediately after misbehavior.
- Punish every act of misbehavior.
- This is also useful with cats.

A discussion of remote punishment would not be complete without mention of relatively low-tech devices. One such device is the ordinary mousetrap. Right-side-up–loaded mousetraps may be used to punish dogs for serious behaviors such as digging under a fence to escape. A loaded mousetrap, carefully placed upside down, flies up into the air when touched and may be enough to frighten a cat. Behavior modification through mousetrap therapy has been used to punish a feline remotely for problems such as digging into flower pots, jumping on counters, soiling a child's sandbox, and urine spraying in specific areas. Most mousetraps must be adjusted so that they can be set and placed upside down and not go off until touched. This usually requires bending the metal tongue that holds the cheese. One can use single mousetraps for small places or arrange a group of them in a line with the intention of achieving a chain reaction. The most interesting arrangement is to stack three or four mousetraps together so that they all go off at the same time (Fig. 3-5). As with any type of remote punishment, it is important that the use of mousetrap punishment be consistent. As soon as possible after some mousetraps have been set off, they should be reset so as to punish repeated misbehavior. After a few days, if there is no evidence of further misbehavior, it may be possible to remove the mousetraps. There are commercially available snappers that have less of a chance of inadvertent injury that may work as well as mousetraps, although they are more difficult to disguise.

Another old-fashioned remote punishment for cats is the water sprayer. The common plant sprayer can be adjusted so that it delivers a stream of water and is relatively quiet so as not to allow it to be identified with the person doing the spraying. To be effective, the cat must be sprayed with the water with complete detachment, and not chased around the house, and the animal should not see the person

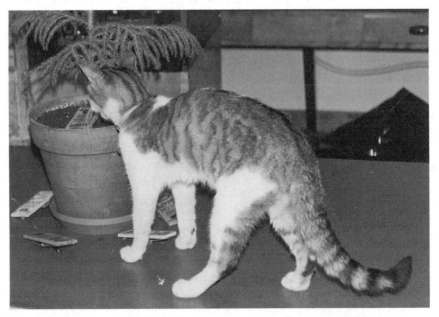

Figure 3-5 Remote punishment. A cat examines the site where upside-down mousetraps have been sprung by another cat.

spraying it. Following the principle of consistency, it may be necessary to physically separate the cat from the object to which misbehavior is directed until the owner is around and able to punish the misbehavior.

When the owner notices the cat engaging in misbehavior, she or he should approach the cat slowly in an unemotional fashion, secretly grab the water sprayer, and spray the cat. When sprayers are left at several convenient locations, it will not be necessary for the owner to dash around looking for the sprayer hoping that the cat will stay at the misbehavior until the sprayer is found. Another option is for the owner to carry around a small squirt gun.

Social Punishment

This type of punishment, referred to as negative punishment, relies on the principle of removing a rewarding stimulus; in behavior therapy this is most commonly achieved by removing social interaction—hence the name *social punishment*. Companion animals, especially dogs, do not like people to abandon them or having to leave a place of fun and social interaction. Thus, one can punish dogs by terminating such pleasant social situations. The advantage of this type of punishment is that it does not involve the direct application of an aversive stimulus. The disadvantage is that it does not have the same immediacy in stopping ongoing behavior as does remote punishment. Social punishment is sometimes referred to as a "time out," when an animal is taken to a room for isolation, such as a utility room or bathroom, for a period of time after it displays some misbehavior.

Whether one is using social punishment in the form of just walking away from the dog or a time-out location, there is always a delay between the punishing effect of social isolation and the behavior that brought on the punishment. Therefore, an audible bridging stimulus, such as a duck call or a toy kazoo, should be used to precede the social punishment. If a bridging stimulus is sounded immediately after the misbehavior occurs, but prior to the social withdrawal, it takes on the aversive properties of the social withdrawal and communicates the exact behavior that is being punished. Several pairings of the bridging stimulus with the social isolation are required to establish a connection between the bridging stimulus and the social punishment. Stimuli that are low-pitched and prolonged have inhibiting effects on behavior,[8,9] and are, therefore, better than clickers as a bridging stimulus for social punishment.

Social punishment may be used with dogs that misbehave by barking or growling at strangers on a walk. Assuming a dog enjoys the walk, one must stage the mis-

---

SOCIAL PUNISHMENT

- Terminate social interaction.
- Reward acceptable behavior.
- Lower motivation for unacceptable behavior.
- Stage misbehavior to optimize effectiveness.
- Use bridging stimulus to target misbehavior.
- Follow rules of consistency and immediacy.

behavior so that a stranger walks up to the dog soon after the walk begins. Upon the first sign of misbehavior the owner then sounds a bridging stimulus (blows a kazoo) and takes the dog back into the house. The reason the dog must be set up for this punishment is that if a stranger were to be confronted at the end of the walk, and the walk terminated at that point, the dog would not necessarily notice that the walk was truncated.

After several staged encounters with strangers within the first minute or two of a walk, it should be arranged so the dog can go on about half of the walks without seeing any stranger and thus without the potential of social punishment. Thus, there is a contrast between walks that are allowed to continue and those that are truncated because of a misbehavior. The problem is resolved when a dog meets strangers and acts in an acceptable manner. This treatment must also be done in conjunction with other behavior modifications, such as desensitization and counterconditioning.

Use of the Nose-Loop Head Halter

With the exception of cats and ferrets, the history of human domestication of animals has invariably involved some type of restraint applied to the head or neck. In the domestication process it was discovered that placing some sort of restraint on the head of horses, cattle, and dogs allowed human handlers to subdue an animal that was larger or more physically adept. The animals could be controlled with relative ease and little confrontation. Control of the dogs has most commonly involved a buckle collar and, when necessary, the choke chain or pinch collar. For dogs that were a risk to other dogs or human handlers, the leather muzzle, and more recently the plastic basket muzzle, has found widespread use. Muzzles are still recommended for certain types of problem behavior discussed in Section II.

In the last couple of decades a new type of collar for dogs was introduced: a head collar with an adjustable nose loop (Fig. 3-6). The head halter is constructed such that when the leash is pulled up (or the dog pulls against the leash) pressure is applied through the nose loop and behind the head. When the leash is pulled there is no pressure on the trachea or other structures in the neck, and no apparent discomfort or pain delivered to the animal. However, the human handler clearly has better control than with any type of neck collar. Aside from facilitating behavior modification, a common use is for dogs that tend to pull against the leash. The head halter gives the handler direct control over the head, and hence the dog is not at a tug-of-war with the handler on the other end of the leash.

Users of the head halter often notice a physiological calming of the dog when the halter is used, perhaps stemming from pressure on the nose loop and behind the head. One school of thought, taking a cue from the acupuncture model, is that the pressure on these areas of the head and neck leads to release of an endogenous endorphin which in turn has a calming influence. Invariably, when caregivers use the head halter in taking a dog on a walk, the dog is more easily led alongside than with a neck collar. When the dog is switched back to a neck collar, the unruly

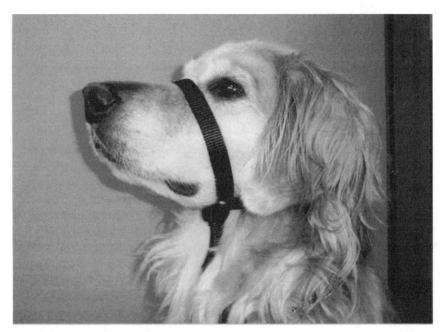

Figure 3-6 Head halter of the type used to gain control of dogs.

behavior often returns at some level, if subsequent training in teaching the dog not to pull is not undertaken.

Some clients will comment that their dog does not "like" their head halter, which is often indicated by a dog trying to avoid having the collar put on. These actions may prompt owners to discontinue the use of the head collar. One study showed no physiological differences between dogs wearing a head collar and those wearing a flat buckle collar, both for the first time.[10] Another study demonstrated that dogs habituated quickly to wearing a head collar, regardless of what type was worn.[11]

Examples of Use of the Nose-Loop Halter

The head halter has found widespread use among behaviorists as an adjunct to behavior modification programs, especially when dogs are exposed to fear- or anxiety-inducing stimuli. For example, a dog wearing the halter can be placed into a sit position with a relaxed leash while anxiety-producing children come into a room at a specified distance. As long as the dog shows no signs of fear or anxiety, these desensitization trials may continue, with the result that the calmness induced by the halter facilitates the desensitization process, somewhat in the same sense expected from an antianxiety drug.

Another use of the halter is to facilitate the assertion of control by members of the family as an aspect of treatment for dominance-related aggression. By having the dog wear the halter continuously throughout the day, or as long as the owners are present, and dragging a lightweight 10-foot leash, a caregiver can more easily grab the leash without being near the dog's head and pull the dog up to a sit position. If this is done repeatedly it facilitates the assertion of control by the person involved. The halter also allows a convenient way to deal with situations where a dog growls when someone attempts to remove it from a bed or couch. One simply grabs the long leash and pulls the dog away from the area of challenge and into an obedient sit position. Use of the halter for correcting behavior should be preceded by a command that gives the dog an opportunity to respond prior to being pulled by the lead. With the use of the head halter it is still recommended that appropriate behavior be rewarded with praise and a food treat. One can also more easily lead the dog into a time-out area.

On a case-by-case basis, the clinician should work with the client to decide whether the dog should wear the halter continuously or at certain times. In many instances of dominance aggression it may be advisable to use the affection-control technique (Chapter 8) first until the dog is showing major improvement, allowing the owner to put the halter on more easily. For predictable fear- or anxiety-producing situations, and where there is no difficulty with putting on the halter, the halter could be used in conjunction with training sessions.

Fitting the Halter

In the use of head halters it is important that dogs associate its use with rewarding events. It is usually recommended that the halter be gradually introduced to the dog while feeding it small tidbits of food through the nose loop so that the appearance and feel of the halter is associated with food treats.

The halter referred to as the Gentle Leader is closely fitted so that the neck strap accepts only two fingers and so that the nose loop cannot be pushed off the end of the dog's nose. It is common for dogs to struggle the first few times they wear the halter by pulling back, twisting, and even spinning on the ground and pawing at the nose loop. The best way to deal with the struggling is simply to stand firmly and pull the leash upward. Every time the dog stops to try to shake its head or paw at the nose loop, one pulls the leash firmly again, and when the dog stops struggling, relaxes the leash. Most dogs will accept the halter within a few minutes of control. One can then be sure to associate wearing the halter with rewarding situations, occasional food treats, and praise and affection. Behaviorists usually find it is advisable to refer to the instructions that come with the product and to fit the halter on a dog in the examination room so that the owner sees how this is to done and how initial struggling is handled. Instructional videos are available to help educate clients. These videos can be played while a client in the waiting room or exam room waits. Technicians should be educated in the proper fitting of the head halters. If one has a pet dog accustomed to the halter, this dog could be used for a demonstration at the office.

References

1. Gustavson CR. Comparative and field aspects of learned food aversions. In: Barker LM, Best MR, Domjan M, eds. Learning Mechanisms in Food Selection. Baylor, Texas: Baylor University Press, 1977:23–43.

2. Gustavson CR, Garcia J, Hankins WG, Rusiniak KW. Coyote predation control by aversive conditioning. Science 1974;184:581.

3. Skinner BF. How to teach animals. Scientific American 1951;185:26–29.

4. Pryor K. Don't Shoot the Dog. Bantam Books,1985;187 pages.

5. Tuber DS, Hothersall D, Voith VL. Animal clinical psychology: A modest proposal. American Psychology 1974;29:762–766.

6. Eckstein RA, Hart BL. Treatment of canine acral lick dermatitis by behavior modification using electronic stimulation. Journal of the American Animal Hospital Association 1996;32:225–230.

7. Wells DL. The effectiveness of a citronella spray collar in reducing certain forms of barking in dogs. Applied Animal Behavior Science 2001;79(4):299–309.

8. McConnell PB, Baylis JR. Interspecific communication in cooperative herding: Acoustic and visual signals from human shepherds and herding dogs. Zeitschrift fur Tierpsychologie 1985;67:302–328.

9. McConnell PB. Lessons from animal trainers: The effect of acoustic structure on an animal's response. In: Bakeson, Klopfer, eds. Perspectives in Ethology, Vol 9: Human Understanding & Animal Awareness. Plenum Press, 1991:165–187.

10. Ogburn P, Crouse S, Martin F, Houpt K. Comparison of behavioral and physiological responses of dogs wearing two different types of collars. Applied Animal Behavior Science 1998;61:133–142.

11. Haug LI, Beaver BV, Longnecker MT. Comparison of dogs' reactions to four different head collars. Applied Animal Behavior Science 2002;79:53–61.

Chapter 4
Hormones and Behavior; Gonadectomy

For thousands of years surgical or other forms of castration were used on male cattle, sheep, goats, and swine as part of routine husbandry practice. The fact that castration was apparently readily adopted by ancient humans is testimony to the effectiveness of the procedure in altering undesirable behavior. Ancient animal caretakers probably were concerned with reducing serious fighting among adult males kept for food and labor, and for reducing the tendency for male animals to be aggressive toward human caretakers. Gonadectomy of companion dogs and cats is a much more recent development. The terms *castration* and *neutering* are used sometimes interchangeably to refer to spaying of females as well as castration of males.

A major motivation for the national effort of neutering pet dogs and cats has been to control the overproduction of unwanted pets. One could, of course, address this goal by vasectomy of males and tubal ligation of females, as in human birth control. Such surgical sterilization, leaving gonadal hormone production intact, has never received serious consideration and neutering of pets is promoted as a humane expression of responsible pet ownership. Given the demographics of pet ownership, this is a reasonable stance. In some other countries, however, gonadectomy is not routinely performed. It is interesting, however, that even among veterinary scientists not much thought is given to any consequences of the widespread physiological effects of removal of gonadal hormones. Two apparent disadvantages are a possible increase in risk of prostatic carcinoma[1,2] and an increased likelihood of progression of cognitive dysfunction in dogs as they age.[3] Admittedly, the behavioral disadvantages of gonadectomy may be outweighed by reducing undesirable behavioral tendencies such as aggressive behavior, at least in the more aggressive breeds, and advancing the goal of convenient pet population control.

In this chapter the behavioral changes that can be attributed to gonadectomy are discussed. With the exception of effects on cognitive function, these changes are in the direction of being desirable from the human standpoint and include a reduced tendency toward several types of aggression, loss of sexual interest, and reduction of urine marking. In a sense, this aspect of companion animal husbandry induces changes in animals that, in nature, would be considered abnormal or maladaptive. Most pet owners are aware of the fact that some animals, especially male cats, would generally be impossible to keep as pets without castration because of the normal occurrence of objectionable masculine behavior, including roaming, fighting, and urine marking. Spaying of females not only prevents pregnancy, but also

prevents these animals from displaying the behavioral aspects of estrus that interfere with the maintenance of pets in urban areas. It is known that although other
hormones—such as the adrenal corticotropic hormone, adrenal cortical steroids,
and thyroxine—affect behavior, the behavioral effects are not pronounced, and
these hormones are not altered clinically with the intent of changing behavior.
Thus, this chapter deals only with gonadal hormones.

Veterinarians and other animal care professionals are expected to know what
behavioral patterns may be altered by gonadectomy, whether it is used for pet population control or therapeutically for altering problem behavior. Clinical retrospective surveys on problem behavior, coupled with laboratory studies on sexual behavior, have provided considerable information about what to expect when adult males
are castrated in an attempt to alter problem behavior. In addition to addressing the
types of behavior that are altered, this chapter examines 1) the probability that a
specific behavior in an individual will be altered by castration, 2) the role of experience in the retention of a behavioral pattern after castration, 3) species differences
between dogs and cats in response to castration, and 4) a comparison of castration
performed before and after adulthood. There are fewer issues to examine with
regard to ovariectomy or ovariohysterectomy in females because adult females generally display fewer objectionable behavioral patterns that are influenced by gonadectomy. The operation usually results in complete and immediate elimination of
female sexual behavior.

The topic of gonadal hormones and behavior is an area where some important
concepts from experimental studies on laboratory dogs and cats, as well as rodents,
bolster information obtained from pet owners regarding the effects of gonadectomy. Some groundwork for discussion of the effects of gonadectomy on clinically
relevant behavior will be reviewed by covering the concept of sexually dimorphic
behavior patterns, dealing with the types of behavioral changes to expect following
removal of gonadal hormones. The discussion then turns to the effects of castration
on clinically relevant behaviors. This is followed by a comparison of males castrated before puberty with the effects of castration on adult males. Some of the
information about the behavioral effects of gonadectomy for females will be discussed although there is much less clinically relevant information available in this
area than with males. Finally, a possible effect of early gonadectomy will be discussed as it relates to cognitive function in aging dogs.

Hormones and Sexually Dimorphic Behavior

A well-established concept in behavioral endocrinology is that developing males
are subject to a surge in testosterone secretion in either early neonatal and/or late
prenatal life, which acts on the brain to bring about sex-specific changes in the
hypothalamus and other areas. This is the so-called organizational effect of hormones. The effects of testosterone in the male brain are through the aromatization
of some testosterone to estrogen, which then brings about the malelike cytoarchitectural changes in brain structure.[4] The basic hypothalamic cytoarchitecture is
femalelike and remains so in females as a reflection of the lack of testosterone (and

estrogen) during early development. This organizational concept was developed from hundreds of studies on laboratory rodents and primates and generally applies to mammalian species, including dogs and cats. The hormonal profiles of dogs and cats during the prenatal period have not been fully characterized. As shown in Figure 4-1, the perinatal surge in testosterone occurs in dogs (and probably cats) in the prenatal period.[5]

When the perinatal brain development period has passed, the tendency toward masculinity in males and femininity in females appears to be irreversibly built into the brain although both males and females still retain the neural circuitry for the display of behavioral patterns typical of both sexes.[6] Even after gonadectomy, the two sexes remain fundamentally different. The administration of estrogen to castrated males does not generally induce much female sexual behavior, nor does the administration of testosterone to ovariectomized females bring on a full display of male behavior. The differences in hypothalamic and other parts of the brain, as they relate to gender, deal with the probability or frequency with which masculine or feminine behavior is displayed, not to an absolute difference between males and females.

Before puberty, when the secretion of gonadal hormones differs very little between the sexes, males still differ from females behaviorally. An obvious difference between juvenile male and female dogs is the urination posture where females use a squat posture and males use the stand-lean urination posture. Sexes also differ in regard to play.[7] Among adults there is a difference in the degree to which the behavior of females and males differ. The leg-lift urination posture of male dogs is highly dimorphic, whereas territorial guarding appears to be much less sexually dimorphic.[8] It is the male sex-typical behaviors that are the most dimorphic that one

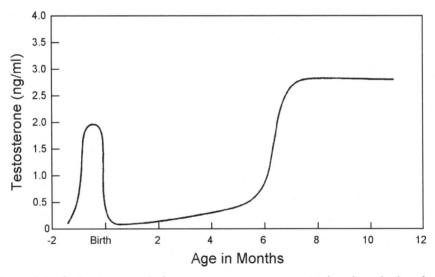

Figure 4-1 Stylized portrayal of serum testosterone concentrations in male dogs from late prenatal life to adulthood (data from Hart and Ladewig 1979[5]). (Reprinted with permission from Hart BL, Problems with objectionable sociosexual behavior of dogs and cats. Therapeutic use of castration and progestins. The Compendium on Continuing Education for the Small Animal Practitioner. 1979;1:461–465.)

would expect to be altered by castration. Consequently, urine marking, mounting, aggression to other dogs, and dominance toward human family members are most readily altered.

When adult male dogs and cats are castrated, all behavioral patterns that are testosterone dependent continue to be displayed for a period of time after testosterone has disappeared from the bloodstream. However, following castration, testosterone almost completely disappears from the bloodstream within hours. The persistence of the behaviors, for sometimes months or years in some individuals, is a reflection of the capability of the brain to continue to mediate this behavior without hormonal support. The persistence is not due to adrenal gland secretion or other sources of androgen.[6]

Observations on females by pet owners reveal that some females display male sex-typical behavior more than other females. Thus, some female dogs engage in leg-lift urination, but most do not. Similarly, some female cats engage in malelike urine spraying, but most do not. In exploring the possible role of perinatal hormones in this difference among females it has been found in rodents that the degree to which females display malelike behavior depends upon intrauterine effects during fetal life. Females that develop prenatally in the uterus between two males can be partially masculinized by diffusion of androgens through the contact of amniotic membranes.[9,10] Another mechanism by which females may be masculinized is by being located in the uterus in the downstream blood flow from male fetuses where they may be affected by blood-borne androgens.[11–13] These studies raise the possibility that enhanced masculine behavior seen in a small proportion of female cats and dogs could be due to fetal intrauterine effects. Limited evidence from a clinical survey was not supportive of this concept with regard to urine spraying and fighting in female cats.[14]

Because behavioral patterns involved in sexual interactions, including mounting, copulatory intermission, and the display of the ejaculatory pattern are so readily influenced by castration, these behavioral patterns have been measured in the laboratory and can be subjected to controlled experiments, which yield useful concepts that may be applied clinically. In all species studied, including cats, dogs, monkeys, and goats, castration is followed very soon by changes in behavior consisting mostly of an increased latency to sexual responses such as mounting the female.[15] The behavioral pattern that is first lost in these animals is the ejaculatory pattern followed later by loss of mounting and interest in females. There are considerable species differences in the rate with which the ejaculatory pattern is eliminated. As illustrated in Figure 4-2, within 5 weeks following castration, about half of male cats no longer displayed the copulatory pattern, for example, whereas in male dogs three-quarters still displayed the copulatory pattern 15 weeks following castration.[15]

Within a species there is considerable variation in the persistence of sexual behavior following castration, with some males no longer responding to females almost immediately after castration and others still responding 1 year later. This persistence of sexual responding in some animals and not others raises the issue of the role of sexual experience in the loss of sexual behavior after castration. All studies conducted in a controlled laboratory setting including those on dogs, show that

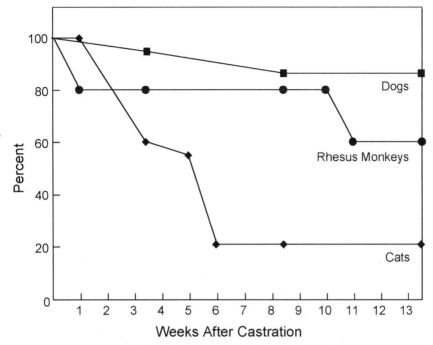

Figure 4-2 Effects of castration in mating behavior of male dogs, cats, and rhesus monkeys expressed as percent retaining the copulatory response for up to 13 weeks after castration. Note that species differences between dogs and cats apparently reflect sensitivity to androgen removal (data from Hart 1974[15]).

sexual experience has no influence on the retention of sexual behaviors after castration (Fig. 4-3).[16] In these studies on hormones and sexual behavior there are three important principles that apply clinically to the effects of castration: 1) there are pronounced species differences in the degree of behavior changes, 2) there are pronounced individual differences within a species, and 3) experience in performing the behavior appears to have no predictive value as to whether the animal will or will not engage in the behavior subsequent to castration.

Effects of Castration on Objectionable Behavior of Adult Male Dogs

The effects of castration have been addressed by asking owners of male dogs that were castrated to assess the degree to which they saw an improvement in problem behaviors. The behaviors that were assessed include urine marking in the house; mounting of other dogs, people, or inanimate objects; and various forms of aggression including that toward another family dog, a human family member, an unfamiliar dog, human territorial intruders, and unfamiliar people outside the home. Also examined was the degree to which the age of the dog and the duration of the problem behavior affected the response to castration.[17]

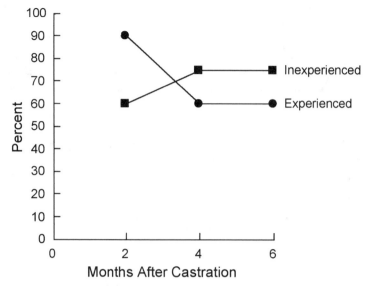

Figure 4-3   Absence of effects of mating experience on performance of mating behavior in male dogs expressed as percent of dogs retaining the copulatory response up to 6 months after castration. Shown is percent of experienced and inexperienced dogs retaining the copulatory response 2, 4, and 6 months after castration. Although experienced dogs had 30–40 matings prior to castrations, inexperienced dogs had only familiarization sessions with breeding females (data from Hart 1968[16]).

The information that may be used as a guideline for advising clients on the likelihood of behavioral change is summarized in Figure 4-4, which shows the percentage of dogs that can be expected to show an improvement of at least 50% or at least 90%. The latter may be considered basically a resolution of the problem. There was a significant effect of castration on all the behavioral patterns with the exception of fear of people or inanimate objects and aggression toward unfamiliar people away from the home. In about 70% of the dogs engaging in objectionable urine marking, mounting, and roaming, there was at least a 50% improvement; in 30% there was a 90% improvement. With about 30% of male dogs showing aggression toward another dog in the family or toward a human family member undergoing at least a 50% improvement, these behaviors were more likely to change than aggression toward unfamiliar dogs away from the home or human intruders with 10–15% of dogs showing improvement at the 50% level. There was no relationship between the effect of castration on problem behaviors and the age of the dog at the time of castration or the duration of the problem behavior prior to castration.

Effects of Castration on Objectionable Behavior of Adult Male Cats

Because tomcats are most often castrated well before adulthood, questions about the therapeutic use of castration to resolve problem behavior in adult males comes

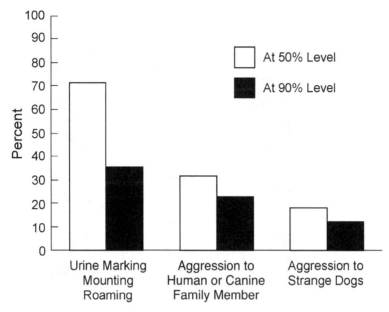

Figure 4-4 Effects of castration in improving problem behavior in adult male dogs expressed as improvement at the 90% level (virtual resolution) or improvement at the 50% or greater level (from Neilson et al. 1997[17]).

up less often than with dogs. Nonetheless, there are occasions when the clinician will be asked about the probability of altering behavior such as urine marking, fighting with other male cats, and mounting in tomcats. In contrast to the available information on dogs, castration is much more effective on cats in eliminating these problem behaviors.[18] In 80–90% of male cats there was a marked improvement in these three behavioral patterns (Fig. 4-5). In the clients surveyed, about one-half reported that there was a rather rapid change (in a week or two after castration), with the other half showing a more gradual change in behavior. When cats were presented with more than one problem behavior, the improvement in one behavior did not necessarily predict a change in the other. Although not systematically explored, there was no indication that those that were older and more experienced in performing the problem behavior were any less likely to be affected than the younger, less experienced males.

Prepubertal Castration

It is common practice for male cats to be castrated before puberty, and this behavior has become more common in dogs. Some research has focused on showing that gonadectomy as early as 7 weeks of age has no serious consequences with regard to increased medical conditions and no differential impact on behavior problems, such as urine marking or aggression, that were severe problems for the owners, than castration beyond 6 months of age.[19,20] Although gonadectomy prior to adulthood, regardless of exact age, seems to make no difference, there may be a mistaken

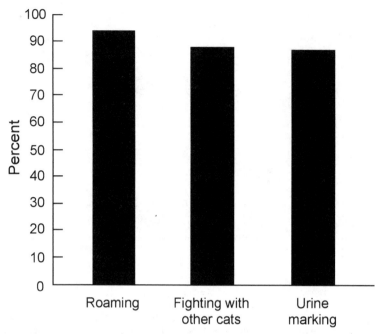

Figure 4-5 Effects of castration in improving problem behavior in adult male cats expressed as percent with marked improvement (from Hart and Barrett 1973[18]).

assumption that prepubertal castration is more effective in preventing problem behaviors, such as urine marking and aggressive behavior, than postpubertal castration in eliminating these behaviors after they have begun. In accordance with concepts from basic research on hormones and sexual behavior and rather extensive clinical information on cats, there appears to be no relationship between the age of male cats at the time of castration and the likelihood of spraying or fighting.[6] The probability of serious urine spraying occurring in cats castrated prior to adulthood was estimated at 10%, which is about the same probability of castration eliminating the behavior after it has started in adult males (Fig. 4-6). The observations on cats, indicating that prepubertal castration does not reduce masculine behavior any more than castration in adulthood, are also paralleled by similar findings in dogs as well as findings from studies on sexual behavior in laboratory rodents.[6]

Behavioral Effects of Ovarian Hormones

There is little clinical or experimental research relevant to the behavioral effects of ovariectomy in adult females. As mentioned, during the prenatal and neonatal development of females there is no significant amount of estrogen or progesterone secreted, and the brain development related to display of female behavior occurs as a function of the absence of testosterone.

In adult female dogs and cats, as in most other mammals, estrogen increases general activity. Females during estrus usually move about more, vocalize more

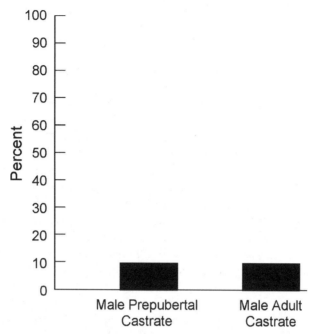

Figure 4-6 Comparison of effects of gonadectomy in cats on prevention of urine marking in males castrated before adulthood with persistence of urine marking in males castrated as adults. Shown are percent of male cats castrated prepubertally, and in which problem urine marking occurred later, and percent of castrated adults in which problem urine marking persisted (data from Hart and Cooper 1984[14]; Hart and Barrett 1973[18]).

frequently, and may act somewhat nervous. The urine and vaginal secretions of females in proestrus are attractive to males. The attractants are undoubtedly noticed by males living in the vicinity of females or by males on their daily treks through the females' vicinity. It is not known whether the attractants are metabolites of estrogen or a secretion added to the urine and vaginal secretions when estrogen secretion is high. There are stories about male dogs being attracted from miles away to the vicinity of an estrous female, presumably by one or more of the sex attractants in the urine. These attractants are probably not so potent as to be detected by males from miles away.

One may hear among dog handlers and dog trainers references to the calming or mellowing effects of allowing female dogs to experience one or more estrus periods. There is no clinical information addressing this issue. One study focused on aggressive dominance in female dogs as a function of the interaction between aggressive temperament and the age at which the dog was spayed. Females spayed before 12 months of age and that had an aggressive temperament seemed to become worse after being spayed, whereas females that had aggressive tendencies but were older than 12 months at the time they were spayed, did not become more aggressive.[21] Progesterone has calming influences, and because spaying removes the source of progesterone production, causing a precipitous fall in progesterone in females during the luteal phase, the sudden removal of progesterone may increase irritable tendencies in young females. After a female has gone through some estrus cycles, and possibly been disciplined for aggressive behavior, the spaying may have less of an impact.

Gonadectomy and Cognitive Impairment

A possible disadvantage of routine, early gonadectomy centers around the indications that estrogen and testosterone may play a role in preventing development of age-related cognitive impairment in dogs. Among other neuroprotective properties, both estrogen and testosterone reduce the accumulation of the beta-amyloid material[22,23] that comprises the neural plaques associated with cognitive impairment in humans[24] and dogs.[25,26] One study compared the progression of cognitive impairment in aging dogs that were neutered with those that were left intact. Gonadally intact male dogs were significantly less likely than neutered dogs to progress from a state of mild cognitive impairment to severe impairment.[3] One would expect estrogen to have a similar protective role in female dogs. If gonadal hormones do have some protective effects with regard to cognitive behavior in dogs, gonadectomy would appear to be important only in aging dogs and even then mostly in the subset of dogs that show mild cognitive impairment. Where age-related cognitive deficits due to gonadectomy may be of interest would be in working dogs where learning and memory are a vital part of their performance.

References

1. Bell FW, Klausner JS, Hayden DW, Feeney DA, Johnston SD. Clinical and pathologic features of prostatic adenocarcinoma in sexually intact and castrated dogs: 31 cases (1970–1987). Journal of the American Veterinary Medical Association 1991;199:1623–1630.
2. Obradovich J, Walshaw R, Goullaud E. The influence of castration on the development of prostatic carcinoma in the dog. Journal of Veterinary Internal Medicine 1987;1:183–187.
3. Hart BL. Effects of gonadectomy on subsequent development of age-related cognitive impairment in dogs. Journal of the American Veterinary Medical Association 2001; 219:51–56.
4. Hutchison RW, Beyer C. Gender-specific brain formation of oestrogen in behavioural development. Psychoneuroendocrinology 1994;19:529–541.
5. Hart BL, Ladewig J. Serum testosterone of neonatal male and female dogs. Biology of Reproduction 1979;21:289–292.
6. Hart BL, Eckstein RA. The role of gonadal hormones in the occurrence of objectionable behaviours in dogs and cats. Applied Animal Behavior Science 1997;52:331–344.
7. Deag JM, Manning A, Lawrence C. Factors influencing the mother-kitten relationship. In: Turner DC, Bateson T, eds. The Domestic Cat: The Biology of Its Behaviour. Cambridge: Cambridge University Press, 1988;23–39.
8. Hart BL, Hart LA. The Perfect Puppy: How to Choose Your Dog by Its Behavior. San Francisco: Freeman Press, 1988.
9. Clark MM, Malenfant SA, Winter DA, Galef BG. Fetal uterine position affects copulation and scent marking in adult male gerbils. Physiology and Behavior 1990;47:301–305.

10. vom Saal FS. Variation in phenotype due to random intrauterine positioning of male and female fetuses in rodents. Journal of Reproduction and Fertility 1981;62:633–650.

11. Houtsmuller EJ, Slob AK. Masculinization and defeminization of female rats by males located caudally in the uterus. Physiology and Behavior 1990;48:555–560.

12. Vomachka AJ, Lisk RD. Androgen and estradiol levels in plasma and amniotic fluid of late gestational male and female hamsters: Uterine position effects. Hormones and Behavior 1986;20:181–193.

13. Krohmer RW, Baum MJ. Effect of sex, intrauterine position and androgen manipulation on the development of brain aromatase activity in female ferrets. Journal of Neuroendocrinology 1989;1:265–271.

14. Hart BL, Cooper L. Factors related to urine spraying and fighting in prepubertally gonadectomized male and female cats. Journal of the Veterinary Medical Association 1984;184:1255–1258.

15. Hart BL. Gonadal androgen and sociosexual behavior of male mammals; A comparative analysis. Psychological Bulletin 1974;81:383–400.

16. ———. Role of prior experience in the effects of castration on sexual behavior of male dogs. Journal of Comparative Physiological Psychology 1968;66:719–725.

17. Neilson JC, Eckstein RA, Hart BL. Effects of castration on behavior of male dogs with reference to the role of age and experience. Journal of the American Veterinary Medical Association 1997;211:180–182.

18. Hart BL, Barrett RE. Effects of castration on fighting, roaming, and urine spraying in adult male cats. Journal of the American Veterinary Medical Association 1973;163:290–292.

19. Stubbs WP, Bloomberg MS, Scruggs SL, Shille VM, Lane TJ. Effects of prepubertal gonadectomy on physical and behavioral development in cats. Journal of the American Veterinary Medical Association 1996;209:1864–1872.

20. Spain CV, Scarlett JM, Houpt KA. Long-term risks and benefits of early-age gonadectomy in cats. Journal of the American Veterinary Medical Association 2004;224:372–386.

21. O'Farrell VO, Peachey E. Behavioural effects of ovariohysterectomy on bitches. Journal of Small Animal Practice 1990;31:595–598.

22. Xu H, Gouras GK, Greenfield JP, et al. Estrogen reduces neuronal generation of Alzheimer beta-amyloid peptides. Nature Medicine 1998;4:447–451.

23. Gouras GK, Xu H, Gross RS, et al. Testosterone reduces neuronal secretion of Alzheimer's b-amyloid peptides. Proceedings of the National Academy of Science USA 2000;97:1202–1205.

24. Ashford JW, Schmitt F, Kumar V. Diagnosis of Alzheimer's disease. In: Kumar V, Eisdorfer C, eds. Advances in the Diagnosis and Treatment of Alzheimer's Disease. New York: Springer Publishing Co., 1998:111–151.

25. Cummings BJ, Su JH, Cotman CW, White R. b-Amyloid accumulation in aged canine brain. A model of early plaque formation in Alzheimer's disease. Neurobiology of Aging 1993;14:547–560.

26. Cummings BJ, Head E, Ruehl WW, Milgram NW, Cotman CW. The canine as an animal model of human aging and dementia. Neurobiology of Aging 1996;209:259–268.

Chapter 5
General Approaches to Behavioral Pharmacology

Enthusiasm is rapidly growing for the use of psychotropic drugs in behavior therapy of dogs and cats, owing in part to the recent availability of such drugs from the human realm that have the potential to change behavior with few serious side effects. Selective use of psychotropic drugs may help aid resolution of some problem behaviors that, for one reason or another, may not be responsive to behavioral or environmental approaches alone. Psychotropic drugs also may help when owners are not able to follow a complete behavior modification program or when the problem behavior needs to be brought under control within a short period of time. However, employment of drugs for problem behavior brings up the possibility that behavioral approaches (environmental management and behavior modification), which are important in long-term resolution, will be neglected and animals and their owners may not be as well served.

There is also the issue of how drugs are actually working to change behavior; in administering a psychotropic drug are we correcting a neurotransmitter imbalance or are we temporarily boosting a neurotransmitter to supranormal or subnormal levels to facilitate a short-term behavioral goal? This latter issue relates to the implications of the illness model (or medical paradigm) versus the ethological model in the use of drugs to treat problem behaviors. These issues, along with the ethics of drug use in animals for problem behaviors are discussed later in this chapter. This chapter also deals with the sources of information for the indications and effectiveness of psychotropic drugs. Chapter 6 covers the uses and indications for specific categories of drugs. The topic of the placebo effect is emerging as very important for not only behavioral pharmacology but the practice of clinical behavior in general and will be discussed first.

The Placebo Effect in Clinical Practice

A major goal of clinical trials is to distinguish real drug effects from improvement imagined by the client or brought about by unscheduled environmental management or behavioral modification introduced by the client. In using drugs to alter animal behavior, these influences together come across as placebo effects.[1] In human medicine the placebo effect is primarily attributed to the patient imagining he or she is better, even to the point where the patient may self-induce physiological changes that might then improve a medical problem.[2] Some studies in fact, suggest that placebos used in a trial of analgesics result in changes in the brain along the lines of those seen with the active drug.[3] Overall, however, reviews of a large number of human clinical trials reveal little evidence of powerful placebo effects.[4]

The extent of placebo effects in animal behavior therapy is just beginning to be understood. Treatment success is necessarily evaluated on the basis of reports by the animal owners rather than by physical examination or laboratory tests, which are the methods of assessing progress in animals receiving drugs for conventional medical problems. Because animals do not know they are being treated, one could argue that there should be a much smaller placebo effect than in humans. However, one could equally argue that animal owners do not see their animals all the time and could easily imagine that the animal has improved more than it actually has. In addition to imagined results, owners who want to see their animal improve are likely to institute behavior modification or environmental management procedures that were not included in the treatment regimen and which would then appear as a placebo effect.[1]

Examples of double-blind, placebo-controlled trials that have been conducted in dogs and cats[5,6] suggest that the percent of clients who could be expected to report improvement in their pets who are given a placebo may range up to 25–50%. If 30% of animals on placebos are reported by owners to show improvement, and drug treatment results in improvement in only 30%, all of the effect may be attributed to the placebo, and there would be no basis for asserting the drug has any therapeutic value beyond the placebo. If there is a 30% placebo effect but drug treatment results in 60% of animals improving, the drug could account for improvement in 30%. Note, however, that 60% improvement is the figure that would be referred to in literature and on the label describing the effectiveness of the psychotropic drug.

The role of the placebo effect in clinical practice is potentially much greater than that which is seen during clinical trials. In clinical trials, an investigator wants to minimize placebo effects to enhance the probability of achieving a statistically significant difference between drug treatment and placebos. However, when a veterinarian treats an individual patient and prescribes a psychotropic drug, presumably along with instructing the client to follow a program of behavior modification and/or environmental management, the placebo effect should be valued. If there is a positive outcome, one will not know how much of the improvement is due to the drug and how much is due to the behavioral approaches instituted or even imagined by the client. There is a tendency to credit the drug for the improvement, even that improvement brought about by behavioral approaches.

Although most veterinarians would be unwilling to prescribe or dispense a placebo, a strong case could be made that veterinarians dealing with problem behaviors should not only be aware of the widespread and inevitable occurrence of placebo effects among their clients, but take advantage of this phenomenon in an ethical and medically sound manner. For one thing, clients should be made to feel confident and secure that they are in the hands of a recognized medical authority. Diplomas, board certifications, and medical instruments in sight generally provide these signals. Careful attention and recording of the client's presenting complaint should reflect greater competence than immediately jumping to a diagnosis, even if the diagnosis is clearly accurate. The clinician should listen carefully and ask suitable questions. The consultation might include questions about what has worked and not worked and about attempted treatments by the client (including use of herbal substances) that the veterinarian might consider to be placebos. Providing a specific diagnosis and prognosis is conducive to improvement, particularly when one wants the client to participate in the resolution of the problem.

The Illness Model Versus the Ethological Model

As argued in Chapter 1, most problem behaviors, which are presented to clinicians for consultation and treatment are normal behaviors, but often unacceptable; this is an aspect of the ethological model. In contrast, the *illness model,* or what may be termed the *medicinal paradigm,*[7] implies that problem behaviors stem from an imbalance of neurotransmitters, hormones, or other biological factors. In the context of the illness model, the use of a psychotropic drug theoretically "corrects" the neurochemical imbalance and normalizes the behavior. Rather than correcting a neurotransmitter imbalance as in the illness model, with the *ethological model* drugs can be considered as elevating one or more transmitters above normal and facilitating behavioral change when used in conjunction with behavior modification. After improvement is seen with this treatment-facilitation approach, the drug is withdrawn, allowing the elevated transmitter levels to return to normal. In treatment-facilitation, drug treatment may be temporary and is used primarily to enhance the effectiveness of behavior modification approaches. The illness model would suggest that one maintain a dog or cat with the problem behavior on the drug indefinitely. The operating principle in this chapter, as throughout the book, generally follows this treatment-facilitation approach related to the ethological model.

Clearly there are instances, even within the ethological model, where indefinite drug therapy may be indicated. One example is urine marking in neutered cats, where the behavior may be so ingrained, at least in the environment in which the cat lives, that drug treatment may have to be indefinite. Other examples are compulsive or stereotypic behaviors where a neurotransmitter imbalance may indeed be present. Aside from these problems, the track record of success with most behavioral techniques without drug treatment is testimony to the philosophy that most problem behaviors are not due to abnormal neurotransmitter amounts or other physiological abnormalities. It has been pointed out that neural mechanisms, including neural transmitters that regulate emotional behavior, have been shaped by natural selection. Drugs that disrupt these mechanisms may impair normal and adaptive behavior. It is the mismatch between the body and current environments that cause most problems, not abnormal functioning of the brain. Just because a drug alters an emotional reaction does not imply that the drug has reversed a brain defect.[8]

Guidelines for Drug Use

Assuming a drug has had positive effects, it is easy for owners to have a false sense of security that the problem behaviors would resolve. The drug-treatment approach is mindful of using drugs to treat other medical or pathophysiological conditions where there is a much more consistent relationship between drug administration and clinical results. There is no guarantee that the drug will continue to control the problem behavior over time, even if some major changes are initially noted. There are virtually no long-term studies to indicate the degree to which drugs will maintain control of behavior for months, let alone years. One may become lax in administering the drug, or there may be changes in neurotransmitter receptors making the drug less beneficial. Currently one should look at drugs as only short-term remedies with a strong emphasis placed on behavior modification, and with the intention of phasing the animals off of the drugs when appropriate.

The use of drugs for problem behavior also differs from the use of other medications in the degree of variability between patients. There is no behavioral problem for which a drug is effective in all animals in attenuating a problem behavior. Effectiveness varies partially because of biological variation in receptors and physiological events related to the metabolism of the drug in individuals. Some variability is probably also due to the diverse effects of environmental stimuli, past history, and early experience in predisposing an animal to engage in a problem behavior. Often some experimentation may be necessary to find the most appropriate drug and dosage. Behavioral approaches, along with administration of the drug, need to be explained to the client so that there is not an overly optimistic feeling that the drug alone, without concomitant behavioral modification or environmental management, will solve the problem.

Another issue to be addressed in considering use of a psychotropic drug for a behavioral problem is whether a drug is even indicated. This requires a diagnosis of the problem and an understanding of underlying causes. House soiling with urine in cats, for example, may be a reflection of urine marking, and a serotonergic drug (along with environmental management) may alleviate the anxiety and resolve the problem. However, problem urination may also reflect inappropriate urination stemming from aversion to the litter box, and strict adherence to hygiene, rather than drug use, is indicated. To treat all urination problems initially with a drug neglects the necessity of making a diagnosis and instituting the appropriate therapeutic approach. An aggression problem in a dog that has both territorial and fear-related components may be intensified by an anxiolytic if the drug diminishes fear, leading the dog to attack strangers more readily. Fear-related and territorial aggression are dealt with behaviorally in different ways.

The issue of administering psychotropic drugs without attending to the underlying causes is particularly relevant when it is possible to alter an undesirable behavior without eliminating the factors causing the problem. Separation anxiety, for example, may be alleviated by an anxiolytic drug producing supranormal levels of serotonin. The problem may appear to be resolved as long as the dog remains on the drug; discontinuation of drug treatment may result in the problem recurring. Thus, there may be a tendency to keep the animal on the drug indefinitely despite the fact that with desensitization and counterconditioning procedures one might well be able to resolve this problem permanently with no necessity for indefinite drug treatment. The ethical issue revolves around the degree to which a clinician should approve the use of an anxiolytic drug without insisting that the client deal with the underlying causes of the problem.

Another caveat concerning psychotropic drugs is that they should not be used to make a diagnosis by response to treatment.[7] A clinician should not diagnose a dog as having separation anxiety solely because it stopped barking when receiving clomipramine, for example. A diagnosis, or at least a reasonable list of differentials, must be made before a medication is prescribed.

Drugs are typically used in three circumstances in behavior therapy. Two circumstances involve instances where behaviors are basically normal, albeit a problem,[9] and involve instances where 1) behavioral approaches alone are usually not adequate, such as with feline urine marking, and 2) one needs to facilitate a behavior modification program that, theoretically, could work alone. The other circumstance is to correct an existing physiological abnormality, such as deficiency in a neurotransmitter system.

Evaluation of Clinical Reports

Given that the issues of behavioral diagnoses, general guidelines, and ethics of drug use are addressed, the use of drugs brings up the topic of selection of the appropriate drug for a particular behavioral syndrome. Some psychotropic drugs approved for human use have involved dogs and/or cats in product testing, but the information is sparse regarding efficacy, adverse side effects, and long-term value in the treatment of problem behaviors of companion animals. This section deals with understanding the basis by which information about drugs is obtained.

Other than safety of the drugs being employed, the overriding issue of concern with regard to progress in the field of behavioral pharmacology is the necessity to separate placebo effects from real drug effects, and it is the task of clinical trials to separate these two aspects. The gold standard for clinical trials is the randomized, double-blind, placebo-controlled clinical trial. Because most drugs used for many problem behaviors in animals have not been subjected to such controlled trials, one is confronted with evaluating the literature that is available.

There are five general types of published studies on use of drugs for problem-solving, ranging from most to least reliable. These are 1) double-blind placebo-controlled clinical trials, 2) open-label or single-blind clinical trials, 3) retrospective case surveys, 4) case reports, and 5) clinical suggestions without any reference to clinical experience. These are discussed in the following sections.

Double-Blind Placebo-Controlled Clinical Trials

This type of trial provides the most accurate information on the effectiveness of drug treatment and is required in the U.S. for approval of a drug for labeling for use in a specific condition. Indications on the label are only for those clinical problems that were tested in the double-blind controlled protocol. The placebo effect may be quantified and distinguished from real drug effects through randomized assignment of animals to two or more groups, utilization of a placebo-control group, and standardization of behavioral modification instructions, if any. In these trials at least two treatment groups are used in a double-blind fashion, in which neither the investigator nor the owners of the animal subjects know which animals are in which groups. Animals in the experimental group receive the drug at the expected effective dose range, usually worked out in preliminary dose-determination trials, which are preceded by efficacy trials and toxicity studies. The control group commonly receives a placebo, usually indistinguishable in appearance from the drug.

For trials in situations where another drug treatment was known to be effective from a previous blinded study involving a placebo, a new drug may be compared with the other drug. This is sometimes referred to as a *positive controlled trial* and the placebo-controlled trial may be referred to as a *negative controlled trial*. In the case of a trial with a positive control, the study outcome should reveal whether the new treatment is at least as good as the reference drug (positive control). Positive controlled trials are usually more acceptable to clients who are naturally not enthusiastic about a 50% likelihood of being placed on a placebo. Selection bias in assigning animals to groups is avoided by a randomization procedure, which may be balanced in terms of age and/or gender of the animals. All participating animal caregivers are given the same information and the same instructions. Evaluation of treatment generally occurs at the end of the trial. If both the new drug and the conventional drug are judged equally effective, the new drug may have advantages if it produces fewer side effects or is less expensive.

Because there are virtually always some individuals that improve on placebo, the main object of negative controlled trials is to determine whether the drug has an effect beyond that of a placebo. One may find, for example, that 40% of animals receiving a placebo improve, whereas 65% receiving the new drug improve. The difference between placebo and drug is 25% in this example, which is an estimation of the number of animals for which the drug was effective and which would not have improved on placebo alone.

In human clinical trials, patients sometimes are able to detect that they are assigned to the drug and not the placebo group based on side effects such as a dry mouth or loss of appetite. This may cancel out the effect of blinding the subjects, leaving the door open for imagined effects. It is sometimes possible for pet owners, as well, to know whether their animal is in the drug group and not the placebo group if the drug is bitter tasting and disliked by the animal, or if it increases appetite. It may not be possible to avoid this type of influence and thus the placebo effect is not always absent, even in the best-designed studies.

The most common protocol for a placebo-controlled trial is the *parallel design,* in which an experimental group and a control group receive treatment concomitantly, and the results are evaluated at the end of the trial, as shown in Figure 5-1. Examples of double-blind trials with negative controls include one on dogs showing no difference between clomipramine and placebo on aggressive dominance,[5] and one on cats showing significant effects of fluoxetine over placebo on urine marking.[10] The double-blind parallel design for a positive-controlled trial was used in a study showing that two serotonergic drugs (fluoxetine and clomipramine) were equally effective in controlling urine marking.[11] A variant of the typical 2 group design shown in Figure 5-1 is a parallel multiple group design where two or more investigational drugs are compared with placebo.

In any clinical trial there is variability from subject to subject, and therefore many subjects are needed in each group. One design that can reduce variability, using subjects as their own controls, is the *crossover design,* wherein treatment for

Parallel - 2 Group

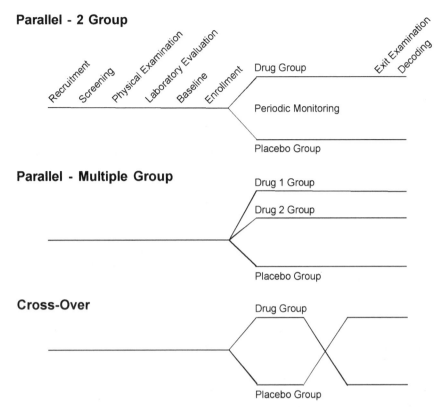

Parallel - Multiple Group

Cross-Over

Figure 5-1 Schematic diagram of various experimental designs for clinical trails. In the parallel trial with two groups, one group is given the trial drug and the second group a placebo. In the parallel-multiple group trial, two investigational drugs, or two doses of one drug, are compared with a placebo. In both types of parallel designs, a proven drug may be substituted for the placebo to compare with a new drug. The crossover design involves reversing treatment at some predetermined point.

each group is switched partway through the trial (Fig. 5-1). Crossover designs cannot be used when the treatment may cause lasting changes in the behavior of the subject, and thus this is not generally an appropriate design for behavioral problems. In a trial testing a drug for separation anxiety, for example, an anxiolytic drug may permanently change an animal's anxiety to being left alone, and a crossover design would not give an accurate indication of the value of drug versus placebo. Crossover designs have been used for compulsive and stereotypic problems that appear to be altered only while the subjects are receiving the drug.[6,12]

Prospective Open-Label or Single-Blind Clinical Trials

The distinguishing feature of this type of trial compared with double-blind studies is that treatment is open-label, meaning that the investigators, and often the animal owners, know which treatment is being given. If the trial involves two different groups, one receiving placebo and one receiving drug, the trial may call for telling the clinicians but not the owners the type of treatment their animal is receiving; this is a single-blind trial. Results are still likely to be confounded by the placebo effect because the investigator, who knows which animals are being treated with drug, may deal with the animal owners in drug and placebo groups differently or be biased in soliciting information from owners. Thus, single-blind studies are not generally any better than open-label studies.[13]

Open-label trials have included examining the effects of a narcotic antagonist on self-licking, self-chewing, and scratching in dogs,[14] and the effects of the anxiolytics, diazepam and buspirone, on urine marking in cats.[15,16] Examples of single-blind trials are comparison of different drugs for the treatment of canine acral lick dermatitis[17] and the effects of the serotonergic, fluoxetine, on dominance aggression in dogs[18] As with double-blind trials, animals enrolled in the most reliable open-label trials should meet specific criteria and the protocol should be planned in advance.

In prospective open-label trials in which all animals are given the new drug, the assumption is that the treatment will be compared to historical treatment, which would be no drug treatment at all. In the previous studies of urine marking in cats, for example, each animal was being used as its own control by referring to the frequency of the behavior prior to drug treatment. It was assumed a reduction in the behavior, if any, reflected the effect of the drug. However, favorable results undoubtedly reflect placebo effect as well.

Retrospective Case Surveys

Conducting a retrospective case survey involves reviewing hospital records with regard to the use of a drug for a particular behavior, and possibly statistically evaluating this information. One may apply specific criteria for determining which cases are included and excluded if this seems to help the predictive value of the information. Unless all cases on record are included, a major concern is that mostly favorable cases are selected. Assuming unbiased case selection, case surveys may provide useful information on the biological variation in animal responsiveness and on the general efficacy of the drug if the number of cases is large enough. One also gets an idea of the possibilities of adverse side effects. The treatment of individual animals which make up the groups surveyed will have been open label, so there will be some placebo effects.

Reports of the effects of castration on problem behaviors are probably the best examples of retrospective case surveys. Here the treatment involves removal of an endogenous hormone rather than administration of a drug.[19,20] Placebo effects are likely in surveys of the effects of castration, but it would be virtually impossible to conduct a study in a blinded fashion.

One of the major problems with retrospective case surveys is that the treatment of animals could have varied as the attending clinicians became more accustomed to using the treatment, with animals treated later in the study faring better than those treated earlier.[13]

Case Reports

Case reports are published accounts of behavioral changes in one or just a few animals being treated, and they usually involve just positive outcomes. There is, of course, little interest in case reports of treatment without positive outcomes. Published behavior cases of the month are the best examples of such useful case reports because they provide detailed information. Case reports provide no information about biological variation among animals and a placebo effect is a major possibility. As mentioned, clinicians tend to implement everything they can to improve a serious problem behavior and they might ascribe the improvement to a drug rather than to the behavioral approaches urged upon the client. Case reports are the only type of information available for many of the uses of psychotropic drugs,[21,22] and although they do not provide reliable information on efficacy and side effects, they are valuable in stimulating further investigation.[23]

Clinical Suggestions Without Outcomes Information

The weakest forms of published information about psychotropic drugs are suggestions from authors and seminar speakers about the use of some drug even while acknowledging that they have had no experience with the drug. For the most part, such suggestions are well meaning and included in papers or lectures for the sake of completeness in discussing groups of drugs. It goes without saying that such information should be taken with great caution.

Conclusions About Evaluation of Literature on Psychotropic Drugs

Behavioral pharmacology as applied to animals differs from other areas of pharmacology because behavior seems to be more prone to environmental influences than organ system pathophysiology in other areas such as cardiology, dermatology, and neurology, and because the results rely on the owner's observations of the animal's behavior rather than on clinical data obtained from direct physical and laboratory examination.[1] Sometimes behavioral data may be reported in discrete events such as the number of urine marks or frequency of growling episodes per day, but more often the owners' reports are in the form of global measures of improvement such as, "The cat is much improved." This is where placebo effects are most likely to confound the interpretation of results.

As drugs are increasingly prescribed for behavior problems, progress in this field is going to depend upon negatively or positively controlled, double-blind studies so that improvement resulting from pharmacologic influences can be separated from improvement resulting from behavior modification or environmental management or imagined improvement on the part of the client. Of course, in the clinical setting, the placebo effect is fully operative and should be welcomed as an important element contributing to the successful outcome of the treatment of problem behavior.

References

1. Hart BL, Cliff KD. Interpreting published results of extra-label drug use with special reference to reports of drugs used to correct problem behavior in animals. Journal of the American Veterinary Medical Association 1996;209:1382–1385.

2. Shapiro AK, Shapiro E. The Powerful Placebo. From Ancient Priest to Modern Physician. Baltimore: Johns Hopkins University Press.

3. Holden C. Drugs and placebos look alike in the brain. Science 2002;295:947–949.

4. Hrobjartsson A, Gotzsche PC. Is the placebo powerless? New England Journal of Medicine 2001;344:1594–1602.

5. White MM, Neilson JC, Hart BL, Cliff KD. Effects of clomipramine hydrochloride on dominance-related aggression in dogs. Journal of the American Veterinary Medical Association 1999;215:1288–1291.

6. Hewson CJ, Luescher A, Parent JM, Conlon PD, Ball RO. Efficacy of clomipramine in the treatment of canine compulsive disorder. Journal of the American Veterinary Medical Association 1998;213:1760–1766.

7. Mills DS. Medical paradigms for the study of problem behaviour: A critical review. Applied Animal Behavior Science 2003;81:265–277.

8. Nesse RM, Berridge KC. Psychoactive drug use in evolutionary perspective. Science 1997;278:63–66.

9. Hart BL, Cooper LL. Integrating use of psychotropic drugs with environmental management and behavioral modification for treatment of problem behavior in animals. Journal of the American Veterinary Medical Association 1996;209:1549–1551.

10. Pryor PA, Hart BL, Cliff KD, Bain MJ. Effects of a selective serotonin reuptake inhibition on urine spraying behavior in cats. Journal of the American Veterinary Medical Association 2001;219:1557–1561.

11. Hart BL, Cliff KD, Tynes VV, Bergman L. Control of urine marking behavior in cats by long-term treatment with fluoxetine and clomipramine. Journal of the American Veterinary Medical Association 2005;226:378–382.

12. Rapoport JL, Ryland DH, Kriete M. Drug treatment of canine acral lick. An animal model of obsessive-compulsive disorder. Archives of General Psychiatry 1992;49:517–521.

13. Pocock SJ. Clinical Trials. A Practical Approach. Chichester, England: John Wiley & Sons, 1983.

14. Dodman NH, Shuster L, White SD, Court MH, Parker D, Dixon R. Use of narcotic antagonists to modify stereotypic self-licking, self-chewing, and scratching behavior in dogs. Journal of the Veterinary Medical Association 1988;193:815–819.

15. Cooper LL, Hart BL. Comparison of diazepam with progestins for effectiveness in suppression of urine spraying behavior in cats. Journal of the American Veterinary Medical Association 1992;200:797–801.

16. Hart BL, Eckstein RA, Powell KL, Dodman NH. Effectiveness of buspirone on urine spraying and inappropriate urination in cats. Journal of the American Veterinary Medical Association 1993;203:254–258.

17. Goldberger E, Rapoport JL. Canine acral lick dermatitis: Response to the antidepressant-drug clomipramine. Journal of the American Animal Hospital Association 1991;27:179–182.

18. Dodman NH, Donnelly R, Shuster L, et al. Use of fluoxetine to treat dominance aggression in dogs. Journal of the American Veterinary Medical Association 1996;209:1585–1587.

19. Hart BL, Barrett RE. Effects of castration on fighting, roaming, and urine spraying in adult male cats. Journal of the American Veterinary Medical Association 1973;163:290.

20. Neilson JC, Eckstein RA, Hart BL. Effects of castration on behavior of male dogs with reference to the role of age and experience. Journal of the American Veterinary Medical Association 1997;211:180–182.

21. Dodman N, Schuster L. Pharmacologic approaches to managing behavior problems in small animals. Veterinary Medicine 1994;89:960–969.
22. Marder AR. Psychotropic drugs and behavioral therapy. Veterinary Clinics of North American Small Animal Practice 1991;21:329–342.
23. Rudorfer MV. Challenges in medication clinical trials. Psychopharmacology Bulletin 1993;29:35–44.

Chapter 6
Prescribing Psychotropic Drugs

Given the recent surge of interest in psychotropic drugs for animal use and the completion of some double-blind trials, which have demonstrated significant effects beyond that of placebos, one could say that behavioral pharmacology is the most rapidly emerging area of companion animal behavior therapy. The categories of drugs that are available for treating problem behaviors in dogs and cats include those that prolong or enhance the effect of the natural brain tranquilizer, serotonin; enhance the inhibitory transmitter, gamma-amino butyric acid (GABA); or enhance the production of the activating neurotransmitters, dopamine and noradrenaline. Interestingly, drugs with different types of influences on brain transmitters may produce what appear to be similar behavioral changes even though the mode of action of each one is different. The approach taken in this chapter is to provide some comments about the mode of action and advantages and disadvantages of drugs from the various categories as well as indications for their use.

Extralabel Use of Psychotropic Drugs

Although drugs should become increasingly available through governmental approval, there will undoubtedly always remain a strong interest in the extralabel use of human psychotropic drugs for dogs and cats. New products are always under investigation and will continue to become available to veterinarians through use in an extralabel fashion. Guidelines for extralabel use provide few restrictions with regard to companion animals aside from adequate labeling on the dispensing container. In the U.S. if there is a drug labeled for a behavioral syndrome in companion animals, the clinician is advised to use this drug per label instructions; theoretically, extralabel drug use is unnecessary. However, if a drug is available for human use, the alternative human drug may be used in an extralabel fashion for economic reasons, because it is considered more effective or has fewer side effects, even though an FDA-approved drug exists for animal use. As with all prescriptions, the American Veterinary Medical Association recommends that the drug container given to the client must be labeled appropriately with the animal's identification, species, and condition being treated. The label must include the name of the drug, active ingredient, prescribed dosage, specified directions for use, dosage frequency, route of administration, and duration of therapy. Furthermore, the label needs to contain the name and address of the prescribing veterinarian. Finally, the label should include cautionary statements or contraindications. These procedures are especially important for extralabel drug prescription. Records should be kept in the veterinarian's office for 2 years. A valid veterinarian-client-patient relationship is required for all drug prescription or dispensing.

Appropriate Types of Use of Psychotropic Drugs

At the present time, psychotropic drugs fill three major roles in behavior therapy. One is resolving problems where the behavior is normal but where the conventional nondrug behavioral approaches typically are not sufficient to alter the problem behavior. An example is the use of a serotonergic drug for urine marking in cats. The second is to facilitate the resolution of problems representing normal behavior and for which behavioral approaches are typically successful, but the client does not have the psychological stamina or time for labor-intensive behavior modification exercises. An example is the use of a serotonergic drug for separation anxiety in dogs. The third is for cases that presumably represent abnormal behavior stemming from a possible deficiency or imbalance of neurotransmitters. An example is the use of a serotonergic drug for acral lick dermatitis in dogs. These types of use are discussed later in this chapter.

When Behavioral Approaches Are Not Sufficient

When clinical experience has shown that environmental management and behavior modification alone are typically not sufficient for resolving a certain kind of problem, a drug may reasonably be offered early in the consultation process. Behavioral approaches need to be recommended as well and are usually an important contributor to the resolution. Probably the best example is in the treatment of urine marking in cats, which is normal but often intolerable in homes. Extensive clinical experience and a carefully controlled clinical trial,[1] involving the behavioral approaches of enhanced vigilance over litter box sanitation and the use of an enzymatic cleaner on urine-soiled areas, show that these environmental measures do not usually resolve the problem, although the frequency of marking may be reduced. Environmental measures and management of intercat interactions can be viewed as increasing the likelihood of a response to the drug and/or enforcing the permanency of the resolution after drug withdrawal. Depending upon the wishes of the client, one may institute both behavioral treatment and drug therapy simultaneously or institute behavioral approaches first to judge the degree of improvement prior to drug administration. The use of a drug in this situation is likely to be long term, requiring months or possibly years of treatment (Chapter 21).

Facilitate Behavioral Approaches in Normal Animals

There is increasing interest in the use of psychotropic drugs to expedite and reduce the effort needed to resolve problems for which behavior modification procedures, such as systematic desensitization and counterconditioning, are generally quite effective. As mentioned, such problems include separation anxiety in dogs. Fear of strange people in cats is another example where it may be difficult to arrange desensitization sessions. In the use of behavior modification there may be more leeway in the exercises required to desensitize and countercondition the response. If the use of a drug leads to a marked reduction in anxiety, desensitization may occur even without staged desensitization sessions, provided the animal still experiences the anxiety-provoking stimulus at some level and desensitizes autonomously (Chapter 3). In this treatment facilitation role the use of drugs should be considered short term. In order to achieve the best outcome, a general guideline is to implement all the desensitization and counterconditioning measures that are appropriate prior to, or simultaneously with, initiating drug treatment.

Taking the example of separation anxiety in a canine patient, the presenting complaint may be that when the dog is left alone it engages in household destructiveness and excessive barking. Nondrug treatment of separation anxiety involves lowering the emotional interaction at times of departure and return, conducting sessions to reduce the overattachment to humans in the home, and desensitization to departures, initially through short separations, that gradually increase in duration. Counterconditioning may be added by pairing an appetizing food treat with the moment of departure to classically condition a positive emotion to departures. With the use of an effective anxiolytic drug, separations of even several hours may not result in as intense an emotional reaction as before, and repeated separations could result in progressive desensitization to departures. Later, with a gradual reduction in drug dosage, desensitization and counterconditioning to departures should be continued. Assuming that the decision is made to use the drug, there should be a clear design set out with an emphasis on the importance of both consistent administration of the drug and conscientious implementation of a behavior modification program.

The lead-in time for full effectiveness of a drug is an important consideration. With the currently available serotonergic drugs one may notice a marked reduction in the problem after 2–4 weeks of treatment. Although the pharmacological literature emphasizes that serotonergic drugs do not have full therapeutic effect for 4–6 weeks, the greatest difference between the serotonergic drug, clomipramine, and placebo in the trial on separation anxiety was after only 1 week of treatment.[2] Because of the lead-in time, some veterinary behaviorists recommend administration of a short-acting anxiolytic, such as diazepam or alprazolam, initially, along with administration of a serotonergic drug.

Correct Presumed Neurotransmitter Imbalance

Like all biological systems, neurotransmitter levels occur along a continuum where extremes can be expected. If a thorough diagnostic workup indicates that the problem behavior is outside normal limits, a psychotropic drug may be viewed as bringing a neurotransmitter agent within more apparently normal limits. For separation anxiety, for example, an animal may be so extremely upset that the behavior is considered beyond normal limits and the typical behavioral approach would not be feasible. In this role drug treatment is likely to be of longer duration than in the drug facilitation role, ranging even to many months or years.

Find the Best Drug

The use of a drug for any behavior problem naturally assumes the drug will actually have noticeable effects on the undesirable behavior. Therefore, it is necessary to try the intended drug of choice to see whether there is an impact on the behavior. If no behavioral change is observed, even after trying different doses and allowing for an appropriate lead-in time, there is no sense in using that particular drug and one should try another drug or settle for attempting resolution with behavioral approaches alone. Remember that drugs should not be used as a diagnostic tool; just because a dog is given clomipramine and stops barking when left alone does not mean it must have separation anxiety. Assuming a drug is found that is efficacious, and then following the drug-facilitation model, the intention should be to phase out the drug in, say, 4 months, while continuing with behavior modification procedures.

Types of Psychotropic Drugs

The drugs available for treating problem behaviors fall into several categories indicated by the following headings. As time goes on, increasing numbers of drugs will receive governmental approval to be labeled for specific behavioral syndromes, and others will be available for extralabel use. Thus, the specific drugs mentioned under each category should be taken as examples of various categories.

The term *tranquilizer* has pretty much been discontinued in favor of terminology referring to mechanism of action (e.g., *serotonin reuptake inhibitors, SSRIs*), biochemical derivation (e.g., *benzodiazepine derivatives*), conventional behavioral action in people (e.g., *antidepressant*), or a combined biochemical and behavioral definition (e.g. *tricyclic antidepressant*). The reader will notice that the term *antidepressant* does not really apply to behavior problems in animals, just as psychiatric conditions such as schizophrenia, bipolar personality, and panic disorder do not generally apply to dogs and cats. These terms refer to specific syndromes in people where verbal reports are an integral aspect of the mental disorder, and there are no clear counterparts in animals. Even the concepts of obsessive-compulsive disorders and hyperactivity need to be modified conceptually to have much meaning in animals. However, the drugs used to treat these psychiatric disorders in humans comprise the mainstay of pharmacological agents available for animal behavior problems. In canine and feline behavior therapy, we are primarily interested in knowing about the mechanism and track record of the drug in resolving some problem behaviors, rather than attempting to match an animal behavior problem to a human psychiatric syndrome.

Serotonin Enhancers

The most frequently mentioned neurotransmitter with pronounced behavioral effects is serotonin. Serotonin tends to have calming and mood elevating effects.

Serotonin, synthesized from tryptophan, is stored in the presynaptic neuron and released at the time of synaptic activation. At the time of synaptic activation, excess serotonin in the synaptic junction is generally taken back up into the presynaptic neuron and used again. It is known that dietary deficiencies of tryptophan may produce lower levels of serotonin and that serotonin can be selectively elevated by increasing tryptophan in the diet relative to other long-chain amino acids.[3] In fact, a few studies have shown that nervousness, reactivity, and aggression can be reduced by elevating tryptophan in the diet.[4] Long-term studies on the effects of tryptophan-enhanced diets are not available, however.

A variety of drugs have their influence through prolonging the action of serotonin at synaptic junctions. Selective serotonin-reuptake inhibitors (SSRIs) reduce this reuptake, thereby increasing the duration and amount of serotonin available to the postsynaptic neuron. Fluoxetine (Prozac®) is the most widely recognized SSRI and one of the most widely prescribed drugs in the U.S. for people and not surprisingly has been given to animals as well. Another commonly used SSRI in humans and animals both is paroxetine (Paxil®). Other drugs enhance serotonin through presynaptic action on neurotransmitters, and still others, notably buspirone (Buspar), increase serotonin through presynaptic activity as well as blocking the reuptake of serotonin. Clomipiramine (Clomicalm®), a tricyclic antidepressant, enhances serotonin by inhibiting reuptake, but it also increases the secretion of norepinephrine and dopamine. Among the serotonin enhancers there are enough differences in the mechanism of action of drugs to suggest some experimentation if the first drug utilized does not give satisfactory results. Table 6-1 reviews some differences, similarities, and side effects of serotonin enhancing drugs.

The prospect of "Pets on Prozac" raises the question that if fluoxetine is effective in reducing a problem, does this mean there was a deficiency of serotonin in the brain? Because there is no reason to believe that a serotonin deficiency is commonly the cause of most problem behaviors, the administration of reuptake blockers would appear to be useful in elevating serotonin above normal, allowing facilitation of behavior modification.

Selective serotonin reuptake inhibitors

The SSRIs have garnered a lot of attention, especially fluoxetine hydrochloride, which has basically replaced diazepam as the most prescribed psychotropic drug in people where the most common indication is depression. Fluoxetine is used in animals, but other SSRIs, including paroxetine and sertraline (Zoloft®), are used as well. All of these drugs have relatively little effect on neurotransmitter systems other than serotonin. A disadvantage, at least in humans, is that it can take 4–6 weeks to get a full effect. This lead-in time is thought to be a result of activation of autoreceptors on the presynaptic neuron from the prolonged availability of serotonin; this in turn prevents additional release of serotonin. After several weeks these autoreceptors are deactivated, which then allows the release of more serotonin to continue. Although the time-course to significant changes in behavior (lead-in time) has yet to be worked out in animals; for the time being, clients should make a commitment to treat an animal for up to 6 weeks to see the full effect of the drug. One

Table 6.1 Serotonin enhancing drugs

Class	Medication (Brand Name)	Reasons for Use	Dog Dosage	Cat Dosage
Serotonin enhancers — Selective serotonin reuptake inhibitors (SSRIs)		Anxiety, urine marking, repetitive behaviors. Some reports of use in aggression.		
	Fluoxetine (Prozac®)	As above.	1–2 mg/kg q24 hours	0.5–1 mg/kg q24 hours
	Sertraline (Zoloft®)	As above.	1–3 mg/kg q24 hours	0.5–1 mg/kg q24 hours
	Paroxetine (Paxil®)	As above.	1–2 mg/kg q24 hours	0.5–1 mg/kg q24 hours
Serotonin enhancers— Tricyclic antidepressants (TCAs)		Anxiety, urine marking, repetitive behaviors. Some reports of use in aggression.		
	Clomipramine (Clomicalm®)	As above. Currently licensed in dogs for separation anxiety in U.S.	2–4 mg/kg q24 hours, or split q12 hours	0.5–1 mg/kg q24 hours
	Amitriptylline (Elavil®)	As above. Somewhat antihistaminic.	2–4 mg/kg q12 hours	0.5–1 mg/kg q24 hours
Benzodiazepines	Diazepam (Valium®)	Anxiety (primarily episodic or panic attacks), urine marking, seizure control.	0.5–2 mg/kg q8-24 hours	0.1–0.5 mg/kg q8-24 hours
	Alprazolam (Xanax®)	As above. Fatal hepatic necrosis reported in cats.	0.02–0.1 mg/kg q8-24 hours	0.125–0.25 mg/CAT q8-24 hours
	Clonazepam (Klonopin®)	As above, plus sleep disorders.	0.1–1 mg/kg q8-24 hours	0.1–0.2 mg/kg q8-24 hours

Azapirones	Buspirone (Buspar®)	Anxiety, urine marking, repetitive behaviors. Some reports of use in aggression.	1–2 mg/kg q8-24 hours	0.5–1 mg/kg q8-24 hours
Monoamine oxidase inhibitors (MAOI)	Selegeline (Anipryl®)	Cognitive dysfunction. Currently licensed in dogs for cognitive dysfunction in U.S.	0.5–1 mg/kg q24 hours	0.25–1 mg/kg q24 hours

trial in cats, for example, showed that although urine marking may be eliminated in some cats within 2–4 weeks, in other cats marked improvement may not occur until treatment continues for 16 weeks or more.[5]

Side effects, such as sedation and ataxia, rarely occur with SSRIs and there is no evidence of physiological or behavioral dependency as with the benzodiazepines. The side effects that are reported for fluoxetine in either dogs or people are loss of appetite, diarrhea, hyperactivity, and lethargy. Fluoxetine has in some cases reduced acral lick dermatitis.[6] The most convincing example of the effectiveness of SSRIs over placebo is with urine marking in cats.[7]

Tricyclic antidepressants

This drug group refers to structurally similar compounds developed initially for use in psychiatry to treat depression, but which have effects on anxiety and other behaviors aside from depression. Of significance to veterinary behavioral pharmacology are clomipramine hydrochloride (Clomicalm®, Anafranil®) and amitriptyline hydrochloride (Elavil®). The most important side effects of tricyclic antidepressants (TCAs) are cardiovascular, cholinergic, and sedative properties. Sedation can be significant with amitriptyline. These drugs may have direct effects on heart rhythm and use of these drugs with canine and feline patients with cardiac problems is contraindicated.[8] Because of the anticholinergic effects, the tricyclics may also produce mydriasis, reduced lacrimation, and dry mouth. These signs generally pose no problems for young, healthy patients, but may lead to complications in compromised or old patients.[8] These drugs also can lower the seizure threshold, so they should be avoided in animals with a seizure disorder. Both amitriptyline and clomipramine increase serotonin by blocking its reuptake but they also block the reuptake of norepinephrine and dopamine, and some effects can be associated with enhancing these neurotransmitters. Of the two commonly used TCAs, clomipramine is the most specific for enhancing serotonin and the least likely to induce cardiac problems.

Although these drugs in humans seem to require several weeks to produce reliable changes, trials with separation anxiety in dogs[2] and urine marking in cats[5] reveal some changes within 2 weeks after the initiation of clomipramine treatment. Stereotypic behaviors such as acral lick dermatitis have responded to clomipramine.[9] Clomipramine had no effect on dominance-related aggression in dogs beyond that of placebo in a blinded, controlled trial[10].

Azapirones

An azapirone is another type of drug that enhances serotonin. The one for which some clinical data are available is buspirone (Buspar). This drug group enhances serotonin levels through presynaptic agonistic effects as well as blocking serotonin reuptake. Buspirone has the interesting effect of increasing serotonergic activity when serotonin is low in the brain, but reducing serotonergic activity when serotonin levels are high.[11] Additionally, buspirone acts to facilitate dopamine release. In treatment of anxiety disorders in humans, buspirone has been shown to be as effective as benzodiazepines.[11]

In cats, an open-label study on treatment of urine marking revealed buspirone was effective in eliminating marking in 55% of animals as long as the cats were on the drug.[12] However, this study did not reveal whether buspirone resulted in a reduction of urine marking beyond that expected of placebo; in this trial the placebo effect could have been quite pronounced. Currently an SSRI would generally be recommended before buspirone. The trial with buspirone did reveal an interesting side effect, possibly relating to altering social dynamics in the home of multicat households. About 10% of treated cats became more aggressive with this drug; some of the aggression could be explained on the basis of reduced inhibition of fear-related aggression. However, the aggressive behavior could also have reflected the release of dopamine.

Benzodiazepine Derivatives

Benzodiazepines achieve the effect of reducing anxiety and fear by an entirely different mechanism than the serotonin-enhancing drugs. Benzodiazepines, which have been available since the introduction of chlordiazepoxide (Librium) in the 1960s, and subsequent introduction of diazepam (Valium®), activate gamma-amino butyric acid (GABA) receptors, thereby mimicking the inhibitory effects of GABA. GABA has inhibitory influences throughout the cerebral cortex and limbic system and even results in some sedation from the action on the reticular activating system. The stimulation of GABA-like activity by benzodiazepines results in anticonvulsive activity, which is utilized in management of seizure activity. The commonly used benzodiazepines are diazepam and alprazolam (Xanax®). There is no question that benzodiazepines reduce fear or anxiety in at least some dogs and cats.[13,14]

A particular advantage of diazepam and other benzodiazepines is a relatively rapid onset of effect, so that one may see antianxiety influences within a day or two after treatment is initiated. Thus, for short-term management of anxiety situations, such as for dogs that are fearful of automobile rides and need to be taken in an automobile only infrequently or for reduction of anxiety to firecrackers once a year, diazepam or alprazolam, rather than a serotonin-enhancer, would be the drug of choice. The rapid onset of benzodiazepines may be taken advantage of in combining diazepam with a serotonergic drug to achieve reduction of fear or anxiety almost immediately. Diazepam would then be withdrawn before major dependency effects occur.

Adverse side effects must be considered in using a benzodiazepine. Diazepam commonly causes temporary sedation and ataxia. Frequently one notices an increase in appetite, which could be a problem in animals that are already overweight. There is a report of hepatic necrosis in cats maintained on oral diazepam for longer than a week or two.[15] Thus, for prolonged use of a benzodiazepine one should evaluate liver function prior to the employment of drugs and reevaluate 3 days after initiation of treatment. Thousands of cats have been given diazepam for treatment of urine spraying and other behavior problems with no indication of hepatic failure. However, in light of the possibility of liver toxicity, liver function evaluation before instituting treatment and periodically during treatment would be advisable. An interesting complication of benzodiazepine is the so-called paradoxical effect where an estimated 10–20% of animals show an increase in anxiety. These medications can also cause disinhibition of aggression; therefore, they should be used with caution in animals known to be aggressive.

Perhaps the biggest drawback for the use of benzodiazepines for usage of 2–6 months or more is that these drugs produce behavioral and physiological dependency. This addictive property is the reason prescription of benzodiazepines falls under the same restrictive classification as barbiturates and narcotics. Withdrawing an animal from long-term treatment with diazepam, even if the withdrawal is gradual, could theoretically produce a rebound reaction, which may bring back the behavior the drug was intended to control.

Phenothiazine Derivatives

These drugs were among the first of the psychotropic medications to be developed and routinely used in human patients and subsequently in animal patients. The group includes a commonly used behaviorally active drug in small animal medicine, acetylpromazine (Acepromazine®). Drugs in this group have their main effect by acting as dopamine antagonists, and were useful because they produced behavioral quieting. However, drugs in this group produce more sedation than the serotonergic and benzodiazepine derivatives. The adverse side effects include anticholinergic influences and alpha receptor blocking, which tends to lower blood pressure, and they should not be dispensed to animals traveling by airplane or without direct human supervision. Phenothiazines also tend to increase serum prolactin, because dopamine inhibits prolactin secretion by the pituitary. Phenothiazines may also produce extrapyramidal motor signs characterized by ataxia and muscle tremors. These effects would be particularly noticeable with long-term treatment. They also can lower the seizure threshold. Because other drugs have more specific effects on anxiety and fears without the side effects characteristic of phenothiazines, this category of drugs is usually not recommended in behavior therapy.

Like benzodiazepine derivatives, one advantage of the phenothiazines is a relatively rapid onset of action, and therefore, they have been used to help animals through difficult short-term emotional situations, such as anxiety seen in exam room situations. However, most animals are able to override the sedative effects and can be more sensitive to noises. Therefore, it is not a very useful drug in these circumstances. In an open-label study of a limited number of dogs, acetylpromazine proved useful in reducing aggressive tendencies of dogs toward other dogs and toward people.[16] If a phenothiazine derivative is used to reduce aggressiveness, even though not recommended, the problem behavior should not be anxiety-related or fear-related, and the intention should be only short-term management of the animal while carefully monitoring the effects.

Monoamine Oxidase Inhibitors

As mentioned in the introduction of this chapter, the use of drugs for behavior problems would appear usually to have the effect of raising one or more neurotransmitters above the normal level to facilitate alteration of behavior to something acceptable to the caregivers. In contrast, the use of a monoamine oxidase inhibitor (MAOI) is primarily for correcting an existing neurotransmitter imbalance, particularly that associated with aging in dogs. As dogs age there are often changes similar to those in humans, including neurological cell death and cytoarchitectural changes along with an alteration of neurotransmitter secretions (Chapter 19). Apparently one of the elements in impairment of cognitive functioning in humans and possibly dogs is depletion of the neurotransmitter, dopamine.[17]

Dopamine depletion comes about through an increase in monoamine oxidase-B (MAOB).[18] A treatment that reportedly alleviates some of the cognitive impairment in dogs is L-deprenyl (Anipryl®; selegiline), which is a selective inhibitor of MAOB. Administration of L-deprenyl results in a decrease in presynaptic dopamine reuptake, which prolongs the action of dopamine. L-deprenyl also increases dopamine-potentiating phenylethylamine in the hippocampus and in the cerebral cortex. In addition to reversing the depletion of dopamine, L-deprenyl has neuroprotective effects through enhancing the survival of dopaminergic neurons.[19] L-deprenyl may also have effects by virtue of antioxidant activity. The legitimacy of using L-deprenyl for treating age-related behavioral changes stems from a placebo-controlled, double-blind trial in which various behavioral signs of cognitive dysfunction were improved in 50–60% of the dogs on 1.0 mg/kg daily compared with only 20–30% of animals that responded to placebo.[20]

Endogenous Opioid Antagonists

This is a group of drugs frequently used in research to learn about the behavioral patterns that are mediated by endogenous opioids. In the brain, the release of opioids is associated with highly pleasurable or rewarding effects. Opioid antagonists, which apparently block these reinforcing effects, have proven effective in altering some clinically relevant behavioral patterns. The drugs that block endogenous brain opioids (mainly endorphins) are naloxone and the longer-acting naltrexone (Trexan®), which is available for clinical use. However, these drugs are often prohibitively expensive and must be given very frequently, thus limiting their clinical application.

In animals there is evidence that confinement-induced stereotypic behaviors—such as cage pacing in zoo carnivores, wood chewing (horses), and tail biting (pigs)—result in a release of brain endorphins. A favored explanation of animal welfare experts is that animals cope with the stress of confinement and boredom by engaging in a behavior that releases endorphins, which then tend to reinforce the behavior. Consequently, opioid antagonists, by blocking the reinforcing effects of endorphin release, reduce the repetitive behavior. A problem with this hypothesis is that after treatment with naltrexone, the repetitive behavior almost immediately stops rather than tapering off gradually as one would expect during extinction of a learned behavior (reinforced by endorphin release). Another problem with this hypothesis is that some problem behaviors, such as tail chasing and acral lick dermatitis in dogs, that do not necessarily occur in confined or stressed animals are also reduced by naltrexone (Chapter 18). Regardless of the mechanism, the behaviors altered by opioid antagonists are reduced only as long as the drugs are administered.

Usually the behaviors return when the drug is discontinued, and this category of drugs has found little clinical application.

Clearly, if the occurrence of a stereotypic behavior, such as cage pacing, represents a kind of coping mechanism for dealing with the stress of the situation, one would have to question the ethics of giving a drug that removes the reinforcing aspects of the coping mechanism without addressing the problem that resulted in the stress initially. If opioid antagonists are given to such animals, a minimum requirement is that a behavior modification and/or environmental management program must be instituted to remove the causes of the behavior so that the behavior will remain normalized after the drugs are discontinued.

Long-Acting Progestins

Progestins were among the first drugs used for problem behaviors of cats and dogs. As early as the 1960s a progestin was reported as effective in suppressing malelike behaviors, especially urine marking, roaming, and mounting in companion dogs and cats.[21] The progestins are synthetic compounds that mimic the effects of the naturally secreted female hormone, progesterone. Progestins are a mainstay of human oral and depository birth control drugs and are used in treatment of breast cancer and benign prostatic hyperplasia. The drugs have long been known for having behavioral effects, and medroxy progesterone acetate (MPA) was found as early as 1970 to suppress pathological sexual behavior in human males and has been since used clinically to treat a variety of abnormal manifestations of sexual drive in human males.[22]

Progestins would seem to have effects through several general mechanisms. One is to suppress the production of testosterone in gonadally intact males through the gonadotropic negative feedback mechanism. Another mechanism is to suppress malelike behavior in animals already castrated. A third mechanism is that of calming properties. It has long been known that progesterone, its metabolites, and progestins—especially in large doses—are nonspecific sedatives and anesthetics.[23,24] The injectable MPA has a very prolonged half life with the effective blood level lasting as long as 3 months.[22]

Of the clinical trials on animals to date, the most extensive data are from reports on cats treated for urine marking.[25,26] Overall, about 40% of cats treated with progestin respond favorably (problem ceased or markedly reduced), and a significantly higher percentage of males than females respond. A small-scale, retrospective study of MPA on intermale aggression in dogs reported that 75% of problem males responded.[27] The potential adverse side effects of progestins have received a good deal of attention. The most serious potential effect is adrenal cortical suppression, with a decrease in resting cortisol and a decrease in cortisol elevation after ACTH stimulation. Other side effects are compromised glucose tolerance and precipitation of diabetes mellitus.[28–30] Mammary gland hyperplasia and tumors have been reported in dogs treated with MPA.[31] An interesting side effect of progestins is appetite stimulation.[32]

Given the value of serotonergic drugs on urine marking in cats, there is no reason to consider using progestins for the problem behavior. Probably the only place the long-acting progestins would appear to have in behavioral pharmacology is for treatment of objectionable malelike behavior when anxiolytics have been ineffective or the owners cannot give oral medications.

Beta-Adrenergic Blockers

A classical concept in the physiology of emotions is that a major contributor to anxiety and nervousness is sensory feedback from visceral organs that are activated during anxiety-provoking situations. There is a peripheral amplification effect in which the more nervous an individual feels, the more severe are the peripheral manifestations adding to the state of anxiety. One way of reducing anxiety, therefore, is to break the feedback cycle through the administration of beta-adrenergic blockers, which reduce the peripheral manifestations of anxiety. The principal drug used in this way is propranolol (Inderal®), but other beta blockers may work as well. Assuming that the concept of the peripheral amplification of anxiety occurs in dogs and/or cats, it would be reasonable, under some circumstances, to use beta blockers in reactions characterized by excessive fear or anxiety. In humans, beta blockers may be used along with other drugs with antianxiety effects, such as serotonin enhancers, in dealing with fears or anxieties. There are no detailed case history reports or surveys on animals offering useful evidence for such treatment.

Central Nervous System Stimulants

The stimulant methylphenidate (Ritalin®) has received attention in human behavioral therapy because this drug is commonly used to treat an attention deficit disorder (hyperactivity) in children, particularly young boys. The drug has the so-called paradoxical effect of calming or slowing down the activity of individuals with this disorder rather than enhancing or activating behavior, as one would normally expect with a central nervous system stimulant. More recently, there has been considerable discussion about whether the drug is overprescribed in human medicine.

In dogs, attention has been focused in the past on a so-called hyperactivity syndrome in dogs that some observers felt was comparable to hyperactivity in young boys.[33] The diagnosis was based on the observation that respiratory and heart rates in some dogs were reduced rather than increased within minutes after injection of the CNS stimulant amphetamine, which has effects similar to methylphenidate. If these vital signs were slowed, the dog was assumed to be suffering from hyperactivity.

Now, with the concerns about drug abuse, one would use methylphenidate rather than a form of amphetamine to "test" for hyperkinesis in dogs. Although a hyperactivity syndrome may exist in dogs, one essential difference between attention deficit disorder in young boys and so-called hyperactivity in dogs is that the condition in dogs is usually diagnosed in animals that have reached maturity, whereas in people the condition is usually restricted to children. Currently one rarely hears about this type of hyperactivity in dogs and methylphenidate seems to have little use in animal behavioral pharmacology.

References

1. Pryor PA, Hart BL, Bain MJ, Cliff KD. Causes of urine marking in cats and effects of environmental management on frequency of marking. Journal of the American Veterinary Medical Association 2001;219:1709–1713.

2. King JN, Simpson BS, Overall KL, Appleby D, Pageat P, Ros C, Chaurand JP, Heath S, Beata C, Weiss AB, Muller G, Paris T, Bataille BG, Parker J, Petit S, Wren J. The CLOCSA (Clomipramine in Canine Separation Anxiety) Study Group: Treatment of separation anxiety in dogs with clomipramine: Results from a prospective, randomized, double-blind, placebo-controlled, parallel-group, multicenter clinical trial. Applied Animal Behavior Science 2000;67:255–275.

3. Sandyk R. L-Tryptophan in neuropsychiatric disorders: A review. International Journal of Neuroscience 1992;67:127–144.

4. Shea MM, Mench JA, Thomas OP. The effect of dietary tryptophan on aggressive behavior in developing and mature broiler breeder males. Poultry Science 1990;69: 1664–1669.

5. Hart BL, Cliff KD, Tynes VV, Bergman L. Control of urine marking behavior in cats by long-term treatment with fluoxetine hydrochloride and clomipramine hydrochloride. Journal of the American Veterinary Medical Association 2005;226:378–382.

6. Rapoport JL, Ryland DH, Kriete M. Drug treatment of canine acral lick. An animal model of obsessive-compulsive disorder. Archives of General Psychiatry 1992;49:517–521.

7. Pryor PA, Hart BL, Cliff KD, Bain MJ. Effects of a selective serotonin reuptake inhibitor on urine spraying behavior in cats. Journal of the American Veterinary Medical Association 2001;219:1557–1561.

8. Simpson BS, Simpson DM. Behavioral Pharmacotherapy. Part I. Antipsychotics and Antidepressants. Compendium of Small Animal 1996;18:10,1067–1081.

9. Hewson CJ, Luescher A, Parent JM, Conlon PD, Ball RO. Efficacy of clomipramine in the treatment of canine compulsive disorder. Journal of the American Veterinary Medical Association 1998;213:12,1760–1766.

10. White MM, Neilson JC, Hart BL, Cliff KD. Effects of clomipramine hydrochloride on dominance-related aggression in dogs. Journal of the American Veterinary Medical Association 1999;215:1288–1291.

11. Tayor DP, Eison MS, Riblet LA, et al. Pharmacological and clinical effects of buspirone. Pharmacology, Biochemistry, and Behavior 1985;23:687–694.

12. Hart BL, Eckstein RA, Powell KL, Dodman NH. Effectiveness of buspirone on urine spraying and inappropriate urination in cats. Journal of the American Veterinary Medical Association 1993;203:254–258.

13. Marder AR. Psychotopic drugs and behavioral therapy. Veterinary Clinics of North America Small Animal Practice 1991;21:329–342.

14. Houpt KA, Reisner IR. Behavioral disorders. In: Ettinger SJ, Feldman EC, eds. Textbook of Veterinary Internal Medicine, 4th Ed. Philadelphia: W.B. Saunders, 1995:179–187.

15. Center SA, Elston TH, Rowland PH, Rosen DK, Reitz BL, Brunt JE, Rodan I, House J, Bank S, Lynch LR, Dring LA, Levy JK. Fulminant hepatic failure associated with oral administration of diazepam in 11 cats. Journal of the American Veterinary Medical Association 1996;209:3,618–625.

16. Hart BL. Behavioral indications for phenothiazine and benzodiazepine tranquilizers in dogs. Journal of the American Veterinary Medical Association 1985;186:1192–1194.

17. Ruehl WW, Hart BL. Canine cognitive dysfunction: Understanding the syndrome and treatment. In: Dodman NH, Shuster L, eds. Psychopharmacology of Animal Behavior Disorders. Malden, MA: Blackwell Science, 1998;283–304.

18. Tariott PN, Schneider LS, Patel SV, Goldstein B. Alzheimer's disease and l-deprenyl: Rationales and findings. In: Szelenyi I, ed. Inhibitors of Monoamine Oxidase B. Birkhauser Verlag, Basel, 1995:301–317.

19. Tatton WG, Greenwood CE. Rescue of dying neurons: A new action for deprenyl in MPtP Parkinsonism. Journal of Neuroscience Research 1991;30:666–672.

20. FDA Freedom of Information Summary, Selegiline. Exton, Pa: Pfizer Animal Health, 1998.

21. Gerber HA, Sulman FG. The effect of methyloestrenolone on oestrus, pseudopregnancy, vagrancy, satyriasis and squirting in dogs and cats. Veterinary Record 1964;76:1089–1092.

22. Hart BL, Eckstein RA. Projections: Indications for male-typical behavior. In: Dodman NH, Shuster L, eds. Psychopharmacology of Animal Behavior Disorders. Malden, MA: Blackwell Science, 1998:255–263.

23. Gyermek L. Pregnenolone: A highly potent naturally occurring hypnotic-anesthetic agent. Proceedings of the Society of Experimental Biology and Medicine 1967;125:1058–1062.

24. Mahesh VB, Brann DW, Hendry LB. Diverse modes of action of progesterone and its metabolites. Journal of Steroid Biochemistry and Molecular Biology 1996;41:401–406.

25. Hart BL. Objectionable urine spraying and urine marking in cats: Evaluation of progestin treatment in gonadectomized males and females. Journal of the American Veterinary Medical Association 1980;177:529–533.

26. Cooper LL, Hart BL. Comparison of diazepam with progestins for effectiveness in suppression of urine spraying behavior in cats. Journal of the American Veterinary Medical Association 1992;200:797–801.

27. Hart BL. Progestin therapy for aggressive behavior in male dogs. Journal of the American Veterinary Medical Association 1981;178:1070–1071.

28. Romatowski J. Use of megestrol acetate in cats. Journal of the American Veterinary Medical Association 1989;194:5,700–702.

29. Middleton DJ, Watson AD. Glucose intolerance in cats given short-term therapies of prednisolone and megestrol acetate or progesterone for four years. Journal of Fertility and Sterility 1985;46:2623–2625.

30. Petersen ME. Effects of megestrol acetate on glucose tolerance and growth hormone secretion in the cat. Research of Veterinary Science 1987;42:354–357.

31. Frank DW, Kirton KT, Murchison TE, Quinlon WJ, Coleman ME, Gilbertson TJ, Feenstra ES, Kimball FA. Mammary tumors and serum hormones in the bitch treated with medroxyprogesterone acetate or progesterone for four years. Fertility and Sterility 1979;31:340.

32. Aisner J, Parnes H, Tait N, et al. Appetite stimulation and weight gain with megestrol acetate. Seminars in Oncology 1990;17:2–7.

33. Corson SA, Corson EO, Decker RE, Ginsburg BE, Trattner A, Conner RL, Lucas LA, Panksepp J, Scott JP. Interaction of genetics and separation in canine hyperkinesis and in a differential response to amphetamines. Pavlovian Journal of Biological Science 1980;15:5–11.

Chapter 7
The Behavior of Sick Dogs and Cats

Although scientists studying animal behavior rarely refer to the behavior of sick animals, veterinarians and pet owners are quite aware of behavioral changes when their animals become sick. Experienced animal handlers and veterinarians recognize the signs of depression, inactivity, and anorexia as the first indications that the animal is becoming sick. The acute onset of these behavioral changes is usually accompanied by a febrile response. There has been a tendency, both among veterinarians and animal behaviorists, to view the behavior of a sick animal as not particularly adaptive and the result of debilitation from a disease process and reduced ability to obtain food and water. Animals acutely ill with a systemic, bacterial, viral, or protozoan infection that are lethargic or depressed, with little interest in eating food or drinking water, may later show signs of dehydration. Animals that frequently groom, such as cats, commonly lose interest in grooming and develop rough hair coats. The sickness-related behaviors of depression, anorexia, and increased threshold to thirst in febrile individuals are not specific to any particular species; the behavior is seen in humans and all mammals, as well as birds. The behavioral signs are also seen with a wide variety of systemic diseases as well as localized infections.

It is now clear that the anorexia, depression, and inactivity of sick animals are not a maladaptive effect of illness but rather a highly organized behavioral strategy that is critical to the survival of the animal if it were living in nature. Perhaps because in veterinary medicine the view of infectious disease is shaped by an orientation on the importance of chemotherapeutic treatment and supportive therapy as well as protection through immunization, it is easy to overlook the fact that animals in nature have been exposed to, and survived, infections of pathogenic organisms through millions of years of evolutionary history.

The perspective represented in this chapter, which has received wide support through a variety of laboratory studies, is that the sick dog or cat should be viewed in the context of its wild counterpart living in an environment without medical or supportive care. When a wild animal is acutely ill with a pathogen it is at a life-or-death juncture, and the behavior associated with being sick can be viewed as facilitating the fever response, putting virtually all of the animal's resources into killing the invading pathogen.[1-3] To understand the behavior of sick animals, the role of the fever response in fighting infectious diseases should be briefly reviewed.

Protective Effect of the Fever Response

When animals are initially infected with pathogens, the febrile response—coupled with a reduction of plasma levels of iron—has the effect of inhibiting the growth of many viral and bacterial pathogens in addition to activating the immunological system. Fever develops because endogenous pyrogens change the hypothalamic thermoregulatory setpoint so that an animal feels cold at previously normal temperatures. To conserve body heat, blood is shunted from peripheral tissues to internal organs and the hair coat may undergo piloerection to increase the insulating value of the pelage. In the most severe cases of fever, body heat can be raised metabolically by shivering.

Endogenous pyrogens are released from fixed tissue microphages, blood monocytes, granular lymphocytes, and phagocytic cells of the liver and spleen when the animal is exposed to pathogenic bacteria, viruses, and protozoa. Interleukin-1 (IL-1) is probably the primary endogenous pyrogen causing fever. IL-1 also lowers blood plasma concentrations of iron and activates nonspecific immune reactions to pathogens.[4–6] Perhaps the best characterization of the fever response is that it is part of a cluster of physiologic reactions, referred to as the *acute-phase response,* which also includes the release of glucocorticoids from the adrenal gland[7] and inflammatory proteins from the liver.[8,9]

A number of experiments have revealed the protective role of an elevated body temperature in fighting disease. Basically, when animals are allowed to develop a fever response there is a higher survival rate from a deadly pathogen than when no temperature elevation is allowed. There is circumstantial evidence, as indicated by studies on elderly human patients, that older animals have a blunted febrile response to infection, and this blunted response has been related to the observation that the elderly have more severe illnesses and higher mortality from infectious diseases than younger individuals.[10–12]

Fever facilitates an animal's ability to fight pathogens in two ways. The first mechanism by which elevated body temperature benefits animals relates to the optimal temperature for pathogenic bacteria and viral growth, which is about the same as the normal temperature of the animals. The febrile response by increasing body temperature has an inhibitory effect of the growth of bacterial pathogens and viruses.[13–15]

Iron is an essential element for bacterial multiplication, and some bacteria that are not inhibited by the febrile temperature or reduced iron alone are inhibited by febrile temperature combined with reduction in available iron.[16,17] It appears as though the release of IL-1, rather than the elevated body temperature, is responsible for the lowering of iron concentration in febrile animals.[18] The critical role of iron in the virulence of some bacteria is receiving increased attention. Recent work on *Staphylococcus aureus* shows how this bacteria counteracts the body's sequestering of iron during infections by liberating heme from red blood cells and importing the released heme across its bacterial membrane where it is utilized as free iron.[19] The protective effects of low blood iron levels possibly explain why physicians and veterinarians embraced blood letting as a therapeutic procedure for more than 2500 years. Prior to the advent of antibiotics, blood letting may have been an effective mechanism for starving bacterial pathogens of iron.[20]

The second way that fever combats infection is that it potentiates immunologic responses so that there is increased bacterial killing by neutrophils, enhanced lymphocyte proliferative response to androgens and mytogens, and greater antibody synthesis.[21–25]

A discussion of the value of the fever response brings up the issue of the evolution of this physiological phenomenon. When prolonged temperatures above 41°C can be associated with tissue damage in the heart, liver, and central nervous system, how can this response level be selected over evolutionary time? Looked at from the standpoint of wild animals, a high febrile temperature that produces some tissue damage may still prove adaptive if the fever is effective at combating an infectious disease and when otherwise the animals would have died. Fever is very costly metabolically and for the response to have persisted in evolutionary development of vertebrates—including fish, amphibians, reptiles, birds, and mammals—there are obviously potential benefits.[25]

Behavioral Changes in Sick Animals

The increased elevation of body temperature seen in the fever response is largely a function of the direct effect of accelerating metabolic processes, resulting in about a 13% increase in metabolic rate for each 1°C rise in body temperature.[26] This translates into an increase in metabolic rate of 30–50% during a typical fever reaction. This metabolic cost is much higher if shivering must be activated. It is this high energetic cost of a fever reaction that relates to the behavioral changes associated with the fever response.[2]

The general behavioral changes that are associated with a fever response are anorexia, increased threshold for thirst, increase in slow wave sleep, and inactivity which are often interpreted as depression.[1–3] On the surface these behavioral changes, particularly anorexia, seem paradoxical because febrile animals need calories to fuel the energetic needs of the elevated body temperature. However, whether a carnivore or herbivore, searching for food in nature is energetically costly and a sick animal would not be very effective at catching prey or, if a herbivore, escaping from predators. What has been selected instead are changes in behavior that reduce activity, conserve energy reserves, and reduce heat lost from convection and conduction by staying in one place and assuming a posture to reduce the exposure of the body surface. By not consuming prey, a carnivore does not take in dietary iron which would otherwise work against the body's sequestration of plasma free iron. An animal would have some probability of surviving even in a dehydrated and nutritionally deprived state, assuming that the pathogen was effectively combated, and subsequently the animal could then go on to recover body condition.

The same endogenous pyrogens that bring about an elevated thermal setpoint appear to mediate the behavioral changes (Fig. 7-1). This includes the suppression of food intake, which lasts only a few days,[27] and enhancement of slow-wave

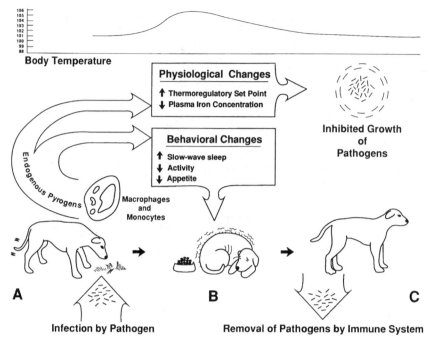

Figure 7-1   Behavior of sick animals. Exposure to pathogens (A) causes release of endogenous pyrogens, which bring about behavioral changes typically associated with sick animals (B). Removal of pathogens allows the animal to recover and behavior to return to normal (C). (Reprinted with permission from Hart BL, Biological basis of the behavior of sick animals, Neuroscience and Biobehavioral Reviews 1988;12:123–137.)

sleep.[28] One might view the occurrence of anorexia, increased sleep and inactivity as a programmed behavioral mode somewhat along the lines of anorexia and inactivity in birds that incubate eggs and in mammals that hibernate.[2] Excessive sleepiness or depression can be viewed as complementary to anorexia because a sleepy and depressed animal is less likely to move around and expend energy that would otherwise be used for metabolic needs of the fever response.

The fever response and the accompanying behavioral signs, triggered by infections with pathogenic organisms are seen in virtually all vertebrate species and with a very wide variety of viral, bacterial, and protozoan diseases. A survey of the common infectious diseases that are characterized by a fever among dogs, cats, horses, swine, cattle, sheep, and humans revealed that in virtually all disease entities in which fever was a noteworthy sign, anorexia and/or depression were present.[2] In dogs the viral diseases of distemper, infectious hepatitis, and tracheal bronchitis, and in cats the diseases of panleukopenia, infectious peritonitis, rhinotracheitis, calcivirus infection, infectious anemia, and cytauxzoonosis, are all accompanied by anorexia and depression. Of course, various diseases produce different reactions in the respiratory, intestinal, and cutaneous systems which then cause other clinical behavioral signs such as coughing, diarrhea, or painful responses that are superimposed on the underlying generic behavioral changes.

There are also important behavioral differences between dogs and cats, not with regard to basic sickness-related behavior, but in the way it is evident to caregivers. Cats lead a relatively sedentary life during the day and the signs of illness may go unnoticed.[29] Cats often eat more irregularly than dogs and anorexia may not be noticed immediately. When free-roaming cats become seriously ill they may leave their home base and take up refuge in hiding places that could be a long way from their homes. Occasionally neighbors may find a sick cat hiding in the shrubbery or in buildings. Sometimes a runaway sick cat may attempt to return to its home just as death approaches and the owner is faced with a cat that has been missing for days or weeks and returned in a state of severe debilitation.

Conclusions and Clinical Implications

The environment of the wild ancestors of dogs and cats exposed them to threats from pathogens and parasites. The threat of debilitating disease may be viewed as responsible for the natural selection of behavioral adaptations that increased an animal's likelihood of surviving and eventually reproducing in this type of environment. There are many behavioral adaptations in animals in nature for avoiding or controlling exposure to pathogens and parasites.[30] When an animal does become acutely ill with an infectious pathogen, it could be at a life-or-death juncture and is putting virtually all of its resources into fighting the invading pathogens. Sickness-related behavior potentiates the fever response by conserving body resources, reducing heat loss, and eliminating dietary iron, which has the effect of slowing the growth of pathogenic bacteria and viruses and facilitating immunological mechanisms.[2] This behavioral mode of sick animals is induced by the secretion of endogenous pyrogens, particularly IL-1. This behavioral mode is seen with fatal diseases as well as those from which animals usually recover. Superimposed on the general behavioral demeanor of sick animals are signs specific to disease causing organisms, such as nasal discharge, respiratory distress, diarrhea, vomiting, or inflammation. Some diseases are characterized by complete anorexia and depression, whereas in others, anorexia and depression may be more subdued, come on more slowly, or vary episodically in severity.

Because of the high level of medical treatment of dogs and cats, the occurrence of full fever is not necessarily critical to survival in the face of an infectious disease. Nonetheless, medical experts now point to the wisdom of allowing fever to occur if not too severe and to use antipyretics when body temperatures threaten to become injurious.[31] It may in fact be advantageous to facilitate a moderate fever in a sick animal, particularly an older one, through environmental means such as raising the room temperature, using blankets, heating pads, or extra bedding.[1] Because anorexia and sleepiness are a normal consequence of fever, animals should not be force-fed immediately upon falling ill unless there is a danger they will go into poor body condition. If and when the animal is force-fed, the food should contain no iron. Although an important aspect of treating sick animals is the use of chemotherapeutic agents, there are increasing numbers of drug-resistant strains of bacteria. A holistic approach to disease management that incorporates the innate, disease-coping behavioral strategy of sick animals seems advisable as an aspect of modern medicine.

References

1. Hart BL. Animal behavior and the fever response: Theoretical considerations. Journal of the American Veterinary Medical Association 1985;187:998–1001.
2. ———. Biological basis of the behavior of sick animals. Neuroscience and Biobehavioral Reviews 1988;12:123–137.
3. ———. The behavior of sick animals. In: Marder AR, Voith VL, eds. Veterinary Clinics of North America: Advances in Companion Animal Behavior. Philadelphia: W.B. Saunders, 1991;225–237.
4. Dinarello CA. Interleukin-1. Review of Infectious Diseases 1984;6:51–95.
5. Dinarello CA. An update on human interleukin-1: From molecular biology to clinical relevance. Journal of Clinical Immunology 1985;5:287–297.
6. Dinarello CA. Biology in interleukin. FASEB Journal 1988;2:108–115.
7. Besedovsky H, del Rey A, Sorkin E, Dinarello CA. Immunoregulatory feedback between interleukin-1 and glucocorticoid hormones. Science 1986;233:652–654.
8. Gauldie J, Richards C, Harnish D, Lansdorp P, Baumann H. Interferon B$_2$ is identical to monocyte-derived hepatocyte-stimulating factor and regulates the full acute phase protein response liver cells. Proceedings of the National Academy of Science 1987;84:7251–7255.
9. Powanda MC, Moyer ED. Plasma protein alterations during infection: Potential significance of the change to host defense and repair systems. In: Powanda MC, ed. Infection: The Physiologic and Metabolic Responses of the Host. New York: Elsevier/North Holland Publishing Co., 1981:271–296.
10. Norman DC, Grahn D, Yoshikawa TT. Fever and aging. Journal of the American Geriatric Society 1985;33:859–863.
11. Wannemaker RW Jr. Key role of various individual amino-acids in host response to infection. American Journal of Clinical Nutrition 1977;30:1260–1280.
12. Weinstein MP, Murphy JR, Reller LB, Lichtenstein KA. The clinical significance of positive blood cultures: A comprehensive analysis of 500 episodes of bacteremia and fungemia in adults. II. Clinical observations with special reference to factors influencing prognosis. Review of Infectious Diseases 1983;5:54–70.
13. MacKowiak PA. Direct effects of hyperthermia on pathogenic microorganisms: Teleologic implications with regard to fever. Review of Infectious Diseases 1981;3:508–520.
14. Small PM, Tauber MG, Hackbarth CJ, Sandie MA. Influence of body temperature on bacterial growth rates in experimental pneumococcal meningitis in rabbits. Infection and Immunity 1986;52:481–487.
15. Carmichael LE, Barnes FD, Percy DH. Temperature as a factor in resistance of young puppies to canine herpes virus. Journal of Infectious Diseases 1969;120:669–678.
16. Bullen JJ. The significance of iron on infection. Review of Infectious Diseases 1981;3:1127–1138.
17. Weinburg ED. Iron withholding: A defense against infection and neoplasia. Physiological Review 1984;64:65–102.
18. Kluger MH, Rothenburg BA. Fever and reduced iron: Their interaction as a host defense response to bacterial infection. Science 1979;203:374–376.

19. Skaar EP, Humayun M, Bae T, De Bord KL, Schneewind O. Iron-source preference of *Staphylococcus aureus* infections. Science 2004;305:1626–1628.
20. Rouault TA. Pathogenic bacteria prefer heme. Science 2004;305:1577–1578.
21. Sebag J, Reed WP, Williams RC. Effect of temperature on bacterial killing by serum and by polymorphonuclear leukocytes. Infection and Immunity 1977;10:947–954.
22. Manzella JP, Roberts NJ Jr. Human macrophage and lymphocyte responses to mitogen stimulation after exposure to influenza virus, ascorbic acid, hyperthermia. Journal of Immunology 1979;123:1040–1044.
23. Banet M, Fisher D, Hartmann KU, Hentel H, Hilling, U. The effect of whole body heat exposure and of cooling the hypothalamus on antibody titre in the rat. Pflugers Archives 1981;391:25–27.
24. Janpel HD, Duff GW, Gershon RK, Atkins E, Durum SK. Fever and immunoregulation. III. Hyperthermia augments the primary in vitro humoral immune response. Journal of Experimental Medicine 1983;157:1229–1238.
25. Kluger MJ. The evolution and adaptive value of fever. American Scientist 1978;66:38–43.
26. Hensel H, Bruck K, Raths P. Homeothermic organisms. In: Precht H, Christopherson, Hensel H, Larcher W, eds. Temperature and Life. Berlin: Springer-Verlag, 1973;503–731.
27. McCarthy DO, Kluger MJ, Vander AJ. Suppression of food intake during infection: Is interleukin-1 involved? American Journal of Clinical Nutrition 1985;42:1179–1182.
28. Krueger JM, Kubillus S, Shoham S, Davenne D. Enhancement of slow-wave sleep by endotoxin and lipid A. American Journal of Physiology 1986;251:R591–R597.
29. Hart BL, Pedersen NC. Behavior. In: Pedersen NC, ed. Feline Husbandry. Diseases and Management in the Multiple-Cat Environment. Goleta: American Veterinary Publications, 1990;289–323.
30. Hart BL. Behavioral adaptations to pathogens and parasites: Five strategies. Neuroscience and Biobehavioral Reviews 1990;14:273–294.
31. Miller JB. Fever. In: Ettinger SJ, ed. Textbook of Veterinary Internal Medicine: Diseases of the Dog and Cat. Philadelphia: W.B. Sunders, 1983;46–50.

Section II
Behavior and Behavior Problems of Dogs

In this section we deal with the most common behavior problems of dogs, which include aggression, separation anxiety and other fear- or anxiety-related problems, excessive barking, inappropriate elimination, roaming and escaping, attention-seeking behavior, problems with feeding, inappropriate sexual behavior, problems with maternal behavior, and compulsive behaviors. To provide an overall understanding of canine behavior and the behavior of the evolutionary ancestor, the chapters give some background on normal behavior related to the problem areas. Although the chapters are self-contained with regard to typical history, diagnosis, and treatment guidelines, frequent reference by the reader to the background chapters of Section I on behavior modification, hormonal control of behavior, and behavioral pharmacology may be helpful. Section I also has a chapter on the medical interview, which is important in providing an accurate history to the clinician and in delivering treatment recommendations.

The evolution of the domestic dog from its wild ancestor has always fascinated geneticists and behaviorists, but the topic has become more interesting with the advent of DNA ancestral tracking. The oldest archeological evidence of an association between the ancestral dog and human is a burial site, 12,000 years ago in what is now Israel, showing a human hand resting on what appears to be a companion dog buried at the same time.[1] More recent research, using mitochondrial DNA tracking rather than paleontological or archeological approaches, now indicates that domestication began as long as 100,000 years ago and was largely centered in Asia.[2]

The genetic aspects of the behavior of the domestic dog reflect millions of years of natural selection of the wolf ancestor, followed by human selection for various behavioral predispositions. Although the most widely recognized effect of human selection was for an extension of puppylike behavior into adulthood, referred to as *neoteny,* more recently other behavioral predispositions are being documented. One is a propensity to pay close attention to where their human companions are gazing and pointing. In fact dogs pick up on such cues much better than wolves, even hand-reared wolves.[3] Presumably because of regulations in the American Kennel Club that restrict registration to dogs whose parents were also registered, current breeds are quite distinct genetically. In a genetic analysis of dogs of 85 breeds involving 5–6 dogs from each breed, 99% of the dogs could be correctly assigned to a breed on the basic DNA profile.[4] Nonetheless, computer analyses revealed groups of dogs that shared some of the same genetic background. The most distinct group, traced back to ancestry in Asia and Africa, is most closely related to the ancestral wolf. This group includes the Siberian Husky, Alaskan Malamute, Shar Pei, Chow Chow, and Akita.

In the discussion of behavior problems of dogs in this section it will be noted in several instances that the behavior under consideration is more likely to be displayed by some breeds than others. This is true of aggression toward human family members, aggression toward other dogs, territorial aggression, excessive barking, and house soiling. The data for these comments on breed predispositions come from a study involving ranking of dog breeds by authorities such as small animal veterinarians across several behavioral characteristics.[5] Although the genetic uniqueness of dog breeds lays the framework for breed-specific behavioral profiles, there is, of course, a great deal of variability within breeds, and comments on breed differences reflect a general overview.

Although one may speak of behavioral characteristics that reflect the evolved behavioral tendencies of the dog's ancestor, the process of domestication has also led to the relaxation of behavioral traits shaped by natural selection.[6] This is seen, for instance, in maternal behavior and some types of interdog aggressive interactions.

The most frequently occurring category of serious behavior problems in dogs is aggression of one type or another. Aggressiveness, however, is not always an undesirable trait. One of the obvious advantages in the initial domestication of dogs was that they had a tendency to protect their adopted human homes just as they would have protected a wolf den. An assertive watchdog or guard dog can be an asset to some people living in a high-crime area. Problems arise because of the inappropriateness of the aggressive behavior. We sometimes expect our dogs to intimidate unwanted visitors, but not to threaten or attack our friends or invited guests.

Although Chapters 8 and 9, which deal with aggression, emphasize the generally natural context of canine aggression, some aggression problems in dogs can be considered abnormal. This sometimes can be true of aggression directed to people or other dogs. The other chapters in this section deal with problems that come up frequently and for which professional guidance is often sought. The final chapter, dealing with selecting and raising puppies, offers some guidance for advising clients. In addition to comments on breed and gender selection, tips on raising dogs to enhance positive behavior and reduce the likelihood of problem behavior are offered.

References

1. Davis SJM, Valla FR. Evidence for domestication of the dog 12,000 years ago in the Natufian of Israel. Nature 1978;276:608–610.
2. Vila C, Savolainen P, Maldonado JE, et al. Multiple and ancient origins of the domestic dog. Science 1997;276:1687–1689.
3. Hare B, Brown M, Williamson C, Tomasello M. The domestication of social cognition in dogs. Science 2002;298:1634–1636.

4. Parker HG, Kim LV, Sutter NB, Carlson S, Lorentzen TD, Malek TD, Johnson GS, DeFrance HB, Ostrander EA, Kruglyak L. Genetic structure of the purebred domestic dog. Science 2004:1161–1164.
5. Hart BL, Hart LA. The Perfect Puppy: How to Choose Your Dog by Its Behavior. New York: W.H. Freeman and Co., 1988.
6. Price EO. Behavioral aspects of animal domestication. The Quarterly Review of Biology 1984;59:1–32.

Chapter 8
Aggression Toward People

Because we live so closely with our dogs as they enter our household social structure (becoming a member of the "pack"), we are necessarily involved in some of the same types of social interactions that dogs display toward their canine pack members or dogs outside of their pack. We may be subject to different levels of aggressiveness as dogs attempt to establish or maintain a position of dominance. More commonly, we use discipline, stern words, or restraint to reinforce our authority. Although we may not consider our disciplinary actions as aggressive, they may represent mild threats or aggression from the dog's standpoint, leading to their responding by showing submissive gestures. As humans, we are less likely to recognize and respond to subtle changes in body language of dogs that signal early signs of aggression, submission, confidence, or fear. Hence, in the typical situation, a stern, low-pitched "No" evokes eye diversion, lowering of the ears, and inhibition of the ongoing behavior, which we as humans may not recognize as submissive or fearful behavior.

Given the prominence of aggressive interactions as a component of social interactions, it is perhaps not surprising that about 70% of canine cases presented to behavioral clinics deal with the problem of aggression.[1,2] Males, because they tend to be more aggressive than females, comprise about 80% of cases dealing with aggression.[3]

The terminology and classification used to describe aggressive behavior of social animals have received attention from animal behaviorists using either a reference to animals in nature or in the laboratory setting and by clinical behaviorists focusing on problems presented by dog owners. In a book dealing with treating problem behaviors, a clinically oriented classification of aggression toward people and aggression toward other dogs is most appropriate. In this chapter encompassing the range of types of aggressive behavior directed toward people for which consultation may be sought, the following are separate headings: 1) dominance-related aggression (also referred to as aggression dominance or dominance aggression), 2) aggression toward young children, 3) fear-related aggression, 4) pain-related aggression, 5) territorial aggression, and 6) abnormal or idiopathic aggression (including potential breed-specific rage). It should be noted that different terminology exists in other sources. Irritable aggression is sometimes a problem in aged dogs; this topic is discussed in Chapter 19.

Although it is most useful to discuss the types of aggressive behavior as discrete diagnoses, in reality it is common for a dog presented for aggressiveness to have two or more types of aggression. The treatment approaches must take into account the multiple types of aggression. The most common multiple diagnosis is a mixture of dominance-related aggressive and fear-related aggression. Frequently the dog appears to be in conflict with regard to aggressive tendencies. Increasingly the term *conflict aggression* is used by clinicians. A dog may show fear-related behavior in the same exam room where the owners are focusing on the aggressive responses toward them. It is important for the clinician to observe the dog carefully in the exam room as family members interact with it, paying particular attention to the dog's body language.

Signs of offensive and defensive, or fear-related, postures, occur on a continuum (Fig. 8-1). Identification of those giveaway aspects of canine body language can help in arriving at an appropriate diagnosis. Ear carriage, and whether the ears are thrust forward in an offensive posture or pulled backward and downward in a fearful posture, is an important feature. Lip raising and whether the head is thrust forward or pulled backward is another important feature. Fearful and submissive dogs are likely to divert eye contact; a dog in an attack mode tends to stare at an opponent. Context is also important in establishing a diagnosis. Just as problems with aggression are likely to reflect more than one type of aggression, there is often more than one feasible therapeutic approach, which is fortunate because it is necessary to tailor advice and recommendations to the client's lifestyle, personality, and available time.

Factors Affecting Aggression Toward People

Before moving on to the specific types of aggression, a review of the genetic, gender, hormonal, social, and learned factors influencing aggression is useful in deal-

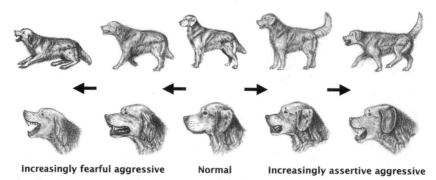

Increasingly fearful aggressive   **Normal**   **Increasingly assertive aggressive**

Figure 8-1 Diagrammatic representation of body postures and facial expressions of dogs involved in assertive aggressiveness and fear-related aggressiveness. The change in posture and facial expression as the dog becomes more assertively aggressive is evident in teeth bearing, open mouth, forward thrust of the body, and tail position. The change in posture and facial expression as the dog becomes more fearfully aggressive is evident in ear carriage, open mouth, retreating body posture, and tail position.

ing with all types of aggression. Also useful are some concepts regarding pharmacological approaches. Finally, as part of the section on factors affecting aggression, a brief discussion of causes of aggression secondary to pathophysiological processes is essential.

Breed Differences

Over centuries of artificial selection of dog breeds for different working and recreational capacities, various types of aggressive tendencies have been enhanced or diminished. Dogs of breeds related to ancestral wolves (see Section II introduction) are more likely than many other breeds to be aggressive, as are guarding breeds that were apparently bred for enhanced aggressive tendencies. Dogs intended for retrieving upland game fowl were bred for diminished aggression. The difference in tendencies toward aggression among breeds is important in the relationship a dog has within the family setting for the problems of dominance-related aggression, aggression toward children, and territorial aggression. A representative sample of breeds most likely and least likely to show the type of aggressive behavior are listed in the sections describing the different types of aggressive behavior toward people. There are, of course, major differences in aggressive tendencies among individuals within breeds that reflect differences in genetic background, early experience in current environment, and personalities of the owners.

Treatment of problem aggression should take into account breed predisposition in giving background information to the client. Frequently, people acquire dogs without knowing of their breed-specific aggressive tendencies. Sometimes, even with attempts to train obedience in a dog, a problem arises because of a mismatch between the temperament of the owner, who may not be sufficiently assertive, and the temperament of a dog that is aggressively assertive. Problem aggression occurring in a breed that is not typically high on that trait might indicate an atypical genetic tendency, and the owner should be cautioned against breeding that dog.

Gender and Hormonal Factors

Among the types of aggression exhibited toward people, dominance-related and territorial aggression are more of a problem in males than in females.[4] This gender difference stems from differences in gonadal androgen secretion just prior to, or after, birth (Chapter 4). The sexually dimorphic difference in aggressive behavior appears to be well established very soon after birth, and even castration within the first 8 weeks after birth does not eliminate these basic differences between males and females.

Aggressive tendencies are activated in adult males by testosterone secretion. Although castration cannot be expected to eliminate differences between males and females, the operation does apparently reduce some types of aggressive tendencies in some males. Clinical findings reveal that castration of adult males appears to resolve problems with aggression toward family members (dominance-related aggression) in about 30% of cases.[5] Territorial aggression toward human intruders is reportedly resolved in about 20% of cases. For each type of aggression, a higher proportion will show improvement by at least 50%. Importantly, age at time of castration, or experience in performing the behavior, is not correlated with whether one can expect changes in aggression.

A frequently asked question about females is whether aggressive tendencies are affected by time of spaying. Specifically, for example, does spaying a female before her first estrus or before she has a litter of puppies make her more aggressive? In general, the answer is no, but there is reason to believe that young female dogs that are already noticeably aggressive may be predisposed toward problem aggression as adults if spayed before 1 year of age.[6] A possible explanation is an abrupt change in hormonal secretions caused by ovariectomy (Chapter 4).

Effects of Early Experience and Socialization

If aggressive tendencies of dogs toward people are a reflection of genetic and hormonal influences, they are equally a reflection of early experience in the socialization of dogs to people. For example, dogs that have not had a chance to become accustomed to young children early in life can be quite fearful of children and this fear may be manifested in fear-related aggression toward children. In a family where a dog may have lived happily with a couple until the couple decided to have a baby, this may be a major problem, especially in breeds known to be predisposed to snapping at children. For people who have no children, and who want to adopt a puppy but plan to have children later, it is wise to have the puppy exposed to children on a regular basis to habituate the dog to children. The absence of early socialization may also play a role in the aggression, especially fear-related aggression, of dogs toward men or even strangers in general if there were few men or strangers in the early life of the young puppy.

As discussed, dogs often interact with people as they would another dog. Thus, the issue of who controls whom invariably comes up. Probably the most important reason for training puppies in puppy classes, and later in more formal obedience classes, is to help facilitate the owners in maintaining control over their dogs. As every veterinarian recognizes, unruly juvenile dogs who start controlling their owners at an early age are often likely to create serious problems for the owners as adults.

Learning

In addition to breed predispositions, gender, hormonal factors, and early social experience, learning plays a role in a dog's tendency toward aggressiveness. If in the process of maturing, a dog learns that a growl, threat, or snap results in some human members of the family backing off and giving the dog its way, aggression will be reinforced and aggressive behavior is more likely to be displayed in the future. The same goes for experience with visitors or strangers to the home; a dog with an inherent tendency to be aggressive toward visitors can be shaped to be more aggressive if the behavior pays off in terms of driving territorial "intruders" away. Learning can also play an important role in reducing or even eliminating aggression, and it is primarily the learning-derived techniques of operant conditioning, desensitization, and counterconditioning (Chapter 3) that are used in resolving these aspects of problem aggression.

Pharmacological Considerations

Given the fact that the majority of problem behaviors in dogs involve aggressiveness with the potential for injury to people, the question of a pharmacological approach naturally arises. However, the use of psychotropic drugs to treat problem aggression is in its infancy. Furthermore, drug companies will be reluctant to become involved in marketing drugs for canine aggression because of the possible huge liability issues.

So far there is little in the clinical research literature to suggest that drugs will be useful in treating aggressive behavior. A double-blind study addressed the effects of a serotonergic drug on dominance-related aggression in dogs in which the dogs enrolled showed no apparent fear and the aggression was judged within normal limits (from the dog's standpoint). These were the types of cases where behavior modification would be considered appropriate. The drug studied, clomipramine, did not reduce instances of aggression beyond that of placebo, as judged by daily scores and global evaluation assigned by the dog owners.[7] In this study there was a pronounced placebo effect; dogs in the drug group had no better improvement than those in the placebo group, suggesting that efforts made by the dog owners, who naturally were looking forward to an improvement in their dogs, were responsible for whatever changes there were in the aggressiveness of the dogs. In another double-blind, placebo-controlled study, it was shown that amitriptyline had no significant effect over placebo in reducing aggression in dogs.[8] The report of a slight reduction in dominance aggression by the serotonergic drug, fluoxetine, in a single blind trial,[9] might be explained as a result of a placebo effect.

This lack of effect of clomipramine for treatment of dominance-related aggression is in contrast with the effectiveness of this drug used at the same dosage to alter signs of separation anxiety and compulsive disorders (see Chapters 10 and 18). Despite the emerging evidence that serotonin is involved in regulating animal aggressive behavior,[10,11] studies of humans suggest that unless there is an indication that the aggression is abnormal, serotonergic drugs cannot be expected to ameliorate the aggression.[12] Augmenting serotonin concentrations in dogs with problem dominance-related aggression may not change the behavior because, for the most part, this behavior is normal.

If or when a drug is developed that does attenuate aggressive behavior in a dog there is no guarantee that the drug will continue to suppress or eliminate aggressive tendencies over a long time. One may become lax in administering the drug, or there may be changes in neural sensitivity to the drug or its metabolites. It is easy for owners to have a false sense of security and put themselves at risk because they are too mindful of using drugs to treat other medical or physiological conditions where there is a much closer dose-response effect or an eventual cure. In the future one should look at drugs, even if efficacious, as a short-term remedy with a strong emphasis placed on behavior modification and with the intention of phasing the dog off the drug as soon as feasible. In addition veterinarians may want to consider extra liability coverage if a medication is prescribed for an aggressive dog.

Aggression Secondary to Other Disease Processes

Diseases of various organs may, on occasion, lead to the onset of aggressive behavior. Aggressive behavior resulting from brain lesions is rare, although it is possible for pressure exerted on the midline hypothalamus by a tumor to result in a gradual increase in irritability or aggression. Such behavioral changes would usually be accompanied by some visceral or metabolic effects as well, such as seizures or a change in water intake or appetite. In some cases of temporal lobe or psychomotor epilepsy, strange aggressive reactions may be seen shortly before or after a seizure attack.[13] Visual or auditory impairment may predispose an animal to some types of irritability because of a dog's inability to see or hear a person approach. An inflammatory process in joints, muscles, or internal organs, such as the prostate gland, may also cause a dog to act irritable and aggressive when handled. The irritability may persist after the resolution of the inflammation because of the sensitization that occurred when handling was painful.

Dominance-Related Aggression

Dominance-related aggression is the most common type of aggression presented to veterinarians and animal behaviorists, representing about 45% of aggression problems.[1] The terms *dominance aggression* and *aggressive dominance* or *dominantly aggressive* are basically synonymous with the term *dominance-related aggression* and are used interchangeably. A person who has been appropriately assertive toward a dog may have a perfectly controlled pet that in an unassertive person's hands would be a severe problem. This problem is often a function of the owner's inability to control his or her dog or the dog's unwillingness to accept the owner's authority, at least in certain situations. It also can be related to inconsistencies in how the owner interacts with their dog. With early advice from veterinarians and puppy training classes, where the importance of maintaining authority over a growing dog is emphasized, the problem can often be avoided.

Not uncommonly, there may be components of more than one type of aggressive behavior in the overall patterns of problem behavior described by the dog's owner. For example, a dog may display aggressiveness when forced to go outside but also shows signs of fear when confronted by the owner. As mentioned in the introduction, the term *conflict aggression* may be used in these instances. For the sake of focusing on causes of the problem and resolution, the diagnostic term of *dominance-related aggression* seems useful and will be used here.

For the majority of cases, dominance-related aggression reflects normal canine behavioral tendencies manifested in a social structure and displayed toward human caregivers. This type of aggressive behavior occurs predominantly in males, which means it undoubtedly reflects the action of perinatal gonadal androgen on parts of the brain mediating aggressive behavior (Chapter 4). In some circumstances a neurotransmitter imbalance may underlie the aggressive tendency and the behavior would be considered abnormal. In such cases, the aggression may not be very amenable to behavioral approaches. However, in most cases, the problem is normal (but unacceptable) and can be controlled with appropriate behavior modification and management, providèd the client is willing and capable of carrying out instructions.

There are breed predispositions in this behavior, with the Chow Chow, Rottweiler, Shar Pei, Akita, Alaskan Malamute, and Dalmatian among those with the greatest aggressive tendencies.[14] Often dogs of the smaller breeds, especially those of the terrier group, tend to be more aggressive toward the owners than dogs of the medium-sized and large breeds.[15] Just because a dog is of a small size does not mean it will be less aggressive.

Typical History

The presenting complaint is usually that the dog displays aggressive responses, including stiffening body posture, staring, dilated pupils, growling, snarling, lip curl, snapping, or outright bites. These responses occur in response to predictable circumstances or triggers. These include discipline attempts, disturbing the dog from resting, reaching for or petting the dog, grooming it, getting it off a bed or furniture, taking away objects that the dog has picked up, taking away food, or putting the dog outdoors. Sometimes the dog even appears to "dare" the owner to confront it by grabbing something like a shoe or glove and displaying the object; when the owner attempts to take the object, the dog growls and threatens. Often, in the hands of a more confident person or a person not in the immediate family, such as a veterinarian, the dog will not display this aggressive dominance.

This problem is clearly a result of the interaction between a person and the dog. Probing the history of dogs presenting this problem often reveals that the dog's behavior is fine "99% of the time." The dog appears to accept the owner's leadership role most of the time, but when it wants to access valued resources, it assumes an aggressive mode and becomes dominant. The dog's dominant aggressiveness may be directed toward only one member of the family, and other members may get along fine with the dog.

Diagnosis

The main differential diagnoses for this problem are fear-related and idiopathic aggression. Territorial aggressiveness is not shown toward family members the dog knows. Although a dog that has been habituated to all members of the family would generally not show classical fear-related aggression toward family members, dogs that have been subjected to aversive handling within the family or inconsistent discipline may display fear-related aggression as well as signs of anxiety toward one or more family members, even in the presence of some triggers of dominance-related aggression. As mentioned, problem dogs are often presented with more than one type of aggressive behavior.

Treatment Guidelines

Successful treatment of this important problem depends upon accurately identifying the circumstances or triggers that evoke the aggressive behavior and on the ability and motivation of the client to follow the clinician's instructions conscientiously. There are three approaches to treatment to keep in mind. First, for reasons of safety, as well as to no longer reinforce inappropriate aggressive behavior, one should avoid circumstances or triggers that evoke aggression until the program of addressing the problem has progressed to the point where the triggers no longer evoke aggressive tendencies. The second approach is to reinforce the control of the caregivers in a nonconfrontational manner using the counterconditioning technique of affection control. The third approach is to desensitize the circumstances or triggers that evoke aggressive behavior using systematic desensitization and counterconditioning. These behavior modification approaches are outlined in the following sections.

Because castration of gonadally intact males has been shown to reduce aggressiveness toward family members, this operation would be indicated for those males that are gonadally intact. As indicated in Figure 8-2, castration of adult males showing dominance-related aggression can be expected to result in virtual resolution in an estimated 20% of male dogs. Aggression will be reduced by at least 50% in 30%

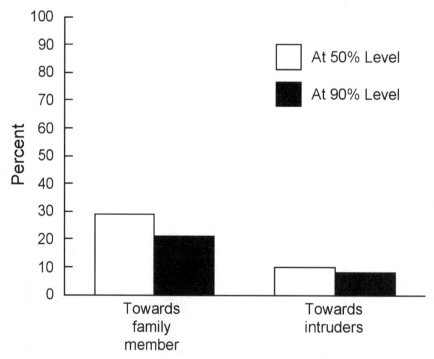

Figure 8-2   Effects of castration of male dogs in improving problem aggression toward human family members (dominance-related aggression) and human intruders. The effects may be at the 50% level, representing at least a 50% improvement, or at the 90% level, representing virtual resolution. Shown are percent of dogs responding at each level.

of males castrated. Although for most dogs castration alone will not make a noticeable difference, there is still reason to believe that the removal of gonadal androgen
might facilitate the behavioral approaches outlined below.

Avoidance of triggers that evoke aggressiveness

Because safety of human members of the family is a primary concern, triggers or
circumstances that evoke aggressiveness should be explicitly written down and the
client instructed on ways that these might be avoided. For example, if approaching
the dog near its food bowl evokes growls or threats, one should place the food in an
area where people are unlikely to approach the dog while it is eating. The same
goes for getting a dog off of furniture or the bed if this also evokes such a threat.
Family members either can make the areas or furniture unavailable or, after the dog
is there, simply act as if they don't care whether the animal is in that position. The
behavior modification discussed in a later section addresses desensitizing the dog
to these areas so that they do not have to be avoided continuously for the rest of the
animal's relationship with the family.

Counterconditioning desirable behavior by affection control

The affection control approach involves withdrawing virtually all affection and
attention from the dog at all times other than when the dog responds to a command,
such as "sit," "lie down," or "stay." The technique is especially effective when dogs
are accustomed to receiving a good deal of affection. The amount of affection to
which a dog is accustomed is often evident in the examination room as the client is
handling the dog.

In outlining the affection control technique it may be useful to suggest that on
the day the therapy begins, the dog not be allowed to sleep in the owner's bedroom
(if this has been the habit) and that affection and attention be withheld for several
hours. Affection control is best obtained by ignoring the dog while it is in the same
room as though it were invisible, not by putting the dog outdoors. This also includes
no eye contact from the owners. After the passage of several hours, the dog is given
a command once, such as "sit," and after the dog obeys, it is rewarded for a minute
or so with affection and possibly food treats. The object is to reinforce obedience
to commands with the positive stimuli of affection and food treats when the owner
wants, not when the dog demands it.

This process is repeated throughout the day at short intervals. For example, at
half-hour intervals, the dog might be given a command such as "come," "sit," or
"down" and, when it responds appropriately, it is given several seconds of affection
and a treat as part of its food ration. Actually, a dog is able to get a day's worth of
social contact, affection, and food this way (but on the owner's terms). The dog is
not rewarded unless it obeys a command. Commands are given frequently, and the
dog is constantly reminded of its subordinate position. The success of this approach
depends on all members of the family stringently withholding affection except
when commands are given to the dog. Food deprivation (e.g., 24 hours), to poten-
tate the effectiveness of food treats, is a useful adjunct if affection control does not
seem to hold that much sway with the dog.

When the procedure begins to have an effect on the dog's attitude, the owners could be advised to be a bit more demanding. They can act like a drill sergeant demanding the dog sit sequentially in 3 different locations before giving affection, or make the dog do a series of different commands, such as "down" and then "sit," etc. Gradually the owners should increase their physical interaction with the dog until they are at a point where they can deal with misbehaviors without fear of reprisal.

As mentioned, for the duration of the training period, the owners should avoid circumstances or triggers that are likely to evoke an aggressive response until the owner's control has progressed to the point that these triggers of aggression can now be confronted. If forcing the dog off the bed has previously evoked a threat or a snap, the owner should find other ways for getting the dog off the bed until the owner's control is such that he or she can give an "off" command and expect it to be followed. However, the dog can be removed from the bed without physical contact. One way would be to have the dog wear a long drag line while in the house with the owners. If the dog is on the bed, the owner says "off" and firmly, unemotionally, and without jerking, pulls the dog off of the bed. The owner's authority over the dog should gradually evolve to the point where all of the predictable triggers of affection can be approached without the owners being subject to any aggression. If the counterconditioning is progressing satisfactorily, it is recommended that the owners introduce the use of a head halter to further reinforce their control over the dog in a variety of situations (Chapter 3).

In household situations wherein only one member of the family has trouble with the dog, all members of the family should completely ignore the dog except the person having the trouble. Only this person should issue commands and reward obedience, and this person should be the only source of affection and food rewards. Likewise, when a dog shows aggressive dominance toward a nonfamily friend, such as a boyfriend, the owner should completely ignore the dog in the friend's presence so that the person out of favor can become the sole source of affection and food treats. The friend in question is instructed to give the dog a command before petting or interacting with the dog. The dog, therefore, learns to respond in a new way to this friend. This approach is potentiated by the owner or family members withdrawing affection from the dog for a few hours prior to a scheduled visit by this friend.

Desensitization of aggression-provoking stimuli

To desensitize a dog to those triggers or circumstances that evoke an aggressive response, one should establish training sessions where the triggers are gradually and systematically approached. If the dog tends to growl or snap when one or more family members come close to its food bowl, it is important to desensitize the dog to stimuli centered around the food bowl. This can be accomplished by picking up and placing an empty food dish back on the floor several times in succession. This should be done in a series of sessions as the dog is asked to sit while the food bowl is placed on the floor and then picked up again. The dog is given praise and a brief bit of affection each time this is done.

The next step is to put a bit of relatively unpalatable food in the dish, giving the dog a command to "sit" as the food is placed on the floor and then lifted off the floor. This is done several times in a row; after each time, the dog is given praise and affection if its behavior is calm and nonaggressive. Gradually over a period of days several pieces of kibble are put in the dish as it is placed down and lifted up again. Following this, if things are going well, something approaching a small amount of its regular food can be placed in the dish and the dish placed on the floor and picked up again in a session of 10 trials.

Another way is to find the distance that the owner can stand from the dog while it is eating out of its food bowl without showing any signs of aggression. At this distance, the owner tosses small pieces of a highly palatable treat into the food bowl. Gradually, over time, the owner steps closer and closer toward the food bowl while the dog continues to remain relaxed during the sessions.

Exercises like this one can be carried on concomitantly with the affection control method of behavior modification. If feeding the dog its normal meals still triggers an aggressive response, the dog can be distracted or out of the room, with the food placed there for the dog to come and eat on its own. The dog is ignored as though human members of the family do not care whether it is eating or not. It is essential that the dog not be given any opportunity to growl or threaten someone that comes by the food bowl. The only interactions between the dog and the people are those in the scheduled trials.

The same routine of desensitization can be used with other sensitive areas, such as when a person attempts to get the dog off the bed or a piece of furniture. The dog can be asked to sit and stay next to the bed when the handler steps a few paces back and calls the dog to come over. When the dog responds appropriately and comes over it can be given praise and a food treat. This procedure should be carried out in a session of roughly 10 trials. The next step may involve placing covers from the bed on the floor and asking the dog to sit on the covers and then stepping away and asking the dog to come over, again rewarding appropriate behavior.

After these floor exercises are going well the dog might be asked to jump on the bed, allowed to stay for a second or two, then asked to jump back down again and sit, at which time it is given an appropriate food treat. Assuming this is progressing well, the dog should be instructed to jump up on the bed for 30 seconds and then called off. This process is continued, allowing the dog longer periods of time until one is ready to approach the dog who has been on the bed the entire night. If there is still any resistance when the dog is asked to leave the bed, one might consider staging an encounter so that there is a sheet or blanket that can be simply pulled off the bed with the dog on it without getting close to the dog. The dog can then be reinforced for sitting.

Use of physical corrections

The question often comes up about simply using a stern "no," a jerk on the collar, or physical correction to meet an aggressive response. When this works, for example, with a puppy, the dog is reminded that it is subordinate to human members of the family and that aggressive threats will be met with appropriate correction.

These direct approaches often occur almost reflexively when a puppy growls or threatens as a family member attempts to groom it, trim the nails, or take away a stolen shoe.

Although such corrections to deal with aggressive tendencies may get the message across in one or two encounters in the hands of an experienced handler, it is no excuse for abusing a dog or carrying corrective measures beyond what is necessary to achieve a change in the dog's behavior. It is perhaps because of an ability to maintain a strong demeanor that experienced dog handlers and veterinarians often have little problem with dogs that are aggressively dominant toward the owners. When handling such a dog, veterinarians may ask the owner to step out of the room, which makes it easier for the professional to handle the dog. Keep in mind, however, that most people seeking the advice of a veterinarian or a consultant seem not to be physically or emotionally predisposed to being very assertive toward their dog. If encouraged to try physical correction they may not be successful, even with a puppy. The problem can become worse as the dog learns that by escalating its level of aggression it can get its way. Thus, while physical correction may be successful in the hands of an experienced dog handler, it is rarely appropriate to recommend when advising dog owners confronted with dominance-related aggression.

Use of a head halter

When treatment of aggressive dominance is going well, the addition of a head halter to the overall program may be beneficial. The use of an adjustable, nose-loop head halter (Gentle Leader®) to control an unruly dog allows the handler to take advantage of the halter's calming properties and thus control the dog's head more easily. After being left on for gradually longer periods of time, the halter can be left on 24 hours a day with a long leash being dragged behind the dog so the owner can easily grab the leash and pull up the dog into an acceptable sit posture on the owner's schedule. The halter can be placed on the dog using food treats and praise. If one has to struggle to place the halter on the dog, use of the halter should be postponed until the dog is more amenable to it after undergoing the behavior modification procedures discussed earlier. Use of the head halter is covered in detail in

---

DOMINANCE-RELATED AGGRESSION

Causes

- Natural tendency for dogs to attempt to be dominant
- Breed and gender predispositions

Prevention

- Follow safety guidelines.
- Avoid triggers of aggression.
- Use affection control: reinforce the obeying of commands.
- Castrate males.
- Desensitize triggers.

Case Study: Dominance-Related Aggression

History

Lola, a 3-year-old female spayed Labrador Retriever with mild hip dysplasia was presented for aggression toward the owners. The owners got Lola at 8 weeks of age. They took her to obedience classes at 6 months of age, where they began to use a prong collar to control her pulling. At 2 years old she began growling at the owners when they approached her while she was eating out of her food bowl. Initially the owners verbally and physically punished these aggressive acts, but Lola's growling increased and she snapped at the owners when they attempted to punish her. She soon began barking and lunging toward the owners if they petted her while she was sleeping on the couch. Her behavior toward other adults and children was generally friendly unless they tried taking food away from her. Her body posture during aggressive episodes, as well as when the owners went to pet her, was one in which the ears were laid back and tail down.

Diagnosis

Dominance-related aggression with components of fear and pain-related aggression.

Treatment

1. Consider a nonsteroidal antiinflammatory medication to reduce the pain from the hip dysplasia.
2. Avoid interactive punishment of aggressive acts.
3. Fit Lola with a head collar to replace the prong collar.
4. Avoid situations that have tended to provoke aggression.
5. Ignore all behaviors initiated by Lola to be petted or given treats.
6. Institute a program of affection control by giving a command to Lola and rewarding obedience; do this frequently throughout the day.
7. Systematically desensitize and countercondition Lola to being handled and having people pass by her when she is eating.

Progress Report

Lola's behavior was improved by 2 weeks. She appeared more comfortable in the owners' presence and did not cower as much. Her obedience to commands improved, and the owners were happy with the head collar. Six weeks after the appointment, Lola was eagerly accepting treats after responding to commands. Lola could be pushed off the couch if she did not come off by voice command.

Chapter 3. In using the head halter the owner should be instructed to give the dog a command frequently, such as "come" and then "sit"; back up the command with a firm upward pull of the halter; and lift the dog's head so that a sit position is gently reinforced. For areas where the dog is likely to resist, the owner should unemotionally grab the leash and pull the dog over into a sit. After major improvement is made, the halter may be removed to see whether it is still necessary.

Aggression Toward Children

A well-mannered dog that has never given anyone a problem with aggressive behavior may develop a nasty temperament toward a new baby or young child in the family. Suddenly the family members are no longer sure that they can trust the dog. The concept of sibling rivalry sometimes comes to mind in this type of problem, especially if the dog was the "only child" until a new baby arrived and the baby has, by necessity, taken up most of the attention.

Typical History

Typically the problem dog has been a perfectly nice and lovable pet with the adults, and even may have gotten along with the neighborhood children who are occasional visitors. Owners who find that the dog occasionally growls at their baby are in a predicament; they may love the dog, but they can take no chances. Successful resolution of this problem allows these people to keep a lovable pet that might otherwise be subjected to re-homing or euthanasia.

The origin of this problem—and the solution, for that matter—relates to the way in which affection and attention shape a dog's behavior. After arrival of the baby, a couple might lavish affection upon their dog, assuming the animal needs assurance that it has not lost favor. However, fearing the dog's potential aggressiveness toward the baby, they remove the dog from the room when the baby is present, reserving display of their affection for the dog for when they are alone with the dog. Thinking that the dog might be "jealous," they might even increase attention and add special food treats; but again, these are given when the baby is not around. The dog develops a dislike for the baby who has come to signal the absence of affection and treats, and when the dog sees the baby it may express its dislike. As time goes on, the contrast in the affection the dog gets when the baby is present and is not present becomes greater. One wonders if, in the dog's mind, it does not feel that were it not for the baby, it would get affection all day long.

Although one could expect this problem with almost any breed of dog, those that have a tendency to snap at children are those where one would expect the most severe problems. Examples of breeds most likely to have a predisposition to snap at children are the Dalmatian, Cocker Spaniel, Chihuahua, Miniature Schnauzer, Lhasa Apso, and Pekingese.[14] Regardless of cause or breed disposition, the overriding issue in treating this problem is to assure safety of the baby or child involved.

Diagnosis

The primary differential diagnoses include fear-related aggression, dominance-related aggression, and predatory behavior. If, because of lack of prior habituation, a dog is fearful of babies or children, the problem becomes one of understanding the origin of the fear and working on a desensitization and counterconditioning program using systematic desensitization, as outlined under fear-related aggression in a later section. Usually the client will be aware of fear-based responses in the dog and the history will reveal whether the baby is a fear-evoking stimulus. For babies and toddlers that are not capable of socially interacting with the dog, dominance-related aggression probably can be ruled out if the baby is not a perceived member of the social hierarchy. Predatory behavior might be suspected if a dog is seen to stalk and approach a moving child with no vocalizations such as growls. The problem addressed here is one in which the aggressiveness appears to be a manifestation of dislike for a baby that has interfered with the dog's relationship with the adults.

Treatment Guidelines

Safety

Parents should never leave their dog and child together unsupervised without a responsible adult present to control any negative interaction. Ways of keeping them separate, but with visible contact, include using baby gates, placing the child in a playpen, or placing the dog in an exercise pen. The parents still need to supervise the child so that he or she does not tease the dog through the bars or throw things at the dog.

In addition to discussing safety of the baby, the first issue to be brought up is the counterproductive use of punishment, especially interactive. The threat of punishment may force the dog not to display overt aggressive behavior when the parents are present, but it is not going to make the dog "like" the baby. In fact, the presence of the baby is likely to signify to the dog that it is apt to be punished. What one wants is for the dog to "love" the child through the judicious use of affection and treats and to induce a positive emotional state in the dog toward the child.

Affection Control

Affection control is similar to the indirect approach to dominance-related aggression because the rewards of affection and food treats are manipulated to get the desired effect. The owner should completely withdraw attention and affection from the dog when the baby is not present. When the baby is present, parents should dispense affection and/or food treats throughout the time the baby is in the dog's environment and especially at the first appearance of the baby. The owners may wish to first give a simple command to the dog. The dog's attention should be directed toward the baby. For some clients, to withhold and deliver affection on a prescribed basis may be very difficult, and in such cases it is useful to explain that this exaggerated treatment is only for a short period and that there are sound theoretical reasons for using this approach. As the clients see that this new behavior modification program has an impact, and the dog's behavior starts to change, the clients can expect to ease back toward a more normal way of interacting with the dog.

To be safe during times when the dog is present, the dog can be put on a lead that is tied to the leg of a piece of furniture so it cannot physically reach the baby. If there is a possibility of fear-related aggression, therapy should stress much more gradual exposure to the baby outside a critical distance, while counterconditioning the dog with affection and food treats when the baby is present. If, in the course of using these suggestions, the dog growls at the baby, one should employ social punishment by having everyone walk out on the dog or calmly, and without any verbal or physical punishment, isolate the dog in a bathroom or utility room for a few minutes. The message one wants to convey is that growling drives everyone away, not only the baby but also the adults who dispense affection.

A question that usually arises when children are the target of any type of aggression is the possibility of euthanasia or finding a new home for the dog. The approaches described here do not involve exposing the baby to being injured by the dog. Of course, baby and dog should not find themselves unrestrained in the same room without direct adult supervision. Usually a dog responds quickly to this treatment program, and one can expect to see progress within a week or two. If after 2 weeks there is no significant improvement, whether due to intractable aggressive tendencies, breed predispositions, or noncompliance by the clients, it is appropriate to bring up the topic of finding a new home for the dog.

If one successfully implements this program, there is still the issue that when babies are capable of moving around, approaching the dog, and contacting the dog, they may not be as gentle as one would like. Children, when they are old enough, need to be taught to approach and pet dogs gently; small toddlers are a different matter. One should work toward desensitizing and counterconditioning the dog to the poking, handling, and hair pulling that sometimes occur with small children; there is no guarantee that children will always be under adult supervision, and there should be a safety margin with regard to the baby-dog interaction. The adults should pair special food treats with gentle poking and pulling, knowing that they are not abusing the dog but helping to "babyproof" the dog with regard to possible future interactions with the baby. Finally, when the child is older and is able to give simple commands, such as "sit," steps should be taken to reinforce the child's control over the dog by having the child give commands before he or she gives any affection or food treats to the dog.

Prevention

The principles used in resolving this type of aggression can also be used in preventing this problem when advice is sought before a baby is on the scene. The focus is on achieving the behavioral goal of having the dog "love" the baby, not just grudgingly tolerate the baby. The attention the dog normally gets throughout the day should be curtailed and affection and attention given freely to the dog when the baby is in its presence. Thus, the baby becomes a stimulus that signals the onset of affection and attention; the dog should then come to welcome the appearance of the

---

AGGRESSION TOWARD BABIES

Causes

- Dog develops dislike of baby since baby takes attention
- Owners punish dog's unfriendly behavior toward baby
- Owners give affection and treats only when baby is absent
- Baby becomes an aversive stimulus

Resolution

- Follow safety guidelines.
- Withhold affection for the dog when the baby is absent.
- Give affection and treats only in the baby's presence.
- Implement social punishment (isolation) if the dog growls.

baby. The greater the contrast in the availability of affection when the baby is present versus when the baby is not present, the more readily the dog will learn to love the baby. Additional information about the aspect of raising puppies is discussed in Chapter 20 on selecting and raising puppies.

Owners that want to be super-prepared for the first baby in a dog's life could be advised to do the same type of affection control in the presence of a life-sized doll, as if it were a real baby. They should prepare the house ahead of time by putting up the crib and introducing baby toys. In addition, they can purchase and play recordings of baby sounds such as crying and screaming. The dog can also be exposed to the odors of babies through clothing (and even soiled diapers).

Fear-Related Aggression

Fear-related behavior is a type of aggressive behavior directed toward specific people or types of people, such as children, adult men, or people in uniforms. Sometimes strangers in general represent the class of fear-evoking people. To cope with its fear, the dog attempts to drive away fear-evoking people by growling when they approach. When growling does not work, the dog might resort to snapping. If, for some reason, snapping ceases to be effective, the dog might escalate its aggression to biting. The reinforcement of behavior that drives away the fear-provoking stimulus can shift the level of aggressiveness to more intense forms.

Typical History

Fear of people, accompanied by aggressive tendencies, is likely to be either a manifestation of lack of habituation to the people to whom the behavior is directed or a result of an aversive experience with a specific person or type of person. Although the aggressive aspect of the fear is a defensive behavior, dogs that are fear-biters are more aggressive in general than those who are just fearful of people and try to escape without acting aggressive.

A carefully explored history usually reveals that the fear-biter tends to move away from people or classes of people to whom it is aggressive. The growling, snarling, and snapping occur when it is not physically possible for the dog to leave, or it does not want to leave, such as when it is standing by the side of the owner or in its own territory. Observation of the dog's behavior in the examination room often reveals a fear component. If the problem is fear-biting toward men, this may be evident with a strange man (e.g., male veterinarian) in the examination room. The dog may hide under the chair of the client. The dog's facial posture is one in which the ears are down, the head held low, and the tail down (Fig. 8-1).

There may be a history of escalation of fear-related aggression, along the lines described earlier from growling to snapping to biting. The more successful the dog is in driving the targeted fear-evoking people away, the more pronounced the aggression can become. Over time, as the dog successfully learns how to cope, the body posture that the dog displays may tend away from that of a fearful dog. If the owner forcefully restrains the dog while a fear-evoking person comes up and handles the dog, this may produce a stronger aversive emotional response to the fear-evoking person.

Diagnosis

The primary differential diagnoses are territorial aggression and dominance-related aggression. The diagnosis should be based on evidence of fear aside from the aggressive tendencies. It is possible that the problem behavior is a mixture of territorial and fear-related aggression. In this case, because there is overlap in the treatment of the two problem behaviors in terms of stimulus exposure and counterconditioning, the treatment regimen should work with both. Although dominance-related aggression is directed primarily toward family members to whom the dog is well habituated, this type of aggression could be generalized toward groomers, veterinarians, and handlers. The distinction between dominance-related and fear-related aggression hinges on signs of fear, both with regard to the dog's posture and with the tendency to leave the target person, as opposed to more offensive aggressive demeanor.

Treatment Guidelines

When it is evident that one is dealing with fear-induced aggression, rather than a desire by the dog to be dominant or protective of a home or family members, it is even more obvious that punishment or severe corrections cannot cure this problem. If the owner restrains a dog while the fear-evoking person approaches and contacts the dog, the dog's emotional response, as mentioned earlier, would tend to be more intense the next time.

While ensuring safety of the volunteers helping with the program, the first step in treating this problem, as with any unwanted behavioral reaction, is to avoid the situations or stimuli that elicit the reaction. The next step is to institute a program that includes systematic desensitization and counterconditioning (Chapter 3). The specific desensitization program involves gradually exposing the dog, in sessions of several trials, to the fear-evoking person and pairing affection and food treats with the graded stimulus to create a positive emotional state associated with the target stimulus. The best way to potentiate the value of affection for counterconditioning is for the owners to withdraw affection from the dog for some time prior to the training sessions.

Training sessions involving exposure to a fear-inducing person should be scheduled daily. Using the example of fear of children, sessions could be staged where the problem dog is brought to a room and instructed to sit beside the owner. Although not necessary, the dog could be trained ahead of time to respond with the head halter, which could be used on the dog during these desensitization sessions (Chapter 3). A child then appears in the dog's visual field at some predetermined distance where the dog shows no emotional reaction—for example, 20 feet (7 meters) away. The child should never be close enough to cause any signs of anxiety or aggressiveness in the dog. Preliminary training could start with a child with whom the dog is familiar and has had positive experiences. The dog's attention should be directed toward the child who has appeared in the room and, assuming the child is beyond the critical distance of causing fear, the dog is petted and given a highly palatable food treat. The child leaves and, after a couple of minutes, reappears. Each appearance of the child paired with affection and a food treat constitutes one trial; a session typically would consist of 10 trials. One or two sessions can be conducted per day. Clients are instructed to give no treats during the day other than during training sessions. Assuming that the dog always remains relaxed, the sessions should involve bringing the child closer and closer to the dog, in measured steps over several days. Assuming progressive desensitization, eventually the child can give the dog a food treat and be the source of affection.

After one fear-evoking child is able to approach and handle the dog without provoking anxiety or any emotional reaction, other children should be introduced and the distance to the dog increased. Sessions with other children should progress faster after the initial set of sessions. During the weeks when training sessions are being conducted, every attempt should be made to prevent the dog from being exposed to fear-inducing children outside of the training sessions because this could cause regression of the training, requiring a return to a previous level of exposure to the stimulus.

If it seems almost impossible for any fear-evoking person to come into the dog's visual field without evoking a fear reaction, use of an antianxiety drug (e.g., fluoxetine, clomipramine) may be useful. A behaviorally effective dose should be obtained, which blocks the fear response. After a change in the fear behavior is noticed, the dog must be maintained continuously on the drug until it is well into the desensitization program. As the sessions are continued, the amount of drug given each day can be gradually reduced. A sample reduction schedule might be to lower the daily dose by 25% every 2 weeks while the training sessions are continued. If the dog acts fearful, the dose should be adjusted upward again for a longer period until more complete desensitization is achieved. It should be emphasized that no medication is currently licensed to treat aggression in dogs, and none has been proven to increase significantly the chance at behavioral improvement, as compared to placebo. It is theoretically possible, in fact, that with fear only partially reduced a dog may snap or bite a fear-evoking person more readily if its fear had been inhibiting some of the tendency to bite.

FEAR-RELATED AGGRESSION

Causes
- Fear of people to whom dog has not been socialized
- Mistreatment by subgroup member
- Reinforced when aggression repels people

Resolution
- Follow safety guidelines.
- Implement social punishment for aggression.
- Desensitize and countercondition to subgroup.
- Avoid spontaneous approaches of subgroup.
- Avoid physical correction for aggression.

Case Study: Fear-Related Aggression

History

Josie, a healthy 7-year-old female spayed Miniature Pinscher, was presented for biting a person when closely approached. The owner, a single woman, did not let Josie interact with other persons or dogs until she was 1 year old, because she was afraid Josie would get a disease from another dog. Josie is usually carried in the owner's arms and rarely encounters other people. Her body language when she encounters people is dilated pupils, ears back, and growling with the lips retracted horizontally. When visitors come to the house, Josie will run from the visitors initially, but later, if she is initially ignored, will warm up to them, jump on their laps, and be friendly. The precipitating incident for the appointment was when Josie was free in the house and bit a workman on the hand when he tried to pet her.

Diagnosis

Fear-related aggression

Treatment

1. Avoid situations where people are likely to reach for Josie.
2. To gain leadership over Josie, apply affection control techniques by frequently issuing commands and reinforcing obedience.
3. Fit Josie with a head collar; use the halter regularly during desensitization sessions.
4. Do not comfort Josie if she appears fearful of people.
5. Systematically desensitize and countercondition Josie to being approached by people using a distance gradient during sessions of 10 trials once or twice a day.

Progress Report

Five weeks after the appointment there was some improvement in her fear of people. The client had not worked on desensitization and counterconditioning, but she no longer comforted Josie when she was fearful. She also carried Josie less. At 9 weeks after the appointment, the owner had started to implement desensitization and counterconditioning techniques; Josie then began to act calm with people reaching for her while being held by the owner. When the owner was contacted 5 months after the appointment, the problem behavior had improved and the owner was then letting adults approach Josie more regularly.

Pain-Induced Aggression

Self-protection against pain is a natural inclination of both animals and people. In the clinical realm, professionals are most likely to see this type of aggression when a dog has suffered from localized pain and has snapped or growled when handled near the painful area. For example, older dogs with arthritis may display this type of aggression. Pain-induced aggression can play a role in intraspecific competition when, during a fight, animals are stimulated to fight more vigorously when bitten by the opponent; this may help the bitten animal suddenly emerge as a winner. During play in juveniles, the escalation of play fighting to serious fighting can be attributed to a painful bite triggering an aggressive retaliation. The elicitation of more intense fighting by pain is the reason one should not attempt to break up a fight by hitting the dogs or using a shock collar. In extreme cases the elicitation of greater levels of fighting by pain is the basis of the despicable practice of dog fighting.

Typical History

In clinical practice, the most common sign of pain-induced aggression is when a dog acts aggressive only when a specific region of the body is touched or manipulated. If the existence of a traumatizing foreign body or inflammatory process is not obvious, the usual approach of using radiographs and other diagnostic techniques to reveal the cause of the pain is in order. Keep in mind that some dogs are sufficiently stoic in the presence of confident owners to suppress aggressive tendencies, but they will show aggression if touched in the painful area by others. Of course, medical resolution of the inflammation and pain-causing problem is the first priority. After the cause of the pain has been resolved, a dog still might act aggressively when touched or handled in the area because pain from handling the area has been conditioned to the area handled. In this instance the aggression can be viewed as a conditioned response and should be amenable to desensitization and counterconditioning.

Diagnosis

The primary differential diagnoses are dominance-related and fear-related aggression. The localization of the stimulus evoking the aggression is a key point in the diagnosis. The challenge comes when the pain-induced aggression is shown toward some handlers or family members but not others.

Treatment Guidelines

For acute pain, it is necessary to remove the source of the pain before expecting much progress. Although with chronic conditions, such as arthritis, recent pharmacological advances have been made to alleviate much of the pain, one cannot expect to remove the source of pain completely. When it seems as though the pain is no longer occurring, or is controlled to the degree possible, the indicated treatment is systematic desensitization plus counterconditioning of handling near the sensitive area (Chapter 3). The desensitization program should begin with staged sessions of trials, using a distance gradient of proximity to the sensitive area or a gradient of pressure over the sensitive area. The distance gradient is usually the most feasible. A trial consists of pairing brief bouts of affection and a food treat with a touch for each of 10 trials comprising a session. After several sessions of 10 trials per session,

---

PAIN-INDUCED AGGRESSION

Causes
- Protective response when painful area handled
- Conditioned response when painful area handled

Resolution
- Follow safety guidelines.
- Remove the source of pain.
- Desensitize and countercondition.

spaced over a few days, the handlers should then be touching closer to the affected area until they are eventually using normal pressure over the affected area. The total conditioning time could take 2 weeks if the program is continued on a daily basis. For a sensitive area near the back leg, for example, one might pet the dog's back and pair a food treat and affection with each petting trial. Then the petting could gradually be moved in steps toward the affected area on the leg. In cases of more extreme reaction, the desensitization may be facilitated with an antianxiety drug (Chapter 6).

The similarities in treatment approaches between pain-induced aggression and fear-induced aggression are quite obvious. Both use systematic desensitization and counterconditioning of the emotional reaction. Desensitization is accomplished by using a gradient of stimulus strength ranging from an initial safe level to the level of full stimulus strength. In both instances, an antianxiety drug may be employed to reduce an aversive emotional reaction to the evoking stimulus and to facilitate a more rapid desensitization process. One must keep in mind that antianxiety drugs may relax some of the inhibitions of aggression directed to a person who might handle the sensitive area, making biting more likely.

Territorial Aggression Toward People

It is possible to have too much of a good thing. This is occasionally true of the territorial guarding behavior of dogs where the territorial protection is appreciated but keeps friends, relatives, and other welcome visitors out of the house or yard. Watchdog barking, another valued trait of dogs, is not necessarily linked to territorial aggression. A dog may be excellent as a barking watchdog but show no aggression toward intruders when they are on the premises. Females in general tend to be as good as males in watchdog behavior, but males predominate in territorial aggression (Chapter 4). Examples of breeds ranking highest in territorial aggression are the Akita, Rottweiler, Doberman Pinscher, Chow Chow, German Shepherd, and Dalmatian.[14]

Typical History

A dog may be perfectly friendly toward strangers away from home but act fiercely aggressive toward those same people when they are in its territory. The pervasiveness of this behavior is due to the dog's natural tendency to protect the territory of the pack. Guarding behavior is reinforced because intruders leave, and for all the dog knows, it has chased away the intruders. Occasionally, owners have rewarded or praised the dog for aggressive guarding and this has also reinforced the behavior. The dog's territory can also be less stationary than its house. Such places are the car and even familiar parts of a walk.

Diagnosis

The main differential diagnosis is fear-related aggression, stemming from fear of strangers. Territorial aggression usually involves no signs of fearfulness. However,

TERRITORIAL AGGRESSION
Causes • Absence of habituation to visitors • Breed-specific and gender-specific tendencies
Resolution • Habituate dogs to visitors using a distance gradient. • Bring the dog under owner control. • Countercondition stranger visits with food and affection.

both territorial and fear-related aggression may occur in the same dog. The latter diagnosis may be indicated by ambivalent signs, such as a dog going back and forth between showing signs of fearfulness and offensive threats. Keep in mind that the territory defended may be broader than the home and often includes an automobile and protective aggression of a caregiver, especially if the dog is held by a leash.

Treatment Guidelines

If the dog shows no fear of the people it is aggressive toward, the most feasible approach involves desensitizing the emotional reaction to strangers. Ensuring safety of the people helping to solve the problem, one can then countercondition the dog to like the people who come within the dog's territory. Basically, the dog is induced to change its attitude toward intruders by positive reinforcement.

Desensitization and counterconditioning are accomplished by staging visits of friends for a specific time. Starting well before the planned visits, the owners should ignore the dog, saving attention or affection for the arrival of friends. Use of a head halter during these sessions may be useful (Chapter 3). At visitation times, the owners, and when possible the visitors, give the dog attention and palatable treats. As the reaction to each visitor becomes more friendly and visitors can dispense treats, the owners should then arrange a visit from the next person along the gradient of familiarity, eventually ending up with strangers. Because the dog receives affection (and food treats) primarily when people visit, it should come to look forward to visitors and lose the territorial intensity.

Although somewhat idealistic, a goal of this reward-based approach is a dog that loves visitors (formerly territorial intruders). For clients who are interested in maintaining some territorial guarding behaviors, an intermediate level of behavior that can be difficult to attain, but perhaps worth trying, is to stage multiple visits to the point where the dog is easily handled.

Idiopathic Attacks on People

This rare type of aggressive behavior is characterized by truly unpredictable and unprovoked attacks on people the dog knows well. The attacks are typically infrequent, often spaced a month or more apart. This is the one type of behavior most easily classified as abnormal with no apparent explanation by reference to adaptive canine behavior or the wild ancestor. The behavior could reflect several causes, including neuropathological lesions, extreme or adverse early experience, and/or genetic predisposition. Because of the inexplicable cause of the behavior, the syndrome has been referred to as *idiopathic aggression.* The syndrome has also been labeled as *episodic* or *dysfunctional rage,*[16] implying an underlying central nervous system abnormality. It should be noted that, although initially there may be no evident triggers evoking the behavior, further delving into the history may reveal subtle, yet predictable, triggers. The association of a syndrome like this with certain breeds, particularly English Springer Spaniels, suggests a potential genetic predisposition. Irritative foci, space-occupying lesions, and subclinical inflammation in the brain could be a cause of this syndrome. Little is known about this type of problem aggression and it is likely that there are several etiologies or syndromes that can bring on unpredictable or unprovoked attacks.

Dogs with this syndrome do not typically display evidence of a clinical abnormality. In some cases, where the animals have been subjected to euthanasia, examination of the brain has revealed no consistent, telltale pathology of the nervous system or other organ systems. With painstaking neuropathological examination, perhaps more could be documented in the way of underlying brain pathology. An imbalance of a neurotransmitter controlling aggression may be a way in the future to understand the biological basis of this and other types of aggression.[17]

Anyone who proposes to treat this behavior is faced with a challenge of interpreting the effectiveness of the treatment. Because the episodes of aggressive behavior may be at widely spaced intervals, this can be risky. How does one know whether the treatment program is effective if the client must wait until an estimated elapsed time for another attack? Because the dogs are invariably well-behaved between attacks, one cannot monitor the effectiveness of treatment. Because the outburst of aggression is unexplainable and treatment difficult to interpret, risk of injury to people is a major concern. This is the one type of aggressive behavior for which euthanasia is usually justified.

Typical History

The typical case is the dog that the owner describes as usually friendly, affectionate, and well mannered. The owners are almost dumbfounded by the attacks in which the dog, for no explainable reason, suddenly turns and attacks (often viciously) a

---

IDIOPATHIC AGGRESSION

Causes

- Genetic or pathophysiological abnormality
- A syndrome with several possible causes
- Neurotransmitter disorder

Resolution

- Human safety is primary.
- Euthanasia is a recommended option.

member of the household or another person. The behavior is unprovoked and unpredictable in that a stimulus that hardly ever bothers a dog, such as petting, evokes an attack and there is no way of predicting when this attack might occur. Often no eliciting stimulus truly may be known. A common triggering stimulus is a trivial command, such as "sit," given in a friendly manner and which would typically be no cause for any type of aggression. Usually the dog gives little or no warning before an attack. The attacks may be directed toward a person's face, neck, or arm. Victims of the attacks are likely to mention that moments before the attack the dog seemed not to recognize them and may have acquired a glazed or distant look in its eyes. After the attack some dogs appear subdued and others act as though they were not aware of what they had done. The attacks initially seem to have occurred sporadically, perhaps about a month apart, and owners may have made up some excuse for the dog, such as it must have been handled in a painful area. When the attacks become more frequent, professional advice is often sought.

Diagnosis

Because one is generally dealing with aggression toward family members the dog knows well, fear-related and territorial aggression can usually be ruled out. Aggression may also be secondary to a seizure disorder or other neurological condition. Pain-related aggression is another differential and should be evident from history and physical examination revealing a specific area of the body which, if handled fairly reliably, provokes aggression; even then one usually notices a warning growl or snap prior to an attack. Attacks associated with pain-related aggression are usually snaps rather than vicious bites.

The main differential diagnosis is dominance-related aggression. The more severe forms of dominance-related aggression are easily confused with idiopathic aggression. Many cases that may appear to be idiopathic aggression are actually more extreme forms of dominance-related aggression where the evoking triggers have not been identified. A careful history should reveal whether attacks are actually unprovoked and unpredictable. The fact that a dog can have both dominance-related as well as idiopathic aggression makes the diagnostic workup more complicated.

Treatment Guidelines

For cases of true idiopathic aggression, probably the best advice to clients, in the interest of their own safety and that of others, is that euthanasia be seriously considered. Some owners, particularly those of small dogs, may insist that treatment be attempted. On the basis that this form of aggressive behavior may reflect abnormal eruption of neuronal activity, some clinicians have found that the anticonvulsant drug phenobarbital is useful in controlling the attacks.[16] The problem with attempting to treat the behavior is that the attacks occur infrequently and are not predictable. As with treatment of convulsive disorders, one would have to treat a dog for several weeks to know whether the treatment is effective and whether the dosage should be adjusted. One must also take into consideration that any apparent improvement in behavior may be due to a transient side effect of sedation. A person could be attacked and injured while the treatment is being evaluated.

References

1. Beaver BV. Profiles of dogs presented in aggression. Journal of the American Veterinary Association 1993;31:595–598.
2. Landsberg GM. The distribution of canine behavior cases at three behavior referral practices. Veterinary Medicine 1991;86:1011–1018.
3. Lund JD, Agger FJ, Vestergaard KS. Reported behaviour problems in pet dogs in Denmark: Age distribution and influence of breed and gender. Preventive Veterinary Medicine 1996;28:33–48.
4. Hart BL, Hart LA. Selecting pet dogs on the basis of cluster analysis of breed behavior profiles and gender. Journal of the American Veterinary Medical Association 1985;186: 1181–1185.
5. Neilson JC, Eckstein RA, Hart BL. Effects of castration on behavior of male dogs with reference to the role of age and experience. Journal of the American Veterinary Medical Association 1997;211:180–182.
6. O'Farrell VO, Peachey E. Behavioural effects of ovariohysterectomy on bitches. Journal of Small Animal Practice 1990;31:595–598.
7. White MM, Neilson JC, Hart BL, Cliff KD. Effects of clomipramine hydrochloride on dominance-related aggression in dogs. Journal of the American Veterinary Association 1999;215:1288–1291.
8. Virga V, Houpt KA, Scarlett JM. Efficacy of amitriptyline as a pharmacological adjunct to behavioral modification in the management of aggressive behaviors in dogs. Journal of the American Animal Hospital Association 2001;37:325–330.
9. Dodman NH, Donnelly R, Shuster L, Mertens P, Rand W, Miczek K. Use of fluoxetine to treat dominance aggression in dogs. Journal of the American Veterinary Association 1996;209:1585–1587.
10. Fuller RW. The influence of fluoxetine on aggressive behavior. Neuropsychopharmacology 1996;14:77–81.
11. Oliver B, Mos J, vanOorschotr R, et al. Serotonin receptors and animal models of aggressive behavior. Pharmacopsychiatry 1995;28:80–90.
12. Constantino JN, Liberman M, Kincaid M. Effects of serotonin reuptake inhibitors on aggressive behavior in psychiatrically hospitalized adolescents: Results of an open trial. Journal of Child and Adolescent Psychopharmacology 1997;7:31–44.
13. Holliday TA, Cunningham JG, Gutnick MJ. Comparative clinical and electroencephalographic studies of canine epilepsy. Epilepsia 1970;11:281.
14. Hart BL, Hart LA. The Perfect Puppy: How to Choose Your Dog by Its Behavior. New York: W.H. Freeman and Co., 1988.
15. ———. Selecting, raising and caring for dogs to avoid problem aggression. Journal of the American Veterinary Medical Association 1997;210:1129–1134.
16. Dodman NH, Miczek KA, Knowles K, Thalhammer JG, Shuster L. Phenobarbital-responsive episodic dyscontrol (rage) in dogs. Journal of the American Veterinary Medical Association 1992;201:1580–1583.
17. Reisner IR, Mann JJ, Stanley M, Huang YY, Houpt KA. Comparison of cerebrospinal fluid monoamine metabolite levels in dominant-aggressive and non-aggressive dogs. Brain Research 1996;714:57–64.

Chapter 9
Aggression Toward Other Dogs

Consider any group of social animals—chickens, cows, rhesus monkeys, wolves—and it is obvious that occasional aggression toward conspecifics within the group is normal. Aggression may be involved when an existing dominance hierarchy is challenged by the maturation of a younger animal or by the aging of an adult. Aggression is commonly displayed toward newcomers to the group. Within a group, body postures and vocalizations displayed by the dominant animals, and submissive gestures by the others, generally keep fighting to a minimum. Although the principles of social interaction seen in nature, especially in wolves, generally apply to dogs, there are some differences created by the way in which humans have selectively bred, raised, and managed dogs. Aggressive tendencies are stronger in some breeds than others as a function of selective breeding over centuries. In raising practices, some dogs may not have had much exposure to other dogs and may not have developed (or refined) social behaviors for settling social conflicts short of fighting. Also, one may interfere with the resolution of canine disagreements by preventing full dominance of one dog by another and unknowingly prolonging aggressive encounters between dogs.

In multiple-dog households, fights may occur between dogs that have an established relationship and get along fine most of the time but are aggressive only in the presence of the owners, primarily as a function of the way the owners interact with them. A different type of problem arises in a household from the absence or instability of a dominance hierarchy between dogs that are fighting.

Outside the family, aggressiveness toward strange dogs may reflect sex-typical predispositions. Dogs of either sex may be very fearful of strange dogs, possibly as a function of little socialization to other dogs in early life (Chapter 20), and act defensively aggressive when approached by strange dogs. Dogs may also be aggressive toward strange dogs as a function of territorial tendencies. In some unfortunate circumstances dogs have been purposefully bred and trained to attack other dogs with no tendency to stop the attack even when the other dog signals submission. This type of aggressiveness, of course, is the profile of dogs used for dog fighting. When offspring of these dogs are placed in homes this type of problem may be brought to the attention of a clinician. The attack of small dogs by large dogs may reflect predatory behavior, which is not typically considered an aspect of aggression; this chapter explores this behavior. Following a discussion of factors affecting aggression toward other dogs, the types of interdog aggression covered in this chapter are: 1) aggression only in the owner's presence, but with an identified hierarchy, referred to in this book, as *dominance-status aggression*; 2) aggression in the absence of dominance hierarchy; 3) aggression toward strange dogs away from home; and 4) predatory aggression toward small dogs. The first two topics cover aggression between dogs within a household and the other topics cover aggression outside the home. Aggression toward other dogs may also involve more than one type of interdog aggression. On some occasions the problem may include aggression toward people as well as other dogs. As with arriving at a diagnosis for aggression directed toward people, evaluation of the body language exhibited by the dog when in an aggressively aroused state is valuable in arriving at a treatment plan.

In all cases involving aggression in dogs, safety of the people and dogs is paramount. In the case of a fight between dogs, clients need to be reminded that in attempting to break up a fight they may get bitten. The owners should never reach between two fighting dogs or grab their collars or scruffs to separate them. If it's necessary to pull fighting dogs apart, some authorities recommend two people pulling on the tails or hind legs of the dogs until they are separated. Using a physical barrier, such as a board, to separate the dogs is safer. Another method is spraying water on the entangled dogs with a garden hose. One must remember not to use anything that causes pain (shock collars, pepper spray, mace) because pain can escalate aggression between the dogs. The larger and more powerful the dogs, the more risky is any attempt to separate fighting dogs.

Factors Affecting Aggression Toward Other Dogs

A discussion of breed differences, gender, hormonal influences, early experience, and the role of social interactions in keeping peace among dogs is useful in dealing with all types of interdog aggression.

Breed Differences

Breed membership may affect aggressiveness toward other dogs. Among breeds that rank high on the tendency to be aggressive toward other dogs are the Rottweiler, Chow Chow, Akita, Scottish Terrier, and German Shepherd.[1] Within breeds, dogs also vary in their pugnaciousness toward other dogs as a function of individual genetic attributes. In some instances breeders have intentionally bred for absence of aggressiveness. Even the notorious Pit Bull breed has its cream puffs as a result of selective breeding away from the fighting tendency. Regardless of breed background, inquiring about the behavior of the dam and sire, as well as of members of previous litters, may offer some guidelines as to whether the aggressive tendencies of a particular dog seem to reflect a genetic influence.

Gender and Hormonal Status

Regardless of breed, there is overall a greater tendency for males to fight with other dogs than for females to fight with other dogs (Chapter 4). Consistent with gender differences in predisposition to be aggressive toward other dogs, castration of males may reduce this tendency. Clinical data[2] indicate that castration more reliably eliminates or reduces the aggression that occurs between dogs in the same household than aggression directed toward strange dogs outside the home (Fig. 9-1). One can expect virtual resolution of problem behavior in about 25% of cases of fighting between dogs in the same home and in 10% of cases of fighting between strange dogs. Improvement, but not complete resolution, occurs with both of these types of aggression in a somewhat higher percent of dogs (Fig. 9-1). Castration may affect aggressiveness in male dogs toward other dogs in two ways: by reducing the aggressive motivation in the problem animal and by altering male-related olfactory cues with the removal of testosterone, resulting in a less tempting target for the opposing male.

Although, in general, females are less aggressive toward other dogs than males are, females that are gonadally intact may act quite aggressive toward other dogs when in estrus or when caring for a litter of puppies. Maternal aggressiveness, driven by a combination of hormonal influences and the presence of puppies, is highly

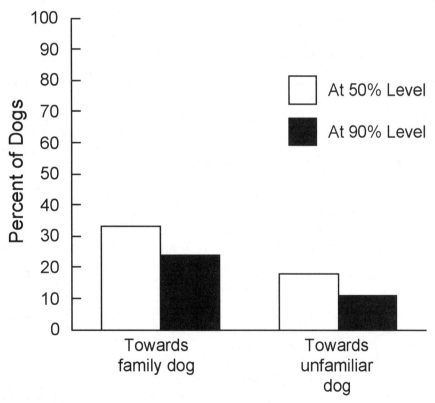

Figure 9-1 Effects of castration of male dogs in improving problem aggression toward other dogs in the family or unfamiliar dogs. The effects may be at 50% level of improvement, representing at least 50% improvement, or at the 90% level, representing virtual resolution. Shown are percent of dogs responding at each level (data from Neilson et al, 1997[2]).

individualistic, and it may be directed toward other dogs or people. This type of aggression is touched upon in Chapter 17.

Role of Early Experience

Through interacting with mother and littermates, and later with other puppies, a dog develops appropriate ways of responding to other dogs. Submissive responses are made to stronger and more dominant dogs, and aggressive responses are inhibited when other dogs make submissive gestures. Dogs also become habituated to other dogs of all shapes and sizes. All of these socialization activities should occur during the socialization period and constitute an important aspect of early experience; comparable experiences in the adult are much less influential.

Without at least some early socialization, dogs may not be habituated to other dogs although they may be well socialized to people. When approached by strange dogs they may be fearful and act aggressive as a self-protective response. One would not expect such dogs to pursue strange dogs aggressively but possibly to act aggressive when approached. If the growling or snapping drives off other dogs, reducing the level of fear or anxiety, the fear-related aggression is enhanced by such reinforcement.

Role of Social Interactions

In most instances where two or more dogs live together, there will be a dominance hierarchy determined by size, gender, seniority in the home, breed-related aggressive temperament, individual genetic makeup, and early experience. Although size is probably the most reliable determinant, the animal that has lived in the household the longest may be the dominant one, even though it may be smaller. Males are often, but not always, dominant over females.

Social position is expressed and reinforced by facial expressions, body posture, eye contact, growls, snarls, and lip curls as well as outright attacks. A subordinate often acknowledges or acquiesces to the signs of dominance by diverting eye contact, turning its head to the side, lowering the tail, and moving away. These same signs of submissiveness are typically shown by dogs toward human family members when the dogs are reprimanded. The social signals exchanged between dominant and subordinate dogs may be so subtle that the owners do not notice. Sometimes owners are not even aware of which dog is dominant. When necessary, dominant dogs can intensify the signals of submissiveness by snapping at or biting subordinates. The extremely submissive sign of rolling onto the back is more likely to be displayed by younger dogs or when a dog is the target of an attack by a much larger and dominant dog.

The reference in this chapter to the dominant dog and the subordinate dog is treated as a clear-cut distinction for the purpose of explanation. This is a useful concept in explaining to clients the source of a problem and the resolution. In reality, dominance is more fluid and may not be absolute. Dominance may be proportionate, with one dog dominant 60% of the time, for example. The dog that is subordinate may acquiesce most of the time, but when a highly valued object such as a rawhide bone is at stake, it may threaten the dominant dog.

Within a household, dominance may be altered over time. This is seen, for example, when a family has an old dog that has been with them for a long time and decides to get a second dog as a puppy for a companion for the older dog and as an eventual replacement. Initially, the old family favorite will be dominant, but as time goes on the younger dog can easily outmatch the older one. Dominance reversal could come about slowly without major confrontation, or the reversal could be triggered wherein one brief fight will settle the new relationship and put the younger dog in charge. This reversal of dominance may occur without the owners realizing that it has happened.

A variant of this reversal of dominance occurs when people adopt a new adult dog that is much larger than the resident adult dog. The new dog, lacking seniority, may remain in a subordinate role at first, but later challenge the more senior dog. Again, the dominance reversal may occur without the owners knowing it. Problems arise when the owners interfere with the social order, putting down the emerging dominant dog and basically disturbing the direction of changes in the dominance hierarchy. The result is more aggression than would occur without the disturbance.

Dominance-Status Aggression

This problem, involving two dogs in the same household, is generally one of the most rewarding to deal with because of the likelihood of resolution with relatively little effort. Typically dogs get along fine except when the owners interfere or are in the vicinity of the dogs. After establishing a diagnosis, one can point out to the clients some new house rules, motivate them to give the plan a chance to work at least over the next 2 weeks, and look forward to hearing about improvement. Behavioral patterns involved in this problem may even be evident in the examination room (Fig. 9-2).

Typical History

Fighting between dogs with an established dominant-subordinate relationship is often provoked by the way the owners interact with the dogs. In the absence of the owners, the dogs are peaceful and show no evidence of fighting. This bit of history alone is usually sufficient to establish that the main cause of the fighting is the owner's interference with the dominant-subordinate relationship that normally keeps peace among the dogs.

One way to look at this problem is that when the dogs are around the owners, especially during greetings, both dogs are focused on gaining attention from the owners. Naturally, the dominant dog expects to be the first to receive attention and it expects the most attention. The subordinate, having an equally strong desire for attention, may try to horn in on the dominant's interaction with the owners. The dominant dog may then growl in an attempt to move the subordinate back, and if this is not successful, reinforce its communication efforts by escalating its aggression, perhaps by snapping. The dominant dog may then be corrected or punished by the owners wanting to treat the dogs equally; soon the subordinate may learn it

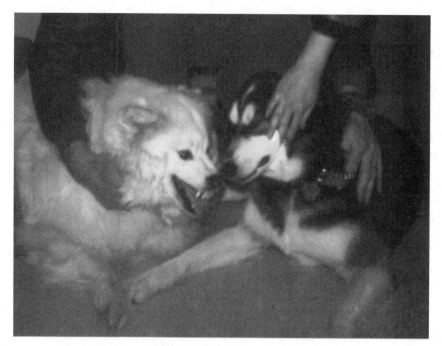

Figure 9-2 Dominance-status aggression displayed by the dog on the left as the dog on the right is brought into close contact with the primary human attachment. The two dogs fought only when interactions occurred with the owners.

is supported or protected by the owners, so it may vie for attention without seeming to pay attention to the dominant dog's threats. The common tendency of people to favor the underdog enhances the problem. They may feel it is appropriate to punish the instigator of aggression, in this case the dominant animal. An aggressive attack from the dominant may result in the owners putting the dominant dog outside while keeping the subordinate inside. This behavior on the part of the owners can escalate the aggression by the dominant dog at the next greeting.

This type of aggressive behavior is common when a family gets a puppy that will grow to a large size to be the companion to a resident dog of smaller body size. The dogs may have long since reversed their dominance relationship, but the smaller older dog may learn that in the presence of the owners it will be supported. It will continue to stand up to the larger dog when the owners are around. In multidog households, this problem can occur between two dogs while the other dogs (either dominant or subordinate to those two) are less involved in the altercations.

Diagnosis

The two principal differential diagnoses are fighting due to dominance-status aggression and absence of dominance hierarchy. Rarely, one may find abnormal aggressiveness in which the dominant dog does not recognize signs of submissiveness and modulate its aggression. In differentiating fighting due to absence of a hierarchy from a dominance-status aggression, the primary sign is that in the latter case fighting almost always occurs in the owner's presence. Abnormal aggressiveness, such as that which could be a reflection of the breeding and raising of dogs for dog fighting, should be considered a possibility when, despite obvious signs of submissiveness and unwillingness of the subordinate to fight with the dominant dog, the subordinate is still attacked by the dominant. This may also be due to lack of appropriate socialization, where the dog cannot recognize such signals. Such abnormal aggression is much more difficult to treat by behavioral means alone, and permanent separation of the dogs may be indicated.

Treatment Guidelines

To treat dominance-status aggression, it is important that the owners understand that social relationships between dogs cannot be handled in the same way as human relationships where individuals are treated equally. It is natural for dogs to accept a dominant or a subordinate role, and it is natural for the dominant dog to reinforce its position periodically with posturing, growls, or threats and for the subordinate to respond by submitting to these gestures. Keep in mind that muzzles should not be placed on the dogs to let them "fight it out." Although muzzles might lower the chance of physical injury, the dogs are in a heightened state of emotional arousal and in a conflict that might not be resolved, resulting in more fighting later. Muzzling only the dominant dog is no solution either, because this can send unrealistic signals to the subordinate dog that it can confront the dominant dog.

The therapeutic approach involves first determining which dog is dominant. The owners may have to experiment by observing the dogs. Signs that one dog is considered to be the more dominant include getting to the food or a food treat first, moving out through the doorway first, gaining access closer to the owners for attention while keeping the other dog away, and gaining access to preferred resting or sleeping spots. In order to establish or reestablish the hierarchy between the dogs, the owners need to be in control. This helps eliminate contradictory signals that the owners give to their pets. The guidelines discussed in Chapter 8 under the treatment for dominance-related aggression toward people are useful. Aside from consistently communicating their social position, the owners also need to reduce the intensity of their greeting responses, so that both dogs are less excited about competing for the owner's attention. This is especially important after an owner's absence from the home. After responding to a command such as "sit," the dominant animal should be treated as the favored dog; it should receive all the respect and privileges that accrue the top dog. This includes receiving attention first and more frequently. During the course of the day the dominant dog should be fed first and when the dogs are taken for a walk, the dominant dog should be allowed outside first.

The subordinate may still try to push the dominant aside to obtain the owner's attention during greetings and at other times of lively interaction with the owners. The subordinate should then be admonished by sending it away, or in major social transgressions, isolated. If any growling occurs, whether by the dominant or subordinate, the subordinate should be verbally admonished ("bad dog") and sent away or removed to an isolation room for about 3–5 minutes, or until the isolated dog is calm. In short, the subordinate dog must learn that it has to respond to the dominant dog's signals when the owners are present just as it does when the owners are absent. Because the dogs get along when the owners are not around, they have obviously developed a way of socially interacting that works.

Favoring the dominant dog may be contradictory to humans' natural tendency to punish the aggressor. This is especially difficult when the subordinate is a favorite. All members of the family and friends should be reminded to support the dominant dog. Your advice may not be readily accepted, and this is why it is necessary to explain the theoretical basis of the recommendations and to suggest that the clients experiment for at least 2 weeks with the new plan. At the same time, ask the owners to exaggerate the differential treatment for the first week or two to impress the dogs, especially the subordinate, that things are now different. Emphasize that the exaggerated treatment is temporary, although the dominant dog will always have to be treated as such with some degree of favoritism.

Dominance-status aggression

Causes

- Dogs have an established hierarchy.
- Owners do not support dominant dog.

Resolution

- Avoid emotional or exuberant greetings.
- Support dominant dog.
- Reinforce owner control.

Aggression Without a Recognized Hierarchy

In this situation, fighting occurs between two dogs in the same household, but the fighting occurs in the owner's absence as much, or more frequently, than in his or her presence. Because fighting brings with it the possibility of injury to the dogs involved, the goal is to help establish and maintain a dominance relationship that keeps peace among dogs. This is best accomplished by orchestrating the owner's interactions to favor the dog destined to be dominant. As an aside it should be noted that in some instances where dogs seem to get along fine, neither dog may be clearly dominant. Therapeutic intervention is indicated where fighting is a serious problem and would be much less a problem if a clear dominant-subordinate relationship existed.

Typical History

Aggression without a recognized hierarchy is a problem that is most likely to occur when dogs, usually of the same sex, are matched in breed and/or size, with one dog not easily attaining dominance. The owners may make the problem worse by being reluctant to encourage one dog to become dominant and the other subordinate, or may suppress aggressiveness by which one dog is attempting to assert dominance.

Often, the dogs have been separated; most dog owners may not be aware of the tendency for dogs to become more aggressive the longer they are separated.

Diagnosis

The principal differential diagnoses are dominance-status aggression, where dogs fight only when the owners are present, and abnormal aggressiveness (covered later), where one dog continues to attack the other even in the presence of obvious and repeated submissive gestures on the part of the other dog. The history about whether the dogs fight only when alone should be sufficient to rule out dominance-status aggression. If the fighting appears to reflect abnormal aggressiveness, this may be evident when a concerted effort is made to institute a dominance hierarchy.

Treatment Guidelines

After reminding the owners to take precautions for their safety and that of the dogs, the clinician should help the owners determine which dog would be dominant if the two dogs were left to their own devices. As mentioned, body size is a major, but not totally reliable, indicator of which dog will be dominant. Other than size, seniority in the family plays an important role. Males are usually, but certainly not invariably, dominant over females, and dogs that are older are generally dominant over juveniles. Of course, eventually dogs reach the point where aging would be expected to weaken their position of dominance. In addition, the temperament of the dogs may play a role. One may have to form a tentative judgment as to which dog will be dominant and then carry on with the following recommendations; in the event that the problem gets worse within a prescribed short time and the predicted dominant dog does not live up to the plan, one should reverse the treatment before injury occurs.

Treatment is focused upon two aspects: having the owners gain or maintain social control of both dogs, and facilitating the establishment of one dog as dominant through treating it as the dominant dog with verbal and physical gestures to communicate to the subordinate its secondary position. Although fighting is still a possibility, the dogs should be allowed to interact when owners are able to keep a close eye on them. The owners should be advised on procedures for safely separating

---

AGGRESSION WITHOUT A HIERARCHY

Causes

- No established hierarchy
- Owners treat dogs equally
- Breed and gender predispositions

Resolution

- Supervise reintroduction.
- Establish one dog as dominant.
- Castrate one or both dogs.

fighting dogs and given safety recommendations regarding the use of head halters, drag lines, and muzzles. If there is any danger of fighting, the dogs should be fitted with basket muzzles. For severe situations, it may be necessary initially to allow the dogs to interact through a fence set up between two rooms. If there is danger of the dogs fighting when people are gone from the home, the dogs should be kept separate.

When using muzzles it is important not to communicate that the muzzle is punishment. Associate the muzzles with food treats given whenever the muzzles are put on. Muzzles should be put on and taken off frequently so the dog cannot predict why a muzzle is being put on. One does not want the placement of a muzzle to be associated only with aggressive encounters. Theoretically, one could just fit the subordinate with a muzzle so it cannot fight back. However, this procedure assumes that the designated subordinate would not provoke the designated dominant dog into fighting, and this might not be the case. Although these behavioral approaches might seem relatively severe to a client, especially if the subordinate dog is a favorite of the family, you can stress that this exaggerated differential treatment is temporary.

In addition to interacting with the dogs to communicate the roles of dominant and subordinate, some physiological means may help tip the balance. If both dogs are gonadally intact males, one may reduce the fighting tendencies of the designated subordinate by castrating him. This procedure also brings about changes in urine smell and possibly other body odors, which can change the stimulus characteristics of the subordinate and possibly reduce the interest of the dominant in being overtly aggressive. Castration of both dogs to reduce fighting tendencies should be attempted if castration of just the subordinate does not work after about 1 month has elapsed. As shown in Figure 9-1, castration can be expected to reduce the severity of this problem markedly in male dogs in about one-quarter of the cases. The use of antianxiety medication should not be expected to be a major help in resolving this problem.

Aggression Toward Strange Dogs

After some mutual investigation and posturing, most dogs away from the home are either indifferent to or interact with other dogs in an amicable way. This is the pattern observed repeatedly in off-leash dog parks, although interactions undoubtedly involve a history of past social interactions. The problem arises in a few dogs that react to strange dogs by fighting; such dogs, of course, should not be taken to off-leash parks. Several factors mentioned in the introduction may contribute to this aggressiveness. These include breed, gender, individual genetic makeup, hormonal status, and degree of early socialization, with fear playing a role in some cases.[3] Although rare, one should not overlook the fact that some lines of dogs have been selectively bred for fighting with other dogs, showing neither submissive gestures when clearly overpowered, nor responding to signs of submissiveness in the other dog. Even among relatively nonaggressive breeds, one may occasionally see abnormal aggressiveness as a reflection of genetic diversity.

Typical History

Aggression toward strange dogs is often directed toward members of the same gender—that is, males toward males and females toward females—although fighting can occur irrespective of the gender of the opponent. As mentioned, interdog fighting is most often a problem in males. There are breed predispositions as well, which are discussed in the introduction to this chapter. A contributing factor is the degree of socialization of dogs to other dogs as puppies, where signals and signs of dominance, submissiveness, or nonaggression are refined. With only limited early exposure to other dogs, social signals might not be perceived or given in a normal fashion and a fight might start with no apparent provocation.

Diagnosis

Some diagnostic possibilities are insufficient early socialization, fear-related aggression toward dogs, male-typical aggressiveness, breed-related aggressiveness, aggressive protection of the owner, and predatory aggression, usually expressed toward small dogs by large dogs. Away from the home, such as at a dog park, interdog aggression could reflect territorial aggression if the dog has visited the area so frequently that the park has become part of its "territory." A sign that one is possibly dealing with a genetic predisposition for fighting may be the complaint that the dog being attacked shows obvious submissive signs even to the point of lying immobilized on his back, and, were it not for the owners pulling off the attacking dog, it is clear that the subordinate would be severely injured or killed. Along with a genetic predisoposition, such behavior may also reflect inadequate socialization.

Treatment Guidelines

Because one is dealing with unknown dog owners and dogs, clients should be reminded about safety of the people and dogs involved. The following approaches may apply to just some dogs; the options are not mutually exclusive and may be used together. Most important is that the owners have physical control when taking their dog on walks in public. In order to help prevent contact from other dogs that might not be leashed, the owner can carry a repellant such as a remote citronella spray (Direct Stop®) to help stop the advancement of the other dog. The owner also should walk the dog during the least busy times on pathways not frequented by many dogs.

With gonadally intact males, castration may remove much of the tendency to fight other males. Currently, available data reveal that approximately 10% of dogs castrated for aggression toward unfamiliar dogs will undergo a virtual resolution, with a higher percentage showing at least some improvement (Fig. 9-1). Castration influences both by lowering the motivation of the problem dog to engage in aggressive behavior and by removing the stimulus odors associated with androgen secretion, making the castrated dog a less interesting target for other dogs to attack.

Regardless of gender and hormonal status, a program of desensitization and counterconditioning is indicated. Staged sessions or encounters should be planned, where a friend brings another dog within view of the problem dog but at a distance great enough so as not to evoke aggressive emotions. One must determine the critical distance where no sign of aggression is evoked. The problem dog is commanded to sit, and its attention is directed to the cooperating dog. It is recommended that a head halter be used with the problem dog during these exercises (Chapter 3). As the problem dog obeys the command to sit in the presence of the other dog, it is given a food treat and praise. The cooperating dog is taken out of view and returned within view again for a second trial. About 10 such desensitization trials would comprise a session. The counterconditioning with food upon exposure to other dogs gradually builds up the positive stimulus value of the cooperating (strange) dog. During subsequent sessions (daily if possible), the friend's dog is brought closer and closer to the problem dog as desensitization continues. When the dog can appropriately interact with the friend's dog, another cooperating dog is introduced at a "safe" distance, and the process repeated. It is important that the problem dog not be exposed to strange dogs up close aside from the desensitization program.

Case Study: Aggression Toward Strange Dogs

History

Willie, a healthy 2-year-old male castrated Malamute cross, was presented for aggression toward other dogs. The owners, a young couple with a 5-year-old daughter, adopted Willie at 1 year of age from the local shelter. They took him to many obedience classes, using positive reinforcement training, and he obeyed commands well. However, Willie played very roughly with other dogs at the dog park. When the other dog would roll over or show other signs of submission, Willie would continue to interact with the dog. If the other dog growled at him, he would sometimes back away; but at other times he continued to interact. Three weeks prior to the appointment Willie had gotten into a fight at the off-leash dog park, causing injuries to the other dog that required medical attention. Recently, he has begun reacting on-leash to large dogs while on walks; his body language is that of leaning toward the other dog and barking when they are about 20 feet away.

Diagnosis

Aggression toward strange dogs

Treatment

1.   Find other ways of exercising Willie other than off-leash dog parks.
2.   Reinforce control over Willie by frequently giving commands and rewarding obedience.
3.   Fit Willie with a head collar so that he can more easily be controlled on walks.
4.   Carry a canister of citronella spray to break up dog fights, should they occur.
5.   When other dogs approach while Willie is on-leash, divert his attention and give a command that conflicts with pulling toward dogs.
6.   Use a systematic desensitization and counterconditioning program for gradual exposure to other dogs, starting with small dogs and working up to large dogs.

Progress Report

At 4 weeks, Willie showed improvement on walks, especially with the use of a head collar. By 8 weeks after the appointment, the owners had started the desensitization and counterconditioning program to other dogs on walks. He had lunged at only two other dogs since starting the program. These times the owners were able to direct his attention easily.

Aggression toward dogs away from home
Causes
• May relate to protection of owner or territory • Inadequate socialization to other dogs • Breed and gender predispositions
Resolution
• Follow safety guidelines. • Avoid unplanned exposures to dogs. • Castrate males. • Implement desensitization and counterconditioning. • Use social punishment with staged exposure to dogs.

Social punishment may be useful where a dog is aggressive to strange dogs it meets on a walk or on other outings. Assuming that walks are very enjoyable, and early termination of the walk aversive, the procedure involves staged outings with a cooperating dog owner where the problem dog meets a strange dog very early in the outing and where growls or threats are expected to occur. The problem dog is to be "punished" by immediate termination of the outing. An acoustic low-pitched bridging stimulus, such as a duck call or kazoo—one that has a unique sound—should be used to associate termination of the walk with the aggressive behavior (Chapter 3). With repeated staged sessions, the dog should eventually associate the onset of its aggression with the sound of the bridging stimulus and subsequent abrupt termination of the outing. Remember not to use direct punishment techniques because these can increase the aggression displayed or can cause the dog to become fearful (or more fearful, if its aggression is based in fear). Future outings should be arranged where it is known the dog will not meet other dogs during the outing and, thus, no aggressive behavior will be evoked and the outing can then continue uninterrupted. The dog should eventually learn that outings in which it shows no aggression allow the walk to continue whereas walks in which aggression occurs are abruptly terminated; the dog's behavior should change accordingly.

Predatory Aggression Toward Small Dogs

In the traditional animal behavior literature, predation is generally not considered a type of aggression because it is not exhibited toward conspecifics. It generally has a behavioral topography different from intraspecific aggression, which is usually preceded by growls, threats, and posturing. In predatory aggression, stalking and attacks are carried out with virtually no warning or internal emotional arousal; warnings or threats prior to a predatory attack would generally be counterproductive to capturing the prey. If a large dog has predatory tendencies to attack small prey, predatory attacks on small dogs could also be a reflection of predatory aggression where apparently the dog does not recognize small dogs as conspecifics.

Typical History

The history often reveals that the problem dog attacks very small dogs without warning and presumably without showing that it recognizes the small dog as a dog. It is common for such dogs also to be known for killing or attacking cats. The tendency may be developmental if in early socialization they were not exposed to a variety of dogs of varying body size. The problem dog is typically well behaved in other ways.

Diagnosis

The main differential diagnosis is aggression toward strange dogs away from home (covered in a previous section). The key elements in the history to distinguish predatory aggression are that the dog attacks only small dogs and does not display this specific type of behavior toward larger dogs. However, it can concurrently display fear-related or territorial aggression toward larger dogs.

Treatment Guidelines

Taking into account the necessity of providing safety for the small dogs in the therapeutic approaches, there are two procedures that illustrate different types of behavior modification. In the first approach the goal is to induce the problem dog to like small dogs by desensitization and counterconditioning. In the second approach the object is to produce a lasting aversion to small dogs with a remote punishment technique. The latter approach should be used only if the first approach has been tried and is unsucessful.

The desensitization and countercondition approach is implemented by repeated, staged exposures to small dogs, perhaps using dogs of friends. The procedure is the same as that outlined for strange dogs in the previous section. One may be able to induce a type of desensitization to the point where the tendency to attack small dogs is reduced and the problem dog comes to recognize them as conspecifics.

Remote punishment is used in instances where the problem dog's existence in the family is threatened, a rapid resolution is required, and desensitization and counterconditioning have not worked. A remotely triggered citronella spray collar may be used to create an aversion to small dogs (Chapter 3). The training sessions should be staged with the cooperation of a friend who has a small dog that would

---

Predatory aggression

Causes
- Small dogs attacked as prey
- Inadequate socialization to smaller dogs

Resolution
- Follow safety guidelines.
- Implement habituation and counterconditioning.
- Implement aversion conditioning using remote punishment.

be a potential target. To be certain that the problem dog does not actually cause any injury to the small dog, the problem dog could be fitted with a basket muzzle and then exposed to the "prey."

The citronella should be remotely triggered as soon as the dog makes a direct predatory-like orientation toward the small dog. If the punishment collar works and the dog is diverted from its attack or orientation toward the small dog, one should stage additional progressive sessions. As with any remote punishment, the principles of immediacy, consistency, and target connectivity should be followed. Irrespective of the outcome the problem dog will have to be watched indefinitely for signs of predatory behavior, and all necessary precautions should be taken around small dogs.

References

1. Hart BL, Hart LA. The Perfect Puppy: How to Choose Your Dog by Its Behavior. New York: W.H. Freeman and Co., 1988.
2. Neilson JC, Eckstein RA, Hart BL. Effects of castration on behavior of male dogs with reference to the role of age and experience. Journal of the American Veterinary Association 1997;211:180–182.
3. Rugbjerg H, Proschowsky HF, Ersboll AK, Lund JD. Risk factors associated with inter-dog aggression and shooting phobias among purebred dogs in Denmark. Preventative Veterinary Medicine 2003;58:85–100.

Chapter 10
Anxieties and Fears

In nature, fears of strange noises and strange animals are adaptive responses because such noises and animals, at least in an evolutionary sense, are sometimes
associated with increased risk of injury or death. Similarly, anxiety or even panic at
the prospect of being abandoned by group members is an adaptive response
because being abandoned, even if not permanently, can be dangerous. It is equally
important that in nature animals habituate to these same fear- or anxiety-provoking
situations if they are repeatedly experienced and not followed by pain or injury. If
habituation to fear-evoking repetitive, but harmless, stimuli did not occur, the animal would be continuously fearful or anxious and unable to survive.

Transferring these concepts from nature to the home environment, we can expect
dogs, and all animals for that matter, to be initially fearful of most novel stimuli,
especially if the stimuli are intense or loud. After repeatedly experiencing the stimuli, dogs, especially puppies, usually habituate, and the fear or anxiety reactions are
eliminated or markedly reduced. Consequently, most dogs may be initially very
fearful of thunderstorms but will eventually show only mild reactions in the presence of thunderstorms.

The same principle of anxiety arousal and subsequent habituation applies to
being left alone. The initial response to being left alone ("abandoned") is one of
fear or strong anxiety, commonly referred to as *separation anxiety* or *separation
distress*. After a puppy is repeatedly left alone and no harm befalls it, the severe
emotional reaction subsides. Most of the habituation to noise stimuli and separation
occurs early in an animal's life unnoticed by the owners. Hence dogs grow up
habituated to vacuum cleaners, children's toys, power tools, lawn mowers, and
automobile rides. Puppies habituate much more easily to strange stimuli and situations than older animals, perhaps because they have not acquired a history of
adverse emotional reactions to such stimuli or situations.

A cardinal rule of the process of habituation is that threatening stimuli, such as
gunshots or firecrackers, are habituated only when repeatedly experienced and no
harm follows. That is, habituation is an active process requiring exposure to the
implicated stimulus; habituation will not occur passively, as happens when a
response is forgotten. Good gun-dog trainers recognize the importance of habituating their dogs to gunshots at a very early age, and training pistols with blank cartridges are a standard item in sporting dog catalogues. The two basic approaches to
habituation are flooding and desensitization, which are covered later in this chapter.

Behavior problems involving excessive anxieties and fears in dogs basically stem from four causes. One cause, as implied earlier, is the absence of prior habituation to the fear-evoking stimulus in the animal's background, especially as a puppy. As adults, the fears may be enhanced because the emotional reaction itself is a source of aversive internal or visceral sensations, which can "prove" to the dog that the fear-inducing stimulus is followed by adverse consequences. Problems involving fear are common in adult dogs, and the reaction may have progressed to the point where the dog may panic and be destructive in attempting to escape from the frightening stimulus or situation. A second cause of extreme or excessive fear stems from the response of the owner. Anxieties and fear reactions can be enhanced by the owners if they provide reinforcement in the form of comfort to the dog when it acts fearful. Thus, a dog that has a fear reaction to thunder and lightning might receive a great deal of comfort and affection intended by the owners to soothe the dog but which actually enhances the fear reaction through the positive reinforcement. Separation anxiety may be enhanced by the owners lavishing affection on a dog just before leaving and increasing the contrast between their presence and absence.

The third cause of excessive fear reactions is that which is acquired through adverse experiences. Being shot with a gun, for instance, is obvious cause for a classically conditioned fear of the gunshot sound associated with the painful experience. Physical abuse may result in a classically conditioned acquired fear of the subgroup of people associated with the mistreatment. Thus, a dog may develop a fear of someone who is innocent but shares physical characteristics with the person that historically had abused the dog. Whereas innate fears are resolved by habituating the innate response, acquired fears are resolved by extinction of the classically conditioned fear response. The term *desensitization* is applied to both processes.

The fourth cause of excessive fear and anxiety reflects a physiological (or organic) basis and is due to an abnormally low behavioral threshold or an abnormally intense reaction to fear- or anxiety-evoking situations. There can be a genetic link to these fear reactions. One example is of a colony of pointers bred specifically to be abnormally fearful, even when adequate attempts are made to socialize them.[1] The problem dog responds in a much more extreme fashion to stimuli or situations than do normal dogs. The use of desensitization exercises, which can usually resolve fears or anxieties, might not work, and such abnormal fears might require long-term anxiolytic drug intervention.

Clinical cases commonly involve several of these processes. Also frequently found are cases where more than one type of anxiety or fear reaction is present. Some attention to conventional terminology, derived from human concepts, is in order. *Anxiety* is an emotional reaction often described as general uneasiness connoting a rather vague reaction. *Fears* are emotional reactions related to specific objects, such as gunshots or children. Fears of objects or situations, which are cognitively understood to be way out of proportion to the actual danger, are referred to as *phobias*. The trouble with applying the term *phobia* to animals is that people can understand, through verbal and written messages, that there is actually little or no danger associated with a certain stimulus or situation, but the reaction is still far beyond that which is reasonable. Because animals do not participate in verbal communications with people, the use of terms like *phobia* or *panic reaction* for extreme reactions in animals do not necessarily refer to comparable reactions in people. Nonetheless, the terms *phobia* and *panic* do convey a sense of extreme reaction in animals and are often used.

General Approaches to Resolution of Fear Reactions

The treatments for fear and anxiety reactions, whether innate (and unhabituated) or acquired and whether a result of separation, inanimate stimuli, or people, are conceptually the same and involve desensitization of the unwanted emotional reaction and counterconditioning of a new, desirable, emotional response. In most instances, the parameters of the fear-evoking stimuli must be precisely identified to be able to treat the problem most effectively. Because the experiences and responses of each problem animal are unique, the treatment program must be specifically designed for each animal.

Flooding

Flooding involves presenting a fear-evoking stimulus at full intensity for a prolonged time or repeatedly. Under some conditions, most notably in puppies and sometimes with animals receiving anxiolytic drugs, flooding results in habituation of the fear or anxiety reaction. In adult animals, or animals with a severe emotional reaction, flooding can make the fear response worse because the physiological reaction evoked by the flooding stimulus is aversive.

Systematic Desensitization

Systematic desensitization involves gradual exposure in an incremental fashion to the stimulus over several sessions of staged trials, starting at a very low intensity level that evokes little or no reaction. The starting level is referred to as the *safe level*. Thus, systematic desensitization differs from flooding because the intensity of the stimulus used to produce desensitization is markedly reduced; the intensity of the reaction evoked is commensurately reduced as well, ideally to an imperceptible level. The animal is desensitized by repeatedly presenting the stimulus at this level and then gradually increasing the intensity of the stimulus through controlled exposures. As mentioned, desensitization for habituation of an innate response or for extinction of a classically conditioned response is the same, requiring stimulus exposure along an intensity gradient.

The intensity gradient may be a function of stimulus duration, stimulus intensity (volume), or stimulus proximity. Finding a way of presenting the stimulus in a gradient fashion can be a major task, and various techniques are discussed later in this chapter under specific problems. For example, one stimulus exposure gradient for separation anxiety is duration of the separation, whereas the gradient for fear of certain classes of people (e.g., children) can be proximity to the fear-evoking people, as well as their movement. The gradient for fear of noises is usually stimulus volume.

Counterconditioning

The most successfully designed programs to resolve fear or anxiety involve pairing something rewarding, such as a favored food treat and affection, with the presentation of graded levels of exposure to the implicated stimulus. These reinforcements produce a favorable or positive internal emotional state that is incompatible with the negative emotional reaction associated with the fear. As long as the aversive stimulus is presented at a level that arouses little or no fear or anxiety, the positive emotional state produced by treats and affection predominates. Thus, desensitization and counterconditioning occur simultaneously. In explaining to clients the processes of desensitization and counterconditioning, the client might be told to think of the sessions as teaching the dog to "enjoy" the aversive stimulus or events. The concepts of systematic desensitization and counterconditioning are explained in more detail in Chapter 3.

Anxiolytic Drugs

Under some conditions, serotonergic drugs or, to a lesser extent, benzodiazepines, which reduce anxieties or fears, may be advantageous for treating fear of loud noises and separation-related anxieties. Although the animal is on drug treatment, stimulus exposure under systematic desensitization and counterconditioning sessions should be conducted regularly. When it is evident that desensitization is occurring, the drug dosage could then be gradually reduced by 25% per week while the animal continues to experience the behavior modification. After the animal is off the drug, it should continue to experience the stimulus. In fact, the intensity of the stimulus can be gradually increased to continue the process of desensitization without drug facilitation.

Separation Anxiety

Dogs, like people, are social animals that naturally experience stress or anxiety when abandoned by companions.[2] Separation anxiety typically first occurs in puppies when they are brought to a new home. When a puppy is left alone, separation distress is seen as continuous loud crying and yelping during the night. Typically, puppies habituate to being left alone at night, although there is a gentle way of habituating them to being left alone (see Chapter 20 on raising puppies).

The separation anxiety that comprises a major problem occurs in older dogs. The growing popularity of doggy day-care centers, where people drop off their dog on the way to work, owe much of their success to the phenomenon of separation anxiety, as well as to the strength of the human-animal bond. Separation anxiety in children may be reduced when we tell them we will be back in a few hours. We cannot explain this to a dog (although we may use the language). When separation anxiety does not occur, it is tempting to say the dog "learned" we will return. A more accurate view is that a dog that does not experience separation anxiety when left alone is habituated to separation as a function of experiencing many departures. In other words, it is the unconscious habituation of emotional responses, through experiencing many departures, that eliminates anxiety, not a cognitive process of a dog "understanding" we will return. When this subtle difference is understood, the prevention of, or resolution of, separation anxiety is more apparent. Both prevention and resolution require repeated exposures to separation, rather than attempting to communicate to the dog to understand we will return or rewarding the dog when we return.

Exposing a dog to repeated separations, starting with short departures that do not upset it and progressively increasing to longer separations, is the standard way of desensitizing a dog's anxiety reaction to separation. Later, by pairing departures with food treats, the departures should take on the positive aspects generated by the treats through counterconditioning. Special treats should be reserved only for departures. The use of videotaping while the owners are gone, both to diagnose the problem and monitor progress, is an important technological advance in dealing with this problem. Although separation anxiety can usually be successfully treated without medication,[2] anxiolytic drugs are now commonly used to treat the problem behavior. Another way of managing separation anxiety is simply to avoid leaving the dog alone.

Typical History

Separation anxiety is usually manifested by the occurrence of several types of misbehavior, which commonly include one or more of the following: chewing furniture, woodwork, or other non-toy items; excessive vocalization; escape behavior; defecating and/or urinating in the house (the dog is otherwise well house-trained); panting and drooling; pacing; and anorexia.[3] Body language often indicates that the dog is emotionally upset as the time of departure nears. Upon questioning, caregivers often reveal that the dog is given a good deal of predeparture affection as well as affection upon returning. The predeparture affection can be counterproductive because it enhances the contrast in the degree of social interaction the dog gets when the owner is home and away.

It is necessary to determine the critical period of time the dog must be alone before anxiety occurs. Videotaping the dog while alone will reveal how long the dog must be alone before it becomes overtly emotional, when the dog is most upset, the duration of the anxiety, and what types of separation-related behaviors occur.

Diagnosis

Although the primary signs of separation anxiety that cause owners to seek help— excessive vocalization, destructiveness, and house soiling—can stem from other causes, one or more of these signs displayed only when the caregivers are away is strongly suggestive of separation anxiety. Because the behavioral signs vary so much, the differential diagnoses vary according to specific signs. A breakthrough in the diagnosis of separation anxiety is the use of videotaping during the time of separation to rule out other causes of the signs. Destructiveness in the house may be unrelated to anxiety or emotional upset and could be due to boredom, playfulness, or even redirected aggression. House soiling may reflect a lack of house-training.

Excessive barking can stem from a number of causes, such as external stimulation from other dogs (Chapter 11), and should be considered in the differential. Non–separation-related barking is usually not contingent upon the owner being gone. It should be noted that more than one type of anxiety-related behaviors can occur at the same time.[4]

Treatment Guidelines

Although discussed separately, the following approaches are recommended to be used simultaneously. It should be mentioned that one study of separation anxiety showed a decrease in owner compliance with the treatment plan when too many instructions were given at one time.[5] Although this is a problem that can be resolved without drug intervention, there is some evidence that administration of an anxiolytic lessens the anxiety, allowing for more rapid, or at least more flexible, behavior modification approaches.[6]

Reducing attachment to owners

An important element in treatment is reducing the extreme attachment some dogs have to their owners by independence training. At a minimum, this could be instructing the dog to sit and walking to another room. For a more advanced stage of this phase, the owners should determine at what distance from them their dog is comfortable and not display any anxiety. At that distance the dog is asked to lay down on a "special" mat or throw rug and is given a special long-lasting food treat, such as a rubber ball stuffed with cheese or a knucklebone, which it gets no other time. This rewards the dog for becoming more independent. Over time the owners should be instructed to place the dog farther away from them while adding movement, such as moving around the kitchen cooking dinner, until the dog can easily be left in another room by itself with the door closed.

Eliminating predeparture and return affection

The owners must be counseled to ignore the dog for 10–20 minutes before leaving the house. They also must wait until the dog has relaxed when they come home before they interact with it. This helps decrease the emotionality associated with these events and reduces the contrast between when the dog is alone and when people are around.

Habituation to predeparture cues

The owners should desensitize their dog to departure cues. Prior to leaving the house, their dog picks up on cues that signal that the owners are getting ready to leave, which initiates anxiety. The owners need to make departure routines unpredictable so that the dog no longer escalates its anxiety level. Before they begin, they must identify situations where the dog begins to show signs of stress. Examples of common departure cues include picking up keys or a jacket, walking to the door, grabbing a purse or briefcase, or wearing certain clothes. The owners need to determine which cues are indicative of departure. After those cues are identified, they should begin the habituation process.

One example is habituating to the sound of keys. During the times that the dog is resting quietly, and when the owners have no intention of leaving soon, they should rattle their keys lightly, completely ignoring their dog, but still watching from the corner of their eye for signs of anxiety. The dog may be anxious at first and then should settle down quickly when it realizes that the owners are not leaving. After the dog quiets, the owners should wait another minute and repeat the process, and then repeat as often as possible so that the dog begins to ignore this trigger. Gradually owners can add other cues, such as standing up after rattling the keys. Again, they repeat this process until ignored and incrementally and gradually add different cues to their repertoire.

Systematic desensitization and counterconditioning

To start the desensitization of a dog to being left alone, the dog should be subjected to a series of separations that are shorter than the critical time for anxiety to occur, as determined by the history or videotaping. The short separations establish a pattern or "track record" so that future separations produce little emotional response. After a series of short separations, counterconditioning should begin by pairing long-lasting treats with the departures (e.g., knucklebone, dried pig ear, nylon bone with holes drilled and stuffed with cheese) or food treats "hidden" around the house or yard in an Easter egg hunt style. To utilize the hidden food technique, one can ask the dog to sit and stay while small food treats are placed around in a dozen or so locations. Then as one walks out the door, the signal "okay" can be given for the dog to start hunting for the hidden treats.

Counterconditioning departures as one walks out the door with food treats creates a positive emotional state to be associated with being left alone. One might say, "We are conditioning the dog to love it when we walk out the door." The departure treat is placed in front of the dog while the dog is required to sit. Just as one closes the door and walks out, the dog is told "okay" and allowed to take the treat. It is important that the treats be highly favored, and it is best if the dog gets no treats unless it is being left alone. If a dog shows no interest in the treat, this is an indication that the departures, even short ones, still produce anxiety and should be shorter. The counterconditioning will be successful as long as being left alone evokes little anxiety.

Procedures must be established for determining whether the dog remains calm when left alone. Again, videotaping is useful. As long as the dog readily goes for the food upon the owner's departure, it is probably not becoming very anxious. Assuming the desensitization and counterconditioning of separations are successful, the duration of separations can be gradually increased by steps, such as 30 seconds, 1 minute, 2 minutes, 5 minutes, 10 minutes, 15 minutes, 30 minutes, 45 minutes, 1 hour, 2 hours, etc., with several sessions of departure training at each step. The separations must be shortened if there is any sign of emotional distress. The use of a drug (see following section), if effective, should allow a more flexible departure training schedule. In fact, with anxiolytic treatment some desensitization to departures undoubtedly occurs automatically even if no prescribed departure program is followed. Nonetheless, counterconditioning departures with long-lasting treats are valuable in the resolution of this problem.

What to do for long unscheduled departures

For a strict desensitization program, the dog cannot be left alone for durations beyond the point achieved in the scheduled desensitization trials. If the owners work during the week and cannot conduct departure training on weekdays, this might mean that the owners should take the dog to work, leave it at a doggy daycare center or with friends, or hire a dog-sitter until the conditioning program is completed. Confining the dog to a kennel (crate) at home without human contact is likely to intensify the anxiety.

Anxiolytic drugs

The use of anxiolytic drugs for this syndrome will undoubtedly become more common because such drugs may reduce the labor-intensive and time-consuming departure training programs. Also, such drugs can allow the dog to be left alone during nonconditioning times if there is evidence that the dog is not overly anxious when left alone. An anxiolytic drug may lower separation anxiety to the point where desensitization to separation occurs automatically without a structured or graded departure program. The anxiolytic, clomipramine, combined with behavior modification, has been reported in one placebo-controlled, double-blind study to produce a faster reduction in signs of anxiety as compared to placebo, when combined with a modest behavior modification program.[6] Telephone follow-up with the dogs' owners 5–16 months after the trial revealed a high degree of variability in outcome, and no adverse effects from extended clomipramine treatment for up to 30 weeks of treatment.[7] Another placebo-controlled, double-blind study found no improvement in signs of separation anxiety, which could be attributed to treatment with clomipramine, although behavior modification, which was quite extensive, was highly effective in reducing the behavioral signs.[8]

While the dog is on the drug, the owners can still carry out the essentials of behavior modification, including cutting back on predeparture affection, pairing

---

SEPARATION ANXIETY

Causes

- Lack of prior habituation to absences
- Change in owner's work schedule
- Lavish affection prior to departures and upon return

Resolution

- Reduce predeparture and greeting affection.
- Avoid separations aside from program.
- Establish desensitization gradient for departures.
- Pair food treats with departure.
- Give antianxiety medication.

Case Study: Separation Anxiety

History

Tuffy, a healthy 7-year-old male castrated Springer Spaniel, was presented for a 4-month history of destruction in the house while the owners were gone. The owners both work full time and had moved to their present single-family home 8 months ago. Tuffy was previously allowed use of the dog door until he escaped the yard while the owners were gone, and the neighbor complained about his barking for hours when he was outside. Inside the house the neighbors could still hear his barking. Among the items destroyed in the house area were a Persian rug, the front door, a window, and some clothing. Tuffy does not engage in destructive behavior when any of the family members are home. However, when they are home, Tuffy consistently follows the owners around the house. In an attempt to control barking when they are gone Tuffy was fitted with a bark collar, which led to some decrease in the barking.

Diagnosis

Separation anxiety

Treatment

1.   Adapt Tuffy to separations in the home with trials of prolonged sit-stays while the owners walk to another room.
2.   Ignore Tuffy's attempts at seeking attention; instead reward him for nonclingy behavior.
3.   Systematically desensitize Tuffy to predeparture cues, such as car keys, by presenting them but not leaving.
4.   Practice departure sessions with graduated departures to desensitize Tuffy's separation anxiety systematically.
5.   Leave chew toys for Tuffy upon leaving.
6.   Give Tuffy the antianxiety medication, clomipramine, which was prescribed.

Progress Report

By 4 weeks, the owners had worked on desensitizing Tuffy to predeparture cues and had worked up to leaving him alone for 5 minutes, with no sign of anxiety. During the therapy program Tuffy was confined to the kitchen area. Eight weeks after the appointment he was able to be left alone in the house for 30 minutes with no barking and no destruction. Six months after the appointment the clomipramine medication was discontinued and Tuffy had no recurrence of signs.

---

departures with a highly desired food treat, and keeping initial departures as short as possible. With serotonergic drugs, such as clomipramine, it is to be expected that the animal may have to be on the drug for 4 or more weeks before full anxiolytic effects will occur. Videotaping the dog's behavior while left alone will provide information about the dog's emotional state when left alone and reveal the effectiveness of the drug. This is especially useful as one starts to phase the dog off the drug.

Fears of Inanimate Stimuli

This type of fear reaction may reflect an innate or an acquired fear reaction. Examples are fears of thunderstorms, bicycles, skateboards, gunshot noise, and loud appliances. Fear of thunderstorms is dealt with as a separate topic later in this chapter. Fear of firecrackers and gunshot noise is probably an innate response but, of course, gunshot fear might be enhanced if the dog is unfortunately hit with a bullet at the time the gun goes off. The strange vestibular stimulation and resultant nausea associated with automobile rides may lead to a fear response to automobile rides. Usually dogs are habituated to these stimuli if they frequently experience them as puppies. A common type of acquired fear is that provoked by the white lab coat worn by veterinarians. This stimulus is often paired with unpleasant or painful experiences, including restraint, palpation, and injections. Thus, fear of white coats tends to continue and become worse as each exposure is accompanied by an aversive experience, and the animal may generalize its fear to anything associated with a veterinary office. Many veterinarians find that taking off the white coat markedly reduces the fear. Some fears of inanimate objects can be avoided in dogs by programming desensitization sessions into the puppy raising (Chapter 20).

Typical History

Clients will usually present a dog with a fear response because they sense the dog is suffering or the fear reaction interferes with family activities. If fear-inducing stimuli can be avoided, dog owners typically will not seek assistance. Indeed, in some instances, it may not be worthwhile to treat a fear. If a fear reaction to fireworks is a problem only 1 day a year, using an anxiolytic at that time might be sufficient. If Fourth of July celebrations go on for weeks, or if a dog is regularly exposed to gunshot sounds from a nearby target range, desensitization may be necessary. The history exploration must be tailored to the specific fears: when, where, and how frequently? One should also obtain sufficient information so that a gradient of stimulus intensity may be arranged where the stimulus intensity ranges from almost nondetectable to fully intense. As part of the history exploration it is necessary to determine the degree to which the reaction may have been enhanced by comforting from the caregivers.

Diagnosis

One task is to determine the specific stimulus or set of stimuli that are related to the fear. Not uncommonly, fears are worse when human family members are away, unless the owners attempt to comfort the dog, thus increasing its reactions; one must be suspicious that the fear is complicated by separation anxiety requiring attention to both problems. In terms of diagnosis, it is nice to know whether one is dealing with an innate fear or an acquired fear (or an acquired enhancement of an innate fear). However, the systematic desensitization technique, coupled with counterconditioning, is the same for both innate and acquired fears.

Treatment Guidelines

The approach to desensitization of fears of inanimate objects or situations can be dealt with through the illustration of fear of gunshot noise. The general approach, that of establishing a gradient of stimulus intensity from weak to full, is the same for all fears of inanimate stimuli using either volume or distance gradient. If a sound recording is used for simulating gunshots, it must be tested to assure that, at its full intensity, the dog shows the problem behavior. The simplest and most effective technique for presenting a graded stimulus for desensitizing a dog to gunshots and firecrackers is to employ a starter pistol of the type used in track events or gun-dog training. The pistols have a solid barrel, fire .22 caliber blanks, and are relatively safe to use. One can even start with a small cap gun when using the gradient. To create a gradient, boxes, blankets and/or heavy towels can be piled over the pistol. Usually eight heavy layers of blankets is an appropriate starting level. The gun is fired from the innermost position. The muffling of the sound must be sufficient that the sound produces no aversive fear reaction.

Systematic desensitization-counterconditioning training sessions should be scheduled with six or seven shots fired during each session (the cylinder holds six or seven blanks). It is best if the sessions are scheduled for the same time each day and in the same place. Later, after desensitization is further along, the time and place should be varied. Starting with maximum muffling, each shot is paired with a food treat and affection (praise), with seven shots comprising one session. Subsequently, a blanket layer is removed every three or four sessions until eventually the unmuffled gun can be shot (human handler wearing ear protection) with relatively little fear response. If necessary, thin towels can be used to provide a finer gradient between blankets. The training session must be set back to a previous level if the dog shows an adverse reaction when some of the muffling is removed. This approach requires patience and consistent effort by the client.

Fear of Thunderstorms

Because most dogs have not been hit by a lightning bolt during a thunderstorm, the fear of thunder probably reflects an innate response, often perpetuated by owner interactions. The fear reaction is usually to a cluster of stimuli, including thunder, lightning, rain, and barometric changes. Fear of thunderstorms can be manifested in a reaction so extreme that dogs will throw themselves through screen doors or glass windows. With such extreme reactions it might be legitimate to refer to the behavior as a phobia or panic reaction.

Most dogs become habituated to these stimuli through repeated exposure, especially as puppies. People who are going to have dogs in locations where thunderstorms are common should see to it that the dogs are exposed, as puppies, to several storms even if the exposure must be intentional; this should result in early habituation to thunderstorms and prevent fear of thunderstorms as an adult. The habituation is facilitated by ignoring any fear reaction and praising calm behavior.

Typical History

Commonly, dogs presented with a thunderstorm fear become extremely anxious— shivering, vocalizing, pacing, running about wildly, and/or chewing up household items during storms. In the classic paper setting the stage for the use of behavior modification procedures for fear of noises in dogs, some dogs were reported to be so terror-stricken by thunder and lightning that they injured themselves in paniclike behavior, such as jumping through screen doors or windows.[9] The natural reaction of owners is to comfort dogs during a storm, and although this is understandable, the affection may reinforce and intensify the dog's fearful behavior.

Diagnosis

The problem behavior is usually easily diagnosed from the client's description of the events causing the problem behavior. The diagnostic task is to determine whether another problem is also involved. A common confounding problem is separation anxiety that may be occurring at the same time.[4] Employment of a videotaping system may reveal whether the behavior is more intense when the dog is alone. If so, separation anxiety may be involved and should be addressed as well. If the response is more intense in the owner's presence, comforting may play a very major role in enhancing the reaction.

Treatment Guidelines

The goal of therapy is to habituate the dog to thunderstorms through systematic desensitization and counterconditioning in scheduled or staged thunderstorm training sessions. The process begins with presentation of the sound of a thunderstorm at an intensity so low it evokes virtually no detectable response. This allows a positive emotional reaction to be produced by the counterconditioning food treats paired with the weak thunder presentation. The most feasible sound presentation system is for the owner to obtain a commercial recording of a thunderstorm, which is available on a number of sound effects recordings. Playing the thunder and storm track once at full, or nearly full, amplitude is needed to verify that the recording creates a fearful reaction. If it does not, one must locate another recording that elicits the fear response. The effective portion of the thunderstorm recording may then be transferred to an audiotape or CD for more convenient repeated use on a tape player for training sessions with several trials. It must be noted that it is difficult to re-create the full effect of a storm by recording alone because of the inability to modulate barometric pressure and the potential atmospheric electrical charge.

Training sessions should be routinely scheduled during the time of year when actual thunderstorms will not disrupt the training. Initially, one should conduct sessions at the same time each day and later vary the time of day. Of course, sessions have to be conducted where a sound system is available. For dogs that are fearful of firecrackers as well as thunderstorms (the stimuli have overlapping characteristics) one could begin desensitization as described earlier for gunshots.

Initially, the dog is taught to sit or lie down in a relaxed fashion for several minutes in the same room with the speakers. The recorded sound may be presented in either of two ways. One way is by turning the storm recording on at the measured "safe" volume for 5–10 seconds; affection and a food treat are paired with the turning on of the storm. The sound is turned off for a minute or two and affection is withdrawn. The sound is then turned on for another 5–10 seconds and again the treat and affection are paired with turning on the sound. This process is continued for about 10 on/off presentations.

The second way of presenting the stimulus is for the storm recording to run continuously for about 20 minutes and about every minute or so (especially after a thunderclap), the dog is given a food treat and affection. After a few sessions with either procedure, the dog should come to "enjoy" the sessions. As the training sessions progress, the owners should gradually increase the amplitude of the recording in measured steps. If the dog shows an obvious fear response, which may be indicated by shivering, panting, and/or a refusal to take a food treat, the training program is advancing too rapidly over the gradient, and the session should be terminated; no comfort is to be given, and the next day the owners should return to a previous safer amplitude. After the dog has had about 30–60 daily training sessions, with progressive increases in sound level to nearly full intensity, and with sessions conducted at different times of the day and at different locations, it may be ready for a more realistic thunderstorm simulation. For the most complete thunderstorm desensitization, a strobe light and water sprayed against the windows can be gradually and sequentially added. During the occurrence of natural thunderstorms, the owners should continue to pair food treats and affection with the storms, especially during thunderclaps and lightning flashes. If the dog is not desensitized by the time the thunderstorm season arrives, one can give a fast-acting anxiolytic, such as diazepam, during the storms.

For dogs that are extremely reactive to any stormlike stimuli, another approach to desensitization is to employ an anxiolytic on a continuous basis for 2 months or longer. One study showed a positive outcome for dogs with thunderstorm phobia using a combination of alprazolam and clomipramine. The owners were asked to fill out a weekly scale of how their dog reacted.[10] The desensitization may be achieved by playing the recording of storms for several hours each day. The sound level is set fairly low and over several days, the intensity gradually increased. The anxiolytic drug is then gradually tapered off. This approach may be used to start a systematic desensitization program that is later continued as in the sessions described earlier.

Fear of Children and Other People

It is natural for young dogs to be fearful of strange people as they would be fearful of strange conspecifics in a wolf pack. However, in the normal growing-up process, most puppies are repeatedly exposed to members of various human subgroups (men, women, children, teenagers) and habituate to them. Problems with fear of certain subgroups can reflect a lack of early social contact with these subgroups, most typically children. In addition, adverse experiences with certain groups of people (e.g., men) can produce an acquired fear of those types of people. Children can be unpredictable in their movement and actions, sometimes causing pain to dogs, whether intentional or not. The barking and growling at uniformed mail delivery people probably does not reflect fear, but rather a territorial behavior that is exacerbated by the repetitious visits to the door by such intruders and the dog's "success" in chasing away these intruders. The treatment approach, systematic desensitization and counterconditioning, is used to eliminate the fear reaction and replace it with a positive response to the previous fear-evoking stimulus. In one interesting case, a dog adopted as an adult became extremely fearful when the owner wore a motorcycle outfit, which included leather jacket, helmet, and boots. Apparently, either through poor socialization of the dog to this unusual outfit or through an experience of mistreatment, the dog had acquired an intense fear of people dressed in classical motorcycle-rider attire. The owner of this dog desensitized the response to this fear by enlisting friends to wear only the jacket or helmet at first and adding other parts of the attire as systematic desensitization continued.

Occasionally, a dog is presented for consultation who has been exposed to only a few people, and the fear is to all people in general except for the immediate family. This problem may arise with dogs raised among many other dogs, but in which contact with people is limited. Fear of people may involve an aggressive component, commonly fear-related aggression; this topic is covered in Chapter 8. As with other fears or anxieties, fear of children and strange adults may be avoided by programming exposure sessions into puppy raising (Chapter 20).

Typical History

In most instances of fear of children the dog simply has had little exposure to children as a puppy. It is important to learn about the boundaries of the stimulus that create the problem and how these might be manipulated along a gradient. Sometimes fear of children involves excessive arm and hand movements, so a gradient can involve degrees of arm waving as well.

Diagnosis

Although useful for complete understanding of the case, a determination of whether a dog was frightened by an adverse experience with a person is not essential to developing a treatment plan. If the fear reaction involves aggressive elements (growling, snapping), one must differentiate fear-related aggression from territorial and dominance-related aggression. There may be a combination of types of aggression, especially with territorial and fear-related aggression.

Treatment Guidelines

Because the desensitization process involves the use of adults or children, one must keep in mind the safety of the cooperating people. A head halter should be used to gain better control. A basket muzzle should be used as appropriate. Two common gradients that are involved in the desensitization of the dog's fear of people are the degree of similarity of the training stimulus to the fear-evoking stimulus and the distance between the training person and the problem dog. When the distance gradient is used, the dog is initially exposed to a fear-evoking person at its "safe" distance, which is far enough away so as to not evoke a reaction. In training sessions, the dog should be repeatedly exposed to a fear-evoking person coming into the area, at the prescribed distance. Treats and affection are paired with the appearance of the person to countercondition the dog to the fear-evoking stimulus. The person then retreats to a position out of sight, comes back in the area a few moments later, and advances to the same prescribed distance; the dog is again given a small food treat in the stranger's presence. The use of affection for counterconditioning is most effective if the owners deprive the dog of affection for some time prior to the training sessions.

As many as 10 such approach trials could be included in one session. Over several sessions, the stimulus person should be exposed to the dog at progressively closer distances. In later sessions, the dog should receive affection and a treat from the stimulus person, who walks toward the dog when deemed safe for the person and for the dog, so that it is not overly fearful. The dog's behavior becomes the guide as to how rapidly owners can progress through the distance gradient in the training sessions. When the desensitization process is under way, the dog's natural inclination toward social interaction may take over. As in resolving all fear reactions, forcing a dog to approach the fear-inducing stimulus or forcing it to stay in one place for the approaching person is counterproductive. Sometimes a dog's fear of people can be so extreme that it is difficult to find a satisfactory starting distance for exposure. An anxiolytic drug may be useful in these situations. Systematic desensitization and counterconditioning training sessions can be established, and while desensitization is occurring, the drug can be gradually withdrawn. Caution must be taken in the use of an anxiolytic in the treatment of fear of people, especially children. In such instances partial reduction of fear might enhance the snapping tendency.

Fear of Other Dogs

Although less common than fear of certain people, fear of other dogs may be a problem for owners who want their dog to interact socially with other dogs. The fear may be manifested as extreme timidity or easily triggered defensive aggressiveness to other dogs.

Typical History

The history of dogs that are excessively fearful of other dogs often reveals that the dog as a puppy was isolated from other dogs during the primary socialization time. It might also have had one or two aversive interactions with another dog during this time. By the time clients bring a fearful dog into the clinic, they can usually identify those situations that will elicit a fear response. Questions can then clarify the particular circumstances (time, place, frequency, range of stimuli) in which the fear is manifested. The presenting complaint may be that the dog seems to avoid (or wants to avoid) contact with other dogs; but when pressed, even by a friendly dog, the problem dog will growl and snap when approached by the other dog. In other instances, the problem dog does all it can to remove itself from the presence of other dogs, avoiding interaction of any type.

Diagnosis

The main differential diagnostic consideration is when the fear response is manifested in aggression. Intermale aggression and offensive aggression toward strange dogs should be ruled out, primarily on the basis of triggering stimuli and absence of a fear component. As with other fear reactions, this problem may occur in conjunction with the other forms of aggression.

Treatment Guidelines

There is no easy way to correct a dog's fear of other dogs, especially when the behavior stems from early experience. If the dog is forced into close contact with other dogs, the problem behavior will become intensified as the social interactions result in unpleasant experiences. The indicated approach is habituation through the process of systematic desensitization to other dogs, using a head halter for better control. An attempt should be made to determine a gradient based on the type of dog-related stimulus to which the problem dog reacts. Counterconditioning the response to other dogs is also useful. Typically one would pair affection and food treats with the repeated appearance of other dogs in staged encounters. Because the owner needs the cooperation of other dog owners in the area, solving this behavioral problem could be complicated. If the owner solicits the cooperation of other dog owners who can keep their dogs under control, the problem dog can be exposed to other dogs over a gradient of distance starting with a "safe" distance.

References

1. Murphree OD, Angel C, DeLuca DC, Newton JE. Links to longitudinal studies of genetically nervous dogs. Biological Psychiatry 1977;12:573–576.
2. Schwartz S. Separation anxiety syndrome in dogs and cats. Journal of the American Veterinary Medical Association 2003;222:1526–1532.
3. Flannigan G, Dodman NH. Risk factors and behaviors associated with separation anxiety in dogs. Journal of the American Veterinary Medical Association 2001;219:460–466.
4. Overall KL, Dunham AE, Frank D. Frequency of nonspecific clinical signs in dogs with separation anxiety, thunderstorm phobia, and noise phobia, alone or in combination. Journal of the American Veterinary Medical Association 2001;219:467–473.
5. Takeuchi Y, Houpt KA, Scarlett JM. Evaluation of treatments for separation anxiety in dogs. Journal of the American Veterinary Medical Association 2000;217:342–345.
6. King JN, Simpson BS, Overall KL, Appleby D, Pageat P, Ros C, Chaurand JP, Heath S, Beata C, Weiss AB, Muller G, Paris T, Bataille BG, Parker J, Petit S, Wren J. The CLOCSA (Clomipramine in Canine Separation Anxiety) Study Group: Treatment of separation anxiety in dogs with clomipramine: Results from a prospective, randomized, double-blind, placebo-controlled, parallel-group, multicenter clinical trial. Applied Animal Behaviour Science 2000;67:255–275.
7. King JN, Overall KL, Appleby D, Simpson BS, Beata C, Chaurand CJP, Heath SE, Ross C, Weiss AB, Muller G, Bataille BG, Paris T, Pageat P, Brovedani F, Garden C, Petit S. Results of a follow-up investigation to a clinical trial testing the efficacy of

clomipramine in the treatment of separation anxiety in dogs. Applied Animal Behaviour Science 2004;89:233–242.

8. Podberscek AL, Hsu Y, Serpell JA. Evaluation of clomipramine as a adjunct to behavioural therapy in the treatment of separation-related problems in dogs. The Veterinary Record 1999;145:365–369.

9. Tuber DS, Hothersall D, Voith VL. Animal clinical psychology: A modest proposal. American Psychology 1974;29:762–766.

10. Crowell-Davis SL, Seibert LM, Sung W, Parthasarathy V, Curtis TM. Use of clomipramine, alprazolam, and behavior modification for treatment of storm phobia in dogs. Journal of the American Veterinary Medical Association 2003;222:744–748.

Chapter 11
Barking: Normal and Excessive

Barking is a normal behavior of dogs, a behavior for which dogs are highly prized and appreciated when they perform the important function of warning family members of intruders. In addition to this natural or instinctive behavior, dogs have been trained to bark on command for treats, and have been bred for barking at foxes, as used historically in the classical hunts of Europe and North America. It is the same behavior that is desirable in some contexts that creates a problem for dog owners in another context. Excessive barking becomes an acute problem when owners are confronted with the option of having to resolve, or markedly reduce, excessive barking due to neighbor complaints. Some cities have ordinances that allow a certain amount of barking but impose penalties on owners when the neighbors complain of barking, especially beyond the prescribed limit. Although problem barking can become threatening to a dog's continued existence in the family, it is one of the more difficult problem behaviors to resolve. Objectionable barking may be viewed as a primary problem and treated directly, or secondary to another behavior problem, such as separation anxiety or fear of loud noises.

There are two aspects to breed differences in barking tendency. Barking at mail delivery people withstanding, the most valued type of vocalization is watchdog barking, especially when dogs are otherwise relatively quiet. Examples of the most reliable breeds for watchdog barking are the German Shepherd, Rottweiler, Miniature Schnauzer, Doberman Pinscher, Scottish Terrier, Pomeranean, Australian Shepherd, and Chihuahua.[1] The other type of barking for which there are clear breed predispositions is for excessive barking. Among breeds considered the worst in such objectionable barking are the Miniature Schnauzer, Chihuahua, Pomeranian, and the terrier breeds.[1] Although there is some overlap of breeds that rank high on both types of barking, it is possible to find breeds that excel at watchdog barking without being high on excessive barking. The German Shepherd, Australian Shepherd and Doberman Pinscher are examples.

Barking is commonly enhanced by the owners, allowing the dog in the house when it barks a lot. The owners may, in fact, have shaped behavior to the most intense and frequent type of barking if they let the dog in only when the barking reaches a very intense level. Social facilitation may lead to excessive barking when another dog sees or hears a neighboring dog bark, whether or not there is visual contact. Somewhat related to social facilitation is barking as part of play. Such barking may occur with dogs barking through a common fence with a neighboring dog much as the two might bark in an open field together. Barking could be a component of territorial aggression toward a neighbor's dog if they are "fence-fighting." In a few instances excessive barking may be a manifestation of compulsive behavior. This would represent an abnormal response, as would excessive barking as an aspect of age-related cognitive dysfunction.

Among the common conditions in which problem barking is secondary is separation anxiety. If one attempts to treat the barking alone, simply because it is the most objectionable aspect of separation anxiety, the problem is not likely to be solved, and may, in some instances, be made worse. Similarly, barking may be secondary to fear of a loud noise such as firecrackers. Like separation anxiety, barking that is secondary to fear of a loud noise is most readily dealt with by treating the fear (Chapter 10).

Typical History

Dog owners often seek professional advice because there have been complaints from neighbors or other members of the family with regard to excessive barking, or they are concerned that such complaints may arise. The clinician should be aware of breed dispositions and tendency toward excessive barking because this information may be needed in the eventual prognosis and consultation with the owners. Realizing that there may be a number of causes of excessive barking, it is necessary to go into the context with regard to when the behavior occurs. For example, does the barking occur only when the owners are gone, suggesting that it is an aspect of separation anxiety? In such instances one would look for other signs of separation anxiety. Does the behavior occur only when other dogs are barking, indicating there is a social facilitation? The same question should apply to barking occurring as a part of playful interactions with neighboring dogs. With regard to learned aspects, one would look for indications that the owners are reinforcing barking, particularly the loudest and most frequent, by allowing the dog in the house when the barking becomes excessive.

Diagnosis

The first task is to determine whether the objectionable barking is secondary to another more general behavior problem such as separation anxiety or fear of certain noises. With separation anxiety the barking would occur only in the owner's absence, and one would expect to see other indications of separation distress. Ruling out barking secondary to fear of loud noises, or as an aspect of separation anxiety, is important because the treatment approach for these problems involves desensitization to the fear-evoking stimulus or separation. These are different therapeutic regimens than barking in response to environmental or social stimuli where the approach could be as simple as environmental management.

The next task is to determine the various factors that go into producing excessive barking, keeping in mind that there is likely to be more than one factor involved. A dog, for example, may be provoked to bark only in response to environmental stimuli—such as passing pedestrians, bicyclists, or garbage trucks in the morning—often in concert with other dogs. If there is a breed predisposition toward excessive barking, the problem may not be resolved to the same degree as it would be in a breed without the same barking predisposition. Because objectionable barking is commonly related to more than one cause, the diagnosis will often reflect more than one type of barking. Correspondingly, the treatment will usually outline several approaches.

Treatment Guidelines

One or more of the following approaches may be employed according to the cause of the problem, discussed above, and the lifestyle of the owners. A dog presented for objectionable barking may be diagnosed, for example, with both separation anxiety and socially facilitated barking and would require a therapeutic program designed for each problem.

Aside from such multifaceted approaches, the first task is to remove the factors that contribute to the onset of the barking. Next one could employ some means of reinforcing nonbarking behavior or at least not reinforcing barking. Finally the use of remote punishment in the form of bark collars that deliver a spray of citronella may resolve a barking problem, when used in conjunction with these other techniques, and when fearfulness does not play a role in the behavior. Here is an area also where simply managing the environment of the dog by scheduling when it is outdoors and able to hear or see bark-inducing stimuli, or bother the neighbors by its barking, may be part of the solution. It might be easier to resolve problems associated with leaving the dog inside than eliminating the barking problem that occurs outside.

Barking Secondary to Other Problems

If the barking is secondary to separation anxiety, this problem should be treated (Chapter 10). It will be necessary to have a dog sitter remain with the dog when it is left alone for long periods, not only to help in the desensitization of separation anxiety but to prevent barking until the separation anxiety problem is resolved. Barking that is secondary to fear of loud noises should also be treated with a desensitization program for the primary problem (Chapter 10).

Response to Environmental Stimuli

Environmental stimuli, such as children playing next door or other dogs running around, may evoke barking that would generally be oriented toward the stimulus. If the stimulus is frequent the barking may be very objectionable. The most effective way to deal with this problem is to avoid exposing the dog to the stimulus. One way is to screen off the area that causes the barking. One might also keep the dog in the house, isolated from the stimulus during those times of day when it is most likely to occur. If there are occasions where children of neighboring homes intentionally, or unintentionally, provoke barking, one might say something to the neighbors about redirecting the factors that evoke barking. This will show the neighbors the dog owner is trying to be responsible and control the barking without unduly confining the dog.

Desensitization to Doorbells and Door Knocking

It is clearly logical that a good watchdog should bark exuberantly at a stimulus that always precedes the arrival of an intruder. Even for dogs that are friendly to visitors, excessive and loud barking at the sound of a doorbell can be unnerving to both the dog owners and the visitors. One approach is to desensitize the stimulus following a standard systematic desensitization and counterconditioning program using a graded intensity of the doorbell. One could stage doorbell-ringing sessions of 10 rings, multiple times per day, with the doorbell muffled by layers of towels or blankets so that the dog is hardly reacting to the sound. A session should begin with the dog called to a place near the door and asked to sit. Immediately after a muffled doorbell ring the dog is given a small favored food treat, assuming it is not aroused or barking. After the pattern of stimulus presentation and counterconditioning is established, one layer of muffling can be gradually removed and the sessions progress. Therapy sessions are continued until all layers of muffling are removed. In the ideal outcome the dog will come to "love" the doorbell and sit quietly for the food treat. During the training period it will be necessary to turn off or completely muffle the doorbell so that the dog is not unintentionally activated by the full sound. For dogs that bark the most actively at doorbell sounds, mild restraint during the training sessions with head halters may be useful (Chapter 3). After the training period the doorbell should be regularly sounded, and food treats given, to maintain the habituation.

Social Facilitation

Social facilitation most often occurs in response to other dogs barking. Sometimes one dog in the neighborhood starts barking and many of the other neighborhood dogs join in. If this is just an occasional occurrence it may present no major problem behavior, but if one lives in an area where another dog regularly engages in barking the clients may have to develop a schedule of putting their dog outdoors only when there is less likelihood of the other dogs provoking it.

Play-Evoked Barking

Some of this may involve the predisposition of dogs to engage in barking in response to attempting play with neighbor children or another dog through the fence. Management of the stimulus by putting up appropriate visual barriers or scheduling outdoor time may be most effective.

Barking Toward Neighbor Dogs

This is seen when two neighboring dogs on opposite sides of an adjoining fence display territorial-type behavior, including intense barking. Treatment includes managing the outdoor schedule of all dogs involved. If the neighbor is unwilling or unable to help, the onus rests on the client. One approach is for the owner systematically to desensitize and countercondition the dog to the presence of the neighboring dog. The dog should be on leash at a distance from the other dog when no aversive emotional reaction occurs, which may be at the far end of the yard or even outside of the yard. Gradual, incremental steps toward the fence line must be taken.

Learned Barking

Diagnosis is a critical factor here in determining the degree to which the barking is maintained by the owner's response. If, when barking, the dog is allowed in the house so as to prevent neighbors from complaining, the behavior is reinforced when it is particularly loud and frequent. If mild barking does not result in getting the dog in the house, the owners have shaped the behavior to the more intense and objectionable form. One of the indications that learning is a cause is if the barking is worse when the owners are home and, thus, able to allow the dog into the house. Dealing with barking that is learned, or enhanced by learning, requires an understanding of reinforcement schedules and the extinction of learned operants (Chapter 3). Basically, one must decide never again to allow barking to pay off. The difficulty is that following the implementation of such an extinction process, there is likely to be a burst of barking preceding the reduction of barking.

There are ways other than barking that dogs can be taught to signal a desire to come in the house. For example, one could hang a bell near the door and train the dog to ring the bell with the paw or nose as a sign that it wants to come inside. Ringing a bell requires more effort than barking, so the sound will occur less often and a gentle-sounding bell should be less disturbing to neighbors and the dog's family as well. An easy way to handle barking to get in the house is to install a dog door and let the dog come and go as it pleases. The doors come with a blocking panel that can lock the dog inside or outside.

Reinforcing Nonbarking Behavior

When a dog barks persistently while the owners are home, this approach might be useful in conjunction with extinguishing learned barking and managing a dog's exposure to bark-inducing stimuli and possibly using a dog door. This approach involves conducting training sessions when barking could occur but is not too likely. When a period of time has passed without barking, starting with a mere few seconds, reward the dog with a treat and praise. If barking occurs, owners' rewards should be withheld for a length of time.

The Use of Bark Collars

Excessive barking has spawned a major industry of bark collars that deliver an aversive stimulus when a dog barks. Theoretically, use of a bark collar is one of the best examples of effective remote punishment; the punishment occurs immediately and reliably after each behavioral act and is directly connected to the misbehavior rather than the person responsible for arranging the punishment.

Given the importance of controlling barking in urban areas and the proliferation of noise ordinances that refer to excessive dog barking, the demand for bark collars has led to a continually evolving area of devices for more reliable and creative remote punishment collars. The important thing to remember is that the collar alone is not going to be nearly as effective if it is not paired with attention to environmental management and behavior modification programs to reduce a dog's motivation to bark excessively, such as those discussed above. Thus, any fear- or separation-related aspects to the barking should be treated with an appropriate behavior modification program; otherwise, the collar may make the dog even more anxious. Bark-inducing stimuli should be managed and nonbarking behavior should be reinforced when feasible. It is only when efforts are employed to reduce barking, and quiet behavior rewarded, that one should consider the use of a bark collar.

Collars differ as to the form of aversive stimulus. The traditional collars deliver an electric shock in response to the vibration or sound produced by barking. A newer collar releases a spray of citronella when barklike vibrations occur. Another type delivers a high-pitched, aversive sound when barking occurs. Some collars deliver a warning sound that precedes a shock, giving the dog an opportunity to first stop barking. Whatever the type of collar, it is important that the punishment be delivered in response to a vibration related to barking rather than by the bark noise itself; otherwise, the problem animal may get punished when another dog barks or an extraneous barklike sound occurs. Some shock collars are triggered only after a few barks, thereby allowing a brief bout of watchdog barking but punishing barking that is excessive. Although theoretically appealing, collars that allow a few "free" barks require a dog to keep track of the number of barks it has emitted and thus may involve a longer time to learn and result in less reliable control of barking. There is some research indicating that the citronella spray collar is at least as effective in suppressing objectionable barking as the shock collar[2,3] and should be recommended instead of the shock collar.

A major problem with bark collars is that dogs learn not to bark when they have the collar on because it weighs more and feels different than a normal collar. Thus owners of problem dogs may have to leave the bark collar on permanently or put it

---

EXCESSIVE BARKING

Causes
- Breed predisposition
- Secondary to separation anxiety
- Acquired because of reinforcement
- Provoked by environmental stimuli
- Social facilitation

Resolution
- Eliminate or treat cause as appropriate.
- Discontinue reinforcement of barking.
- Screen off provoking stimuli.
- Use remote punishment (bark collar).
- Reinforce nonbarking.

on when the chances of barking are high. In the ideal situation, with the owners employing appropriate environmental management, systematic desensitization, and/or other behavior modification program to reduce the likelihood of barking and reinforce nonbarking behavior, the bark collar would eventually no longer be needed. As a start in this direction one can frequently put on and take off the bark collar, being sure to put it on when the likelihood of barking is low. This makes it more likely the dog will associate the punishment with the barking rather than the collar. A dummy collar could be used at some times when barking will not occur (e.g., at night) so the real collar can be charged. As mentioned, the goal should be to shape a dog's barking behavior so that eventually the bark collar is not necessary.

References

1. Hart BL, Hart LA. The Perfect Puppy: How to Choose Your Dog by Its Behavior. New York: W.H. Freeman and Co., 1988.
2. Juarbe-Diaz SV, Houpt KA. Comparison of two antibarking collars for treatment of nuisance barking. Journal of the American Animal Hospital Association 1996;32:231–235.
3. Wells DL. The effectiveness of a citronella spray collar in reducing certain forms of barking in dogs. Applied Animal Behavior Science 2001;73:299–309.

Chapter 12
Excessive Activity and Destructiveness

The problems discussed in this chapter are commonly referred to as misbehaviors much as are jumping on people or not coming when called. However, the diagnostic concerns merit a discussion of relevant normal canine and breed-specific behaviors aside from just implementation of behavior modification to resolve or ameliorate the problems. For example, most people expect puppies to be very active. In fact, when a person has children, puppies are an excellent source of entertainment; a puppy should win out over a computer game anytime. But when an adult dog is continually buzzing around, people find the behavior almost intolerable. Activity level may be a reflection of breed membership. Breeds that are high on activity level include the terrier breeds, Pomeranian, German Shorthair Pointer, Weimaraner, Dalmation, and English Springer Spaniel.[1] Because a high level of activity is typical for some breeds of dogs, the best we can do in some instances is to enhance the problem dog's quiet periods and not increase the problem through reinforcing a high activity level. In addition to developmental and breed predispositions, excessive activity in rare circumstances may reflect a syndrome referred to as *hyperactivity* or *hyperkinesis,* which appears to be an abnormality associated with a neurological disorder that shares some similarities with the neurological disorder known as attention deficit disorder in preteen children, especially boys.

Household destructiveness, like excessive activity, may reflect normal puppy behavior. In adults, destructive behavior may be a manifestation of separation anxiety or, rarely, a type of compulsive behavior. Like excessive activity, a complaint of destructiveness requires a carefully executed history. Both of these problems are discussed in the following sections.

Excessive Activity

Typical History

An excessive activity problem may be presented to a clinician as part of a suite of problem behaviors, including objectionable barking and destructive behavior. Each of these problem areas may be dealt with separately or one may look for an underlying basis. Although the dog owner will focus on the many situations in which the dog is overly active, it is important to find out when and where the dog is calm on its own as well. The application of behavior modification principles to enhance quiet behavior will be based on expanding the times when the dog is good by rewarding this appropriate behavior and decreasing the amount of time when it is overly active.

Some clients may have heard about the canine hyperactivity syndrome and wonder about the application of this syndrome to their dog. The first observations of hyperactivity in dogs were by a psychiatrist who discovered that if such dogs were treated with the stimulant amphetamine, the hyperactivity was suppressed so that handlers could socialize with the dogs and work with them in obedience training.[2] As mentioned, this syndrome is rare and considered likely only after completely ruling out other possibilities. The central nervous system stimulant methylphenidate (Ritalin®) has been used with dogs, but there are no clinical trials reporting efficacy or time course to response.

Diagnosis

The first task is to determine whether one is dealing with puppylike activity or the innate tendencies of some breeds to be very active. The second is to rule out a pathophysiological cause such as excessive secretion of the thyroid hormone. The third task is to assess the degree to which the behavior seems to be enhanced by owner reinforcement and could be resolved by behavior modification procedures. The unlikely possibility of hyperkinesis may be considered. One should take a conservative approach and diagnose a dog as hyperkinetic only after more likely diagnoses, such as a lack of control by the owner, have been ruled out.

Treatment Guidelines

Excessive activity, like that typical of puppies and adolescent dogs, strikes some people, who are accustomed to the slow pace of an older dog, as abnormal. Usually the owners of such dogs do not realize how active a young Golden Retriever or Boxer can be, and they believe the dog may be abnormal when, in actuality, the behavior is typical. One approach to problems of this type is to help the owners realize that their dog is normal and that they may be enhancing the behavior by giving the dog attention when it is particularly active. Second, the dog should have regular opportunities to engage in acceptable types of physical activity, such as jogging or playing, as well as opportunities for mental stimulation through training. The best schedule is a predictable, energy-intensive outing or session with the owner every day, not just when convenient, as well as short, frequent, structured obedience sessions.

As for the use of behavior modification, when the dog's activity or play becomes very objectionable, the owner should employ social punishment with a bridging stimulus (Chapter 3) such as sounding a low-pitched howl and walking away. If there are times during the day, or in certain places, when the dog is relatively quiet, it may be amenable to using behavior modification to increase the likelihood of calm behavior. For example, the dog may be calm at first for a half-minute after it is told to "be quiet," or if a particular member of the family is petting it.

The principle of successive approximation can be used here to countercondition calm behavior. If, for example, the dog is calm for 20 seconds when someone calmly says "be quiet," this can be used as a starting point. The dog is asked to be quiet when the owners know it is likely to be quiet. Food treats and verbal praise are given to the dog when it has been calm. Over several days a longer duration of being calm is required before rewards are given. Depending upon the success of the initial conditioning sessions, the goal of having the dog remain calm for a half-hour or more can be approached. If the excessive activity seems to reflect a breed or individual predisposition, behavior modification procedures can be expected, at best, to decrease the frequency of excessive activity but not to eliminate the problem.

As for the canine hyperactivity syndrome, in those rare occasions when extra-label treatment with methylphenidate may be indicated, the clinician should adjust the dosage according to the needs of each individual dog. The behavior should be closely monitored with daily observation forms. Keep in mind that occasionally the diagnosis of hyperactivity in a dog has been used as a ploy for access to amphetaminelike drugs in drug-abuse instances.

Destructive Behavior

Digging holes, chewing on furniture, and clawing into the side of a house are common complaints. When these behaviors are displayed by puppies we tend to attribute it to normal puppy behavior and cope by keeping targeted objects out of reach until the puppy grows up. In an adult dog, destructive behavior is a different matter. Adult dogs are large enough to do serious damage and, if uncorrected, the behavior is likely to persist. Destructive behavior is also one of the hallmarks of separation anxiety. Aside from this separation anxiety, the easiest form of destructive behavior to treat is that which happens predictably each day and where an effective behavior modification program can then be designed around this predictability.

Typical History

Of prime importance is the history regarding when the objectionable behavior occurs and when the dog is good. Does the behavior occur only when the owners are gone, or does it happen when they are present? Reprimands or other direct punishment, for example, can cause the dog to learn not to engage in the behavior in front of the owners. What is the history of response by the owners when the dog is destructive? The owner may find, for example, that departures in the morning, particularly if the dog was taken on a walk prior to departure, are much more likely to lead to misbehavior. There may be some other factors involved, such as the presence or absence of other dogs. Sometimes loud noises, such as airplanes taking off or noise from a nearby construction site, stimulate a dog. If this is the case, the anxiety produced by the loud stimulus will have to be addressed in eliminating the destructive behavior. As mentioned, the easiest situation to handle is when the behavior is predictable and consistent. When the destruction is sporadic and unpredictable, additional background observations may be useful. Is the dog's destructiveness limited to one area, such as repeatedly digging a hole in the same place or is the behavior directed to a myriad of locations? When the destructiveness is directed at a different area each time, this may be an indication that emotional anxiety may underlie the behavior.

Diagnosis

The treatment of destructive behavior hinges upon an analysis of the dog's emotional state during acts of destructiveness, analysis of when the destructiveness occurs, and the type of destructiveness. A dog left alone may be tearing into things as an outlet for boredom because the exercise is intrinsically rewarding. Alternatively, there may be some tangible rewards, such as food scraps for a dog that gets into garbage cans. These motivating factors would not appear to involve anxiety or fear.

If the dog appears very anxious and upset when left alone, the behavior may represent an aspect of separation anxiety, and the destructiveness must be dealt with as secondary to the anxiety. Separation anxiety, and its related destructiveness, are dealt with in Chapter 4. One useful clinical sign in diagnosing separation anxiety is whether the dog displays several types of behavioral manifestations, such as excessive barking, house soiling, and anorexia, in addition to destructiveness.

Treatment Guidelines

In many instances, one may utilize behavior modification to enhance the good behavior. For example, if a dog is digging holes in a number of places around the yard, it might be possible to condition the dog to dig where the owners would find it acceptable. One or two digging centers can be created by first making a sandy digging spot and then hiding a bone or chewable treat below the surface. Eventually the dog finds the bone by digging in the area. Next time the bone should be buried deeper and at subsequent times deeper and deeper. Two or three bones could be spread out and buried. Bones could be hidden only sporadically to reinforce digging behavior on an intermittent basis. Meanwhile if the dog digs a hole in an unacceptable place, remote punishment might be tried. By working with punishment of the occasional digging and intermittent reward of acceptable digging, one may successfully train a dog to dig only in the one allowable corner of the yard.

A somewhat more labor-intensive type of behavior modification may be used for household destructiveness, where one can also attempt to condition a dog to display good behavior by designing a gradient of increasing duration when the dog is left alone. To begin, with the owner should supply the dog with acceptable and appealing objects on which to chew. The objects should be easily differentiated from unacceptable chewing targets; thus, an old shoe will not work as an acceptable chew toy if the dog is drawn toward chewing good shoes. It might be typical for a dog to be good if left alone for 10 minutes but to chew on unacceptable objects if left alone for 2 hours. Initial departures are designed to be short enough to preclude any destructiveness by the dog. Good behavior of the dog when it is left alone is rewarded by food treats and affection upon return of the owner. The departure durations are then gradually increased as long as the dog continues to be good. If destructiveness does occur, the owner should completely ignore the dog for a period of time upon return and the next time conduct a training session of shorter duration. The goal is for the dog to be reliably well behaved for as long as 8 hours. By gradually moving along the departure gradient, the duration of time the dog can be left alone is increased. The dog might be provided a cue, during training sessions, to which acceptable behavior can be associated. Tuning the radio to a program not normally listened to is appropriate. Between training sessions the dog must be physically prevented from being destructive whenever it is necessary to leave the dog alone for periods longer than those of the training sessions.

These departure sessions are somewhat similar to those used with separation anxiety. With separation anxiety, food treats are given at the moment of departure to countercondition the anxiety associated with the separation. Antianxiety medications may be used to reduce the emotional distress. With destructiveness not related to separation anxiety or fear-inducing stimuli, food treats are used at the end of the departure to reinforce good behavior and medication would not be indicated.

If a cause of the behavior is related to boredom or a need for activity, a regimen of exercise, short obedience training sessions, and regular interactions with the owners may aid in therapy and prevent recurrence after the behavior is controlled. However, extra exercise or attention sessions should be scheduled only if they are a daily routine, and not just on weekends and the occasional weekday. Inconsistent interactions may evoke undesirable destructive behavior as the dog becomes more frustrated in its attempt to find an opportunity for exercise. During training sessions the dog should not have access to the places where destructiveness occurs until the problem behavior is resolved.

An aspect of environmental management to reduce the likelihood of destructive behavior when the human family members are gone is to supply the dog with several acceptable chewing objects or robust entertainment centers, such as a rolling cube that dispenses treats or food-filled rubber toys. One should confirm, however, that the dog is entertained by these toys. The toys should be rotated on at least a weekly basis to maintain some degree of novelty.

Remote punishment is particularly indicated when the problem is directed to a specific item or place (Chapter 3). If the misbehavior varies so that there is a different target each time, remote punishment is inappropriate. For example, a dog may dig repeatedly in one area of the yard or chew in one specific place on a fence. By using a motion-detection repelling device connected to a sprinkler system or an aversive spray emitter (citronella) near the object which is repeatedly chewed, one is appropriately utilizing remote punishment. As a low-tech approach one may place loaded mousetraps on the spot in the yard which is repeatedly dug for large dogs. The punishment is delivered immediately after the misbehavior and the punishment is directly related to the target area. If one has the opportunity to spy on a dog every time it has an opportunity to be destructive, one could tie a bunch of tin cans together and string them up above the area where the misbehavior occurs. The tin cans could then be released at the onset of misbehavior. Keep in mind that interactive punishment such as verbally admonishing or physically correcting a dog is counterproductive. Even when such interactive punishment occurs immediately after the misbehavior, the connection between the behavior and the punishment is probably obscured, and the animal can develop a fear of the person delivering the punishment.

References

1. Hart BL, Hart LA. The Perfect Puppy: How to Choose Your Dog by Its Behavior. New York: W.H. Freeman and Co., 1988.
2. Corson SA, Corson EO, Kirilcuk V, Kirilcuk J, Knopp W, Arnold LE. Differential effects of amphetamines on clinically relevant dog models of hyperkinesis and stereotypy: Relevance to Huntington's Chorea. In: Barbeau A, ed. Advances in Neurology, Vol.1. New York: Raven Press, 1972;681–697.

Chapter 13
Escaping and Roaming

Central to the concept of dealing with escaping from kennels, yards, and other enclosures, or roaming from the home, is the commonly held notion that the life of some dogs left alone during the day is rather boring. Dogs adapt surprisingly well to long periods of being left alone if there is a schedule of predictable outings and interactions with human members of the family. As creatures of habit, dogs usually accept a consistent routine—for example, morning and evening walks—and they will usually not excessively vocalize or attempt to break out of their enclosures. Although this arrangement is obviously not as much to a dog's liking as a more open habitat, most dogs can accept confined living quarters.

Confined dogs are, however, too often subjected to erratic routines. Never being let out to play on weekdays, but being taken out on and allowed to play with people in the house on weekends, is asking a lot of the dog's biological clock. Lacking a routine, the dog is unable to predict when outings will occur and this may lead to repeated attempts to escape. As a dog digs and chews at a fence, and even jumps and throws itself at the fence, the owner may become inconsistent in behavior toward the dog. The dog may be punished one time, but the next time the escape attempt may be reinforced by taking the dog inside the house until the fence is repaired.

When dogs attempt to escape from an enclosure and fail, the escape behavior is not reinforced and they soon give up. However, if the enclosure is not perfectly secure, a vigorous escape attempt may pay off; further attempts at escaping are to be shaped into being even more intense. Minimal patching on such an enclosure will probably fail to prevent the dog from escaping again. The dog will try a little harder the next time because it was only the most vigorous attempts at escaping that were reinforced before. If the enclosure is made absolutely secure after two or three escapes, the dog will make many attempts to escape, but the behavior will eventually be extinguished. Extinction of escape behavior will be more rapid if the enclosure is made absolutely secure immediately after the first escape rather than after several escapes.

With regard to roaming, few people live in rural settings where they can safely allow their dogs to run free. But dogs with such access to wide-open spaces may take advantage of this freedom and repeatedly roam for several hours or days at a time. To understand the roaming behavior of dogs, it's useful to remember that the wild canid ancestor had a home hunting range of several square miles that may have included several den sites. Members of the pack may wander off for several days. The wolflike form of wandering has some implications for the situation of a dog living in a home or even on a farm. A dog's natural home range may be the size of a small town. Although we might believe it to be abnormal for a dog to roam far from home, the dog may find this quite natural. The dog has not forsaken its pack-like bonds with the family for wanderlust; it is just traveling about in its home range.

Roaming in dogs may have its intrinsic rewards just as in wolves. For one thing there may be an exploratory drive that is second nature to the species. Another cause is the powerful attraction of an appealing mate. Roaming for this reason is more likely in gonadally intact rather than neutered males. Females in proestrus or estrus may roam for equally obvious reasons. Availability of food at the distant place is also a possible reward for roaming; or a dog may be drawn to distant social activity. When the home base is quiet, a playground with school children could be too much to resist. For similar reasons, a dog may also be attracted to the company of other dogs living some distance away.

Escaping From Enclosures

The most frequent example of this problem is the escape from yards or kennels. In addition to the nuisance caused to the owner, a dog may injure itself in the process of escaping or be in danger of being hit by a car after escaping. Although one may argue that life in a kennel is less than ideal, much can be done to make it acceptable and also prevent escaping. For example, following a successful escape, if the owner does only a slightly better patch job each time—as chewed wood is replaced or reinforced by chicken wire fencing, making it only a little more difficult for the dog to chew through—the dog may be conditioned to persist in escaping until it gets through the next patch job. If the wire fencing is then replaced by hardware cloth, more effort is required, and the dog must take more wear and tear on its teeth and jaws to get out. But if the dog escapes again, the owner may finally put up chain-link fencing. Now, however, the dog's moderate escape attempts may have been shaped to that of fierce biting and pulling, allowing some dogs to break through the chain-link enclosure. Normally dogs will not go through chain-link fencing, but they can perform some unbelievable acts of strength and endurance if their behavior is shaped.

Typical History

Not uncommonly, the presenting problem is a dog that has become an escape artist in breaking out of enclosures. The escaping dog may have ripped and torn at the fence to the point where the feet may be lacerated or teeth broken. If traumatic injury to the mouth is the presenting complaint, clinicians should be alerted to the possibility that there may be a behavior problem to control as well as a medical one. The escapee may briefly visit other dogs and return home where it awaits its owner's return. Perhaps, because the enclosure had a new hole, the owner let the dog in the house during the repair period, thereby adding further reinforcement to the persistence of the problem behavior.

Diagnosis

The main diagnostic challenge is to differentiate escape behavior that is secondary to separation anxiety or a fear reaction to loud noises from a problem motivated by escape from an aversive situation and/or the reinforcement of escape behavior. If escaping is intensified by separation anxiety, resolution of the problem requires following treatment guidelines for separation anxiety (Chapter 10). In some instances fear of loud noises, such as those occurring with fireworks or starter pistols near a track field, may play a role in evoking escape attempts if the problem occurs only during times when these loud sounds occur. Again, one must treat such fear prior to addressing the escape problem as a separate issue.

Treatment Guidelines

If separation anxiety or other fear problems are likely to be the cause or contributor to the problem, it is important to treat these problems first. In fact the escape problem is likely to be resolved after separation anxiety is resolved. A component of the treatment program for separation anxiety will be to not leave the dog alone in the enclosure until the anxiety has decreased. A complicating factor may be that the enclosure itself has acquired an aversive property and evokes anxiety, which means the dog may now have to be desensitized to the kennel or enclosure.

If separation anxiety is not involved as part of the escape problem, it is necessary to make the enclosure totally escape-proof to extinguish the escape behavior. Ideally, the enclosure is made secure immediately after the first escape so as not to reward a more intense form of escape behavior and increase the animal's resistance to extinction. As mentioned, the more extensive the history of escape behavior, the longer it will take to extinguish the behavior.

For escape attempts that are limited to one or two specific areas of the enclosure, remote punishment may be of some value in creating an aversion to the area. Setting mousetraps around the escape area can produce a snap, and a loud noise may be effective in dogs with a low or moderate motivation to escape. For the more ambitious escape artists, one could use a remotely activated fencing system around the perimeter, as discussed in the next section.

Aside from securing the enclosure, the most important guideline is to maintain a routine in removing the dog from the enclosure. This means maintaining a schedule of walks and feeding and even visiting the dog in the enclosure in the same manner every day of the week. If one can only walk a dog for 15 minutes a day during the week, this schedule should not be increased on the weekend even if the owners have more time on the weekend—at least until the problem is resolved.

The enclosure should also be made as enticing as possible. Ways to accomplish this are by leaving food-dispensing toys around and, for dogs that escape from enclosed yards, hiding or scattering food around the enclosure, so that the dog is continually "hunting." This method may be made more effective if the dog is fed

---

ESCAPE BEHAVIOR IN DOGS

Causes

- Environment outside rewarding
- Inconsistent outing schedule
- Enclosure not secure

Resolution

- Make enclosure secure.
- Schedule routine outings.
- Do not give attention for escape behavior.
- Administer remote punishment for escape attempts.

---

less of its food in its food dish. Although toys other than food-dispensing types may be entertaining, dogs often play with their toys only when people are present and interacting with them. To help toys be more effective, the owners should rotate the toys on a regular basis.

Many people seeking consultation will have attempted punishment of some kind when their dogs get out. Such punishment is usually interactive punishment, such as verbal admonishment or even hitting, which does little to alter escape behavior. Remote punishment is much more effective because the aversive stimulus is directly related to the behavioral act and the escape behavior is punished instantaneously. Keep in mind that remote punishment always is most effective if the motivation to engage in the misbehavior is reduced. Thus, it is necessary to establish and maintain a routine of outings and make the environment more interesting before employing punishment.

Sometimes the question comes up as to the potential value of acquiring another dog to provide company for the problem dog and presumably reduce the boredom. The experience of some clients is that this does indeed solve the problem, although almost as many clients have found the problem persists. The best advice is that another dog is a good idea if the owner would like another dog, not as a solution to the original dog's problem.

Use of anxiolytic drugs may come into the picture if separation anxiety or fears of loud noises are involved. Aside from fear or anxiety-motivated escape, an anxiolytic may flatten the emotional arousal involved in intense, emotionally charged escape attempts. The dog can be phased off of the drug after a routine has been in practice for a month or more.

Roaming

This problem may occur in dogs that leave a home or yard that is not enclosed. Roaming may also be involved when a dog escapes from enclosures and then wanders off rather than staying home. If coupled with escape behavior, attending to and treating the roaming may reduce the motivation for escaping.

Typical History

The typical case is a dog that wanders off for several hours or even days. Roaming may be a problem just certain times of the year or under special circumstances. The history should focus on when the dog roams; why the dog roams, which may be evident by examining distant attractants, exploratory drive, or sexual motivation; and to where the dog roams, especially whether it is several locations or just one distant location.

Diagnosis

Aside from separation anxiety and fears of loud noises, which are ruled out if the wandering is not correlated with departures of human family members or the occurrence of loud noises, roaming is generally not confused with other problems. Aside from ruling these out, the diagnostic task is to determine the reasons for the roaming. For example, is the dog returning to a territory that was the location of the previous home? Is it because everyone in the family is gone during the day so that the only social contact for the dog is several blocks away? Is it because someone at a distant location is feeding the dog? The role of sexual motives in roaming of gonadally intact males and females in proestrus or estrus has been mentioned. The reasons for roaming affect the choice of therapeutic approaches. If one can remove the motivation or source of the attraction, solving the problem will be greatly simplified.

Treatment Guidelines

The indicated treatment approaches will usually involve more than one approach. Unless there is an obvious, nonsexual attraction, such as a playground or food source, one should suspect sexual motives in any gonadally intact male. Roaming is one of the indications for castration (Chapter 4). Castration can be expected to resolve a roaming problem in some but not all males (Fig. 13-1).

Rewarding good behavior is especially important but easy to overlook when focusing on preventing the roaming behavior. Even with the use of remote punishment one needs to reinforce staying-around behavior frequently. If the dog had typically run away during the day, one can arrange for the delivery of food at unpredictable times during the day so there is a chance, at any time of the day, the dog may get a food treat for just hanging around. A good reward is some nutritious favored food, like bits of chicken, beef jerky, pieces of cheese, or steak-flavored treats.

The use of appropriate punishment invariably arises. Dog owners undoubtedly feel ambivalent when they catch the wandering dog and must decide whether they should punish the dog, welcome it with open arms, or act indifferent. Punishing the dog may cause it to run away from the owner when attempting to catch it the next time. Yet, to pet the dog and welcome it into the car seems like reinforcing it for roaming. It is probably safest to be indifferent when catching the dog and bringing it home.

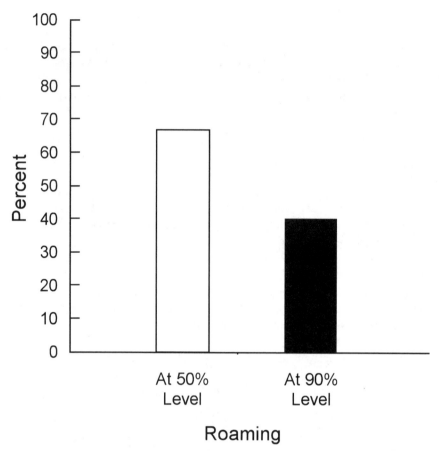

Figure 13-1 Effects of castration of male dogs in improving roaming behavior, expressed as 90% improvement (virtual resolution) or improvement of 50% or more (data from Neilson et al. 1997[1]).

Some punishment at the hands of people may be useful, however; if the dog visits a specific household, those people should be asked to never reinforce the behavior. In addition to not feeding, playing with, or letting the dog into their house or yard, the people at the location to where the dog roams may be persuaded to direct a blast from a garden hose toward the problem dog, creating an aversion to the place to which the dog goes. Presumably, the dog will avoid a location that is punishing and thus be more likely to choose to stay home.

Finally, the buried perimeter has gained favor to deal with roaming dogs. This method of controlling roaming represents an ideal use of effective remote punishment. The buried perimeter wire triggers a warning sound and then either a spray of citronella or a mild electric shock through a special collar worn by the dog when the dog approaches the property boundary.

Most fencing systems stress the importance of following behavior modification and environment management procedures before activating the system. Probably not stressed in literature enclosed with the perimeter wire systems is the importance

ROAMING BEHAVIOR IN DOGS

Causes
- Attraction of distant places
- No reward for staying home

Resolution
- Eliminate distant attractions.
- Castrate intact males.
- Punishment at the destination.
- Install buried perimeter wire.
- Reinforce for staying home.

of lowering the motivation to roam in the first place before activating the perimeter fence system. As for installing the perimeter wire, it is imperative that the buried wire have visual landmarks that a dog can associate with the potential of being shocked. The use of existing landmarks, such as trees or boulders, supplemented with small flags around the boundary, is the typical arrangement. The dog owners must behave as though a sturdy structural fence stands where the buried wire runs. It is also important to establish a nonwired, clearly marked gate through which the dog and owner can safely pass. Ideally the gate would be a real structural gate that is clearly in an open or closed position. In many instances one or more doors of the house comprise "the gates" through which a dog can be taken for a walk or in the car.

There are a couple of concerns regarding the use of these systems. One is that if a dog successfully escapes the yard, it may be deterred from crossing back into the yard because it will receive the aversive stimulus activated upon crossing the border. Another major concern involves dogs that are aggressively territorial. Without a visible fence, visitors can unknowingly enter the dog's territory and potentially activate an aggressive display.

Reference

1. Neilson JC, Eckstein RA, Hart BL. Effects of castration on behavior of male dogs with reference to the role of age and experience. Journal of the American Veterinary Medical Association 1997;211:180–182.

Chapter 14
Urination and Defecation Problems

House soiling is one of those areas where a diagnostic workup is especially important. First, there is the issue of whether one is dealing with problem urination, problem defecation, or both. It is necessary to differentiate house soiling as a primary behavior problem from medical conditions where house soiling is secondary, such as urinary incontinence stemming from a weakened urinary bladder sphincter or the frequent and urgent need to defecate secondary to bacterial enteritis. House soiling could be secondary to another behavioral problem, such as separation anxiety. House soiling may be a primary behavior problem if it reflects an absence of or interruption of house-training, submissive urination, or urine marking. This chapter deals with household defecation and urination that are primarily problem behaviors under the headings of inappropriate urination and defecation, submissive urination and urine marking. In this light, some discussion of the den sanitation concept and process by which dogs are house-trained is in order.

Den Sanitation Predisposition

This is an area of animal behavior where much misunderstanding arises. When we house-train a dog, we are not actually teaching it new eliminative habits, but simply relying on the dog's instinctive tendency to keep its den and rest areas clean. In this respect the dog is no different than a number of other fastidious species, including cats, rabbits, skunks, and even swine that eliminate in selected areas in order to keep their sleeping, eating, and resting areas clean. The reason nesting or denning animals are innately fastidious about the sleeping and resting areas relates to the fact that, in the wild ancestor, feces invariably carried eggs of internal parasites. If feces were deposited where animals slept, ate, or rested, infective larvae, which hatch from the fecal-borne parasite eggs, would contaminate the pelage of the lounging animals or their packmates. When they groomed, the animals would then infest themselves with the parasites.[1] Contaminated food eaten in a fecal-soiled den would lead to infection as well. Den sanitation also involves avoidance of soiling sleeping areas with urine. Although in nature urine carries few pathogens or parasites, urination in the den would lead to a moisture buildup, which would bring on problems with bacterial or fungal overgrowth. Therefore, contamination of the den by urine was also undoubtedly selected against. Occasional contamination of a den with urine is not as potentially devastating as contamination with feces, and probably the den sanitation tendency is stronger for feces than urine.

Naturally, the young animals are most at risk, and over evolutionary time parents that had the most sanitary eliminative habits had healthier and faster-growing off-spring than less sanitary parents. Hence, the fastidious eliminative behavior has been "hard-wired" through natural selection.[1] The den sanitation tendency even carries over to the cleanup a mother dog performs with her newborn puppies. When she licks the anogenital areas of her puppies as elimination is occurring, this keeps the nest clean (recently passed feces do not contain infective forms of parasites so the mother is not reinfected). To complement the system, newborn puppies reflexively defecate and urinate only when licked by the mother.

The ease with which dogs are house-trained makes them favored pets. In fact, a great many dogs are probably house-trained in spite of their owner's rather clumsy attempts to assist in the process. The house-training of puppies is discussed as well in Chapter 20. Clearly dogs are more easily house-trained than children. Human babies, like young and even adult primates in general, do not innately keep sleeping and resting areas free of urine and feces. House-training is a classic area for people to be anthropomorphic. When "accidents" occur we may assume the dog knows it has been bad and we proceed with punishment. With our children, we almost always take the time to explain verbally the particular acts that upset us. But there is no comparable way to explain to a dog that has defecated on the living room carpet why it is being punished. Some of the common acts of punishment, such as rubbing an animal's nose in the soiled area or angrily pointing to a mess several hours old, hinder the house-training process rather than help.

There are breed differences in the apparent ease with which dogs may be house-trained. Owners seeking advice in acquiring a dog may be interested to know that some breeds are more easily trained than others. Among the more easily house-trained are the Chesapeake Bay Retriever, Golden Retriever, Australian Shepherd, Collie, Shetland Sheepdog, German Shepherd, and Doberman Pinscher.[2] On the domestic scene, the increasing use of drugs for treating parasites may also potentially lead to relaxation of the innate den sanitation behavior. Thus, the occasional canine parent without the fastidious behavior produces young that are as healthy as the most fastidious parents but which carry genes for weakened den sanitation. When a dog with weakened den sanitation behavior is confronted with the task of identifying the entire house as a "den," one can see how training may become difficult.

It is important to remember that house-training is an extension of a dog's innate behavioral tendencies, which enable it to generalize that the entire house is its den. It has been known for a long time that the tendency of dogs to keep their nest clean is evident as soon as they are capable of leaving the nest.[3] In the newly adopted puppy, this behavior is seen when it is placed in a small pen. If it eliminates at all, it will generally be on the side of the pen away from the resting and feeding areas.

Some dog owners desire a dog to be trained to eliminate in only some areas of a backyard. This is a realistic goal, but it generally requires some staging. One should take the dog to the preferred spot—such as a corner or preferred substrate such as leafy or mulched areas—when the likelihood of elimination is high. It might be, for example, when the dog awakens after a long rest or finishes eating. The dog should be praised and rewarded for using the preferred area. When droppings are found on the lawn, at least part of the droppings should be placed in a preferred area to establish the odor cue of a toilet area. For male dogs one might provide a marking stump to lure the dogs from unintended potential marking targets.

Inappropriate Urination and Defecation

This section deals with problem elimination associated with incomplete house-training or problem elimination in a previously house-trained dog. Either or both defecation and urination may be involved. One should obtain a history and/or medical workup sufficient either to rule in or rule out the possibility of a pathophysiological basis. Sometimes there may be a medical disorder that initially led to the problem but, even though resolved, the problem behavior remains. For example, with prolonged diarrhea, the normal diurnal visceral rhythm for defecation urges may be disrupted, leading the dog to continue to soil the house at night. After the diarrhea is resolved, a toilet area may have been established so that the house is now divided into "den area" to be kept clean and "non-den" area to be soiled. In addition to enteritis and urinary cystitis, house soiling can stem from food allergies, arthritis (making it painful to move to the toilet area), and insufficient tone in the urinary bladder or anal sphincter muscles. One should next rule out problem elimination associated with other behavior problems, namely separation anxiety, various types of fear-related problems, and age-related cognitive dysfunction.

Typical History

House soiling reflecting incomplete house-training or interruption of previous house-training tends not to occur in the owner's immediate presence, but the dog will use the house as a toilet area during the night or when the owners are away. For a dog that was previously house-trained, a common problem is that it cannot make it through the night without soiling some part of the house, such as the living room or hallway carpet. When crated for a few hours, the dog usually does not soil the area. Thus, the dog may soil the living room at night, but if crated or tied to a bed all night, it will not eliminate until allowed outdoors. Sometimes the house soiling also occurs during the day out of view of the owner. One or more favorite toilet areas may have been established. This history should be explored as to how well the dog was previously house-trained and factors that may have led to the onset of house soiling.

Another possibility is that the house soiling reflects a background in which the dog had been kenneled or confined for a long period of time without appropriate opportunities to eliminate away from sleeping and eating areas. This may be seen in dogs from animal shelters or dogs that have been kenneled for long periods. In fact, one of the challenges for animal shelters in preparing dogs for "re-homing" is to establish or reinforce a den sanitation behavior so the newly adopted dogs are less likely to house soil the new home. House soiling may also be seen in dogs that are, at least somewhat, neglected by their owners and kept confined for inordinate amounts of time in crates, small dog runs, or even tethered close to an object such as a tree.

Diagnosis

The possible behavioral causes of fecal house soiling, other than difficulties in house-training, are separation anxiety and age-related cognitive decline. With regard to urine house soiling, submissive urination and urine marking are possibilities along with separation anxiety and cognitive decline. The time and circumstances when elimination occurs should rule out separation anxiety and submissive urination. Urine marking is usually directed onto "target" objects by leg lifting. Problem elimination due to cognitive decline, indicated by the correlation with other markers of cognitive decline, is dealt with in Chapter 19. If the dog soils the bed even if taken out recently, one should strongly consider the possibility of incontinence.

Treatment Guidelines

Some dogs diagnosed with inappropriate urination include those that, because of management or environment, were never, or only partially, house-trained. More common are those who were previously house-trained but seem to have lost the house-training, either partially or completely. The guidelines for house-training of adult dogs not previously house-trained, as well as those previously house-trained, are discussed in the next section.

House-training the adult dog

House-training actively involves training of both the dog and the owner. From the naive dog's standpoint, it may be difficult to perceive the entire house as the den. If permitted free, unsupervised access, untrained dogs might naturally consider areas away from where they sleep and eat—such as the living room, family room, and dining room—as toilet areas.

To make the house-training task easier, with the goal of encouraging the dog to hold its urine and feces until taken outside to eliminate, one should begin by restricting the animal to one small room or a part of a room, especially if the owner is unable to supervise the dog completely. A collapsible exercise pen is a possibility; this enclosure then becomes the "den." A bed should be provided in this area along with food and water. When the owners want their dog to interact with the family, the dog must be under complete supervision so that it does not sneak off into another room to eliminate. One way to achieve this is to tether the dog to the owner with a long line tied to the owner's waist or belt. Another way is to tether the dog to a piece of furniture close to the owner. This helps allow the owner to be aware of the dog's body language, which may be signaling that it is time to eliminate, as well as prevent the dog from sneaking into another room to eliminate unnoticed.

INAPPROPRIATE ELIMINATION IN ADULT DOGS

Causes
- Medical problem or behavioral senility
- Disturbance of normal house-training
- Weak den sanitation predisposition

Resolution
- Treat medical or primary behavioral causes.
- Reinstitute house-training.
- Schedule frequent trips to the outdoors test.
- Clean soiled areas.
- Implement remote punishment near soiled area.

The dog should be taken outdoors frequently, especially when the tendency to eliminate is high, such as after consuming a meal, awaking from a nap, or after a play session. The dog should also be rewarded for the act of appropriate elimination outside. This should be done with calm, quiet, verbal praise and perhaps a small food treat, although the act of eliminating is self-reinforcing. Rewarding a dog, especially for eliminating in the most appropriate locations, is useful.

For the human part of house-training, the dog trains the owner to be aware of signals to go out. The dog may stand by a door or emit a vocalization. For caregivers that quickly catch on to the sometimes subtle signals and act immediately to let the dog out, this aspect of training seems to progress rather easily. Part of the caregiver training is to suppress the urge to physically punish a dog that has house soiled. By yelling at or hitting the dog for eliminating inappropriately, the dog might learn that it should never eliminate in front of its owner, with the worst situation being a reluctance even to eliminate outdoors in the presence of the owner. The dog can also develop a fear of the owner expanding to beyond just the act of eliminating. That said, it is sometimes possible to use remote punishment to create an aversion to a specific area the dog repeatedly soils. Techniques including the use of upside-down plastic carpet runners, contact paper with the sticky side up, or electronically triggered alarms, are discussed in Chapter 3.

Previously house-trained dogs

Most commonly a partially house-trained dog soils the house at night. The first task is to confirm whether the dog still has the ability to make it through the night without urinating or defecating in the house. This can be quickly explored by tying the dog close to its sleeping area (this might be on or near the owner's bed) for a night or two. If the dog soils the area close to the bed (but is not incontinent) under these circumstances, some manipulating of the dog's intestinal system may be necessary. The owner may need, for example, to get up at midnight to take the dog outdoors. The midnight excursions can then be gradually advanced, over a period of a couple weeks, to the early hours of the morning and eventually to the normal wakeup hour. Successful training of the intestinal system should be possible if there is no persisting gastrointestinal disorder or incontinence.

Submissive Urination

Submissive urination is an example of a problem that often perplexes clients who are not familiar with this aspect of normal canine behavior. The complaint is that the dog urinates in front of people, usually family members, when they approach it, especially during a greeting from an absence. The first thing to realize is that urination upon the approach of a dominant individual (pack member) during greetings is normal for puppies. In the ancestral wolfpack, this is a type of submissive behavior that has the function of inhibiting aggressive approaches from dominant individuals. In other words, this is a form of communication that implies something like, "look, I am submissive just in case you have any doubts." A vicious cycle can be started by owners of puppies who scold them for submissive urination. Because shouting and physical punishment are perceived as aggressive responses by the puppy, the young dog urinates even more to show submissiveness to reduce the aggression.

Typical History

A typical complaint is that the owners know the dog is house-trained, but they cannot understand why the dog urinates when it seems the most happy to see them. Most dog owners will recognize that this type of house soiling is not a reflection of absence of house-training. The behavior is more prevalent in females and young dogs. Often the behavior is worse around exuberant people and during enthusiastic greetings. It is necessary to determine what circumstances, and which types of people, evoke the behavior. For example, exuberant greetings may evoke the urination, whereas quiet greetings may not.

Diagnosis

Although this is a type of house soiling, the context is very specific as are the triggers—most commonly, the return of the owners after an absence. The main differential diagnostic considerations are separation anxiety, inappropriate urination (described above), and urinary bladder dysfunction, all of which can usually be ruled out by details in the history.

Treatment Guidelines

The owners should be educated that direct punishment can make the problem worse because the dog is urinating because it is submissive and possibly fearful. As a start, owners should completely ignore their dog when they come home until it has calmed down, which avoids the emotional arousal. While the dog is ignored, the owner can unemotionally let the dog outside to urinate, which at least decreases the amount of urine voided. When the dog is greeted, it should be done in a very low-key manner, even somewhat indifferently. The owner can also come into the house through a different door, because this may be less evocative.

   If the rather simple steps above are not sufficient, the next step to handling this problem involves habituating the dog to greetings and social interactions with the

---

SUBMISSIVE URINATION

Causes

- Natural response to preclude aggression by dominants
- Interactive punishment exacerbates
- Prominent during greetings

Resolution

- Tone down greetings.
- Practice greetings first where problem is minimal.
- Use social punishment with bridging stimulus.
- Desensitize by staging multiple greetings.

---

human family members. The systematic desensitization model is followed so that a series of training sessions involving staged and repeated greetings is scheduled, starting with the least threatening situation and progressing to those that are presumably most threatening. Counterconditioning can also be employed by calmly offering a food treat during the greeting process when urination does not occur.

Additional progress may be made by employing social punishment at the onset of submissive urination that occurs during any greeting. When the problem dog submissively urinates upon the approach of family members they simply turn and walk away without any interaction with the dog, as though the urination "drove them away." When, during other greetings during the staged trials, no urinations occur, the people continue to enter the home, calmly pet the dog, and offer a food treat. Thus, the dog experiences a contrast between behavior that drives the caregivers away and behavior that allows them to stay. Such social punishment avoids the disadvantages of direct punishment, but the owners at least can feel they are not just doing nothing. As soon as habituation has progressed so that the dog does not urinate during greeting encounters in one setting, trials can be scheduled in situations more likely to evoke urination. This might mean changing the time of day or place when greetings are made.

Urine Marking in the House

Owners of male dogs are well accustomed to seeing them urine mark trees and posts along the way whenever they take a walk with the dog. When a dog uses this type of territorial marking inside the house a major problem arises. This can become one of the most difficult problem behaviors to resolve. Given that territorial marking in nature consists of depositing and renewing an olfactory mark on one or more specific objects, it is perhaps surprising that urine marking inside the house is not more common. Most male dogs that are house-trained usually do not urine mark in the house. This makes sense because in nature the close-in territory already has an abundance of odor cues, and it would be disadvantageous for males to deposit urine in a den and keep the area moist. Experimental evidence shows that the urine marking tendency is much higher in novel areas than in a dog's home area.[4] Urine marking behavior is almost completely sexually dimorphic; only rarely do females urine mark in the house. Urine marking in the house is a problem behavior where castration would appear to resolve the problem in about 40% of cases (Fig. 14-1). Interestingly, castration does not appear to affect urine marking markedly in outdoor areas.[4] It appears that outdoors, where there is no denlike feeling, and where the olfactory and visual stimuli evoking markings are very strong, and castration has little effect.

Typical History

Most owners seeking help with this problem will have noted an onset of urine marking after their dog has gone through puberty. The behavior is often evoked by a visit from another male dog in the house, the sight of another dog walking down the street, or new objects in the house, such as a visitor's luggage or even bags of

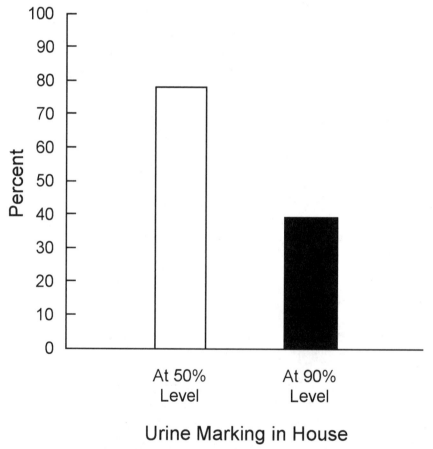

Urine Marking in House

Figure 14-1 Effects of castration of male dogs in improving problem urine marking behavior in the house, expressed as 90% improvement (virtual resolution) or improvement of 50% or more (data from Neilson et al. 1997[5]).

groceries. The effect of the arrival of a new dog in the home may be so great that even a well–house-trained dog may start urine marking household furniture.

Diagnosis

The deposition of urine on vertical surfaces, such as the corner of a wall or piece of furniture, is a dead giveaway for diagnosis. However, not all urine marks end up on vertical surfaces. In these instances, the main diagnostic considerations are separation anxiety and absence of house-training. With separation anxiety, one should be able to discover other signs of separation distress, and there would be problem urination only when the owner is away. In differentiating this problem from lack of house-training, the main factor would be that the dog is well house-trained most of the time and the in-house urine marking occurs only when the dog is provoked by environmental stimuli and/or other dogs or odors.

Treatment Guidelines

As mentioned earlier, castration is effective in eliminating house urine marking in dogs showing this behavior in about 40% of males with about 80% showing an improvement by at least 50%.[5] No study has focused upon breed differences in problem urine marking although there appears to be a feeling that terrier breeds are most likely to be problem markers.

When castration is not effective, or when a castrated male takes up urine marking in the house, two approaches are possible. In environmental management, one could think of visually blocking the provoking stimuli outside the house such as access to a window where other dogs are seen. If only a few places are targeted for marking, one may block access to these areas or create an aversion to these areas by remote punishment using electronic alarms, upside-down plastic carpet runners, or upside-down contact paper. Although there are no published accounts of the success of drugs in eliminating urine marking, the administration of an anxiolytic drug might be useful in situations where environmental management and behavior modification are not effective. Long-acting progestins have, in some cases, suppressed urine marking in castrated males and might be considered in dire situations, but only if anxiolytic drugs have no effect (Chapter 6).

References

1. Hart BL. Behavioral adaptations to pathogens and parasites: Five strategies. Neuroscience and Biobehavioral Review 1990;14:273–294.
2. Hart BL, Hart LA. The Perfect Puppy: How to Choose Your Dog by Its Behavior. New York: W.H. Freeman and Co., 1988.
3. Ross S. Some observations of the lair dwelling behavior of dogs. Behaviour 1950; 2:144–162.
4. Hart BL. Environmental and hormonal influences on urine marking behavior in the adult male dog. Behavioral Biology 1974;11:167–176.

5. Neilson JC, Eckstein RA, Hart BL. Effects of castration on behavior of male dogs with reference to the role of age and experience. Journal of the American Veterinary Medical Association 1997;211:180–182.

Chapter 15

Attention-Seeking Behavior

Attention-seeking behavior problems can usually be handled with dramatic success. What's more, if you resolve the problem, your client will think you are a diagnostic genius, especially if someone else has wrestled with the problem unsuccessfully. Diagnosis depends upon determining what the dog does when it believes no one is around. With the widespread availability of videotaping, one can often determine what a dog does when no one is around to deliver attention, and making a diagnosis is fairly easy. Yet this problem appears to be frequently underdiagnosed.

What are attention-seeking problem behaviors? They can range from what seem to be medical problems, such as anorexia or self-mutilation, to repetitive behavioral patterns, such as tail chasing and snapping in the air that are suggestive of compulsive disorders. One thing that all these responses have in common is that performance of the behavior results in a payoff, usually in terms of extra attention from the owners. The initiation and maintenance of the behavior depends on the dog receiving the reinforcements of attention, affection, or social contact.

Because dogs have the ability to learn an infinite variety of behaviors, attention-seeking behaviors almost defy categorization. Behavioral acts originally diagnosed as compulsive may be primarily attention seeking rather than a reflection of a true neurotransmitter imbalance. Unusual acts such as chasing shadows, barking at light beams, or snapping at imaginary flies can be attention seeking, as can a variety of would-be medical problems, including lameness, paralysis, muscle twitching, diarrhea, and vomiting. Even anorexia can be attention seeking—for example, when a dog receives special food and hand feeding as the owner pleads with the dog to eat. In some cases the behavior may be quite evident in the examination room (Figs. 15-1 and 15-2). At other times the examination room setting may be distracting enough to inhibit the behavior.

Most times a behavior such as acting lame or coughing has a genuine medical cause to begin with, but because the behavior results in more attention than usual, the dog retains the behavior long after resolution of the medical problem. A classic example is for a dog to feign lameness for attention. A dog that has injured a foot often receives more affection and sympathy while it is injured. Because being lame pays off in terms of more attention and affection, the dog learns the value of pretending to be lame after the injury has healed. In some instances a dog may be "found out" when it forgets which leg was supposed to be "injured," and favors the wrong leg. Many times this problem could have been prevented by not giving

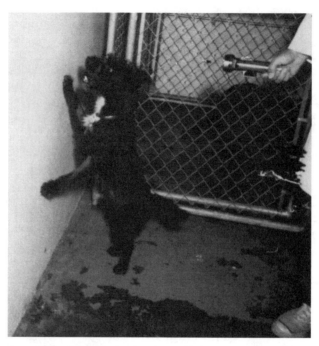

Figure 15-1 Attention-seeking behavior. This dog would chase and bark at shadows or moving spots of light—in this instance, the light from a flashlight.

excessive attention to the injured or sick animal. Sometimes a dog puts on an attention-seeking act in the presence of one member of the family, but then drops the act in the presence of other members that ignore the attention-seeking behavior.

Attention-seeking behavior is typically found in the household situation in which the dog is already heavily indulged with affection. Although this may seem a little illogical, it is the dogs that demand the most attention that will go to some effort to gain even more. In other words, it is probably impossible to satiate most of these dogs with too much attention. Attention-seeking behavior also frequently occurs when there is more than one dog in the family. There is invariably some competition between dogs for attention from the human side of the family. If one of the dogs happens onto a gimmick that results in receiving more attention than its competitor, it will tend to stay with the behavior as long as there is a payoff.

Typical History

Dog owners may have been referred to a behaviorist because clinical tests and a physical examination by a referring veterinarian have revealed no pathophysiological cause for this behavior. The owner will usually complain about a problem behavior that occurs so frequently they find it aversive. When considering an attention-seeking diagnosis, one should ask questions about what the owner does when the animal displays the behavior in question. Giving comfort and affection are obviously suspect, but also just looking at the dog is attention. Even shouting

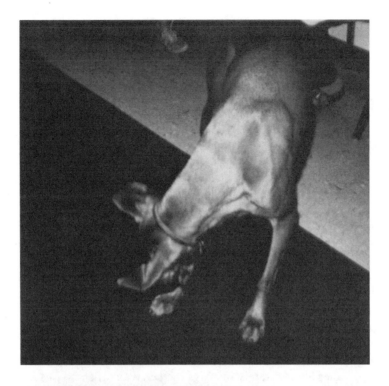

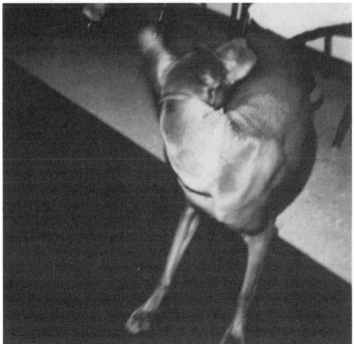

Figure 15-2 Attention-seeking behavior resembling a neurological problem. This dog made repeated movements back and forth between the postures seen in the top and bottom photographs.

can be reinforcing because it is better than being ignored. About the only thing an owner can do that could not be construed as reinforcing is to completely ignore the dog or walk away when the problem behavior is occurring.

Diagnosis

The first alternative diagnosis to come to mind is a medical problem causing the behavior in question. A careful diagnostic workup for the possibility of a medical cause is indicated. Although the lynchpin of this diagnosis is that the dog displays the behavior in question only when it believes someone is around to observe it, the diagnosis of attention seeking is often suggested by the process of exclusion after conducting a physical examination and clinical tests. Thus, lameness that persists in spite of every indication that the leg is normal, or a postural twitch that persists when a neurological examination yields nothing abnormal, suggests the diagnosis of attention-seeking behavior. At this point one has the choice of pursuing further clinical tests or exploring the possibility of an attention-seeking cause directly before further medical workup. Clearly a few days spent on exploring the attention-seeking possibility can be more cost effective than a series of diagnostic imaging procedures, if the animal's health is not in jeopardy.

The diagnosis of attention-seeking behavior requires a bit of detective work to determine whether the dog rarely displays the behavior when no one is around to reward it. One approach is to hospitalize the dog. Some dogs that display their acts in front of their owners will act perfectly normal in the hospital. If the act continues in the hospital, have hospital personnel sneak up on the dog and watch it when it does not know it is being watched. One can use a wall-mounted mirror to observe the dog at a distance. If the dog displays the behavior only when there is a person present, this is fairly conclusive evidence for the existence of an attention-seeking motivation. A behavioral pattern that is secondary to a disease, or that is truly compulsive, will generally be displayed whether a person is around or not.

Generally, the test for diagnosis of attention-seeking behavior will be conducted at the owner's home. The most reliable home-based diagnostic test is to set up a video camera. When the problem behavior occurs, the owners can walk out, turning on the video camera as they leave the house completely. An occasional display of the problem behavior when the dog is alone does not rule out an attention-seeking component. Performance of the behavior 95% of the time when people are around, and 5% of the time when they are not, would be consistent with an attention-seeking diagnosis, because animals can maintain a learned response in the face of no reinforcement as long as reinforcement is given intermittently.

If videotaping is not feasible, another option is for the owners to leave the house and pretend to leave in the car as soon as the problem behavior begins. They then need to sneak back to spy on their dog. The dog may have to be kept in one room so it can be easily seen from outside the house. If the owners can see the dog is behaving normally when the dog does not know they are around, the diagnosis is pretty clear.

Treatment Guidelines

There are three elements involved in treating the problem. One is to attempt to extinguish the attention-seeking behavior by completely removing reinforcement. The second is to reinforce desirable behavior, sometimes using a type of distraction to initiate a bout of good behavior. A third element is to use social punishment, in the form of leaving the dog alone, when the problem behavior occurs.

Before instituting these therapeutic measures, recognize that owners are often reluctant to believe the problem is behavioral and not due to a brain tumor. Therefore, it is usually necessary to explain fully what has been going on. If the owners have been able to videotape or spy on the dog and can see for themselves that the behavior does not occur when they are not around, this is often enough to convince them to follow the instructions. The client may be dumbfounded or feel betrayed to learn that the dog has successfully played such a trick on them. This actually makes it easier for the client to begin ignoring the behavior. If the dog has been hospitalized and not displayed the behavior for an entire week at the hospital, this information may also convince the owners. Dealing with attention-seeking anorexia requires special consideration and is discussed under a separate heading.

Owners may also have a difficult time understanding this diagnosis because they believe they give their dog plenty of attention. It is your job to explain that their dog has learned how to get even more attention when the dog wants it. For those owners who wish to have a more medically sophisticated sounding diagnosis, the alternative wording "audience-affected repetitive behavior" could be used. The treatment approaches are detailed in the following sections.

Extinguish Undesirable Behavior and Reinforce Desirable Behavior

These aspects of the treatment are very important and, when done together, can rapidly alter the behavior. Step one is to ignore the dog absolutely and completely when attention-seeking behavior occurs. If the behavior is going on most of the time, the owners will have to ignore the dog persistently. When good behavior occurs, such as sitting and being still, the owners should give affection, attention, and even food treats to reinforce the desirable alternative behavior. Ignoring a family pet is very difficult for a lot of people. An approach that frequently works with reluctant owners is to suggest they try an experiment for 1 or 2 weeks. There will usually be substantial progress in 1 week, and owners will then be willing to continue to follow your advice.

Ignoring a dog displaying the problem behavior and rewarding good behavior are often not intuitive for a lot of people, and it is usually just the opposite of what was occurring before. Previously, when the dog was engaging in the problem behavior, it got attention; when it was lying still, it was left alone. Under the treatment plan, a contrast is created between acceptable behavior that begets attention and the problem behavior that begets indifference and neglect. The more the contrast can be emphasized, the more readily the behavior will be altered.

On some occasions, a distracting stimulus can be very useful in evoking good behavior. This might involve the surreptitious use of a water sprayer when the problem behavior starts. This works best if two people are in the room and one can squirt a dog without being seen. When the problem behavior stops for a few minutes, the owners can then reward good behavior. Whether or not such a distraction is used along with the process of extinction, the object is to get the dog to behave appropriately more and more frequently, or for longer durations, so that good behavior can then be reinforced with affection. The owners must be more progressively demanding of longer periods of good behavior over time.

Socially Punish the Problem Behavior

The previous technique will often reduce the behavior to sporadic occurrences but may not entirely resolve the problem. When the problem behavior is occurring only sporadically, social punishment is useful. At the onset of the problem behavior, the owners should immediately leave the dog alone by getting up and leaving the room, closing the door behind them and returning only when the dog has stopped the behavior. The idea to be communicated to the dog is that the behavior "drives away" the human family members. The use of a low-pitched bridging stimulus is useful (Chapter 3).

Attention-Seeking Anorexia

The diagnosis for this form of attention seeking behavior is almost always reached by the process of exclusion where a thorough medical workup reveals no explanation for the anorexia. The behavior of a dog in avoiding food as a reflection of attention-seeking anorexia requires special consideration. The reinforcement is usually in the form of an owner pleading to the dog to eat. The dog is shunning one reinforcement, food, to obtain another reinforcement, attention. The diagnosis is based on how much attention is lavished on the dog to get it to eat, and on the absence of illness to explain the behavior. Owners have often tried other methods to get the dog to eat, such as top-dressing the food with broth, changing the brand or type of food, and making homemade meals for their dog. A tip-off might be if the dog eats when fed by someone who pays little attention to it, but does not eat, or is perceived not to eat, when cared for by the owner.

The treatment of ignoring the behavior must be balanced against the danger of the animal losing weight. Probably the best approach is to proceed by offering the

---

ATTENTION-SEEKING BEHAVIOR

Causes

- Attracts attention from owner
- Two (competing) pets in family
- May stem initially from medical problem

Resolution

- No attention for problem behavior
- Social punishment with bridging stimulus
- Attention for good behavior

dog small dishes of the food while basically ignoring or being indifferent to the dog. When behavior is in the direction of eating, such as just smelling or tasting the food, the dog is petted, or at least given verbal praise. When it turns away from the food, the owners should turn away from the dog. The idea is to reinforce any behavior related to eating. If the dog does not smell the food but only looks at it, this behavior may have to be reinforced. When the dog smells, tastes, or eats just a little food, the criterion for reinforcement can be made more stringent, and one should demand eating a larger amount before offering affection to shape the appropriate behavior. The success of the program requires that attention throughout the day be withdrawn so that the dog gets attention only for good behavior related to eating.

Chapter 16
Problems with Feeding Behavior

Owners are often concerned about the eating habits of their dogs. Sometimes dogs consume inappropriate objects such as pieces of wood or rocks. Coprophagy, consumption of cat or dog feces, is especially objectionable to dog owners. For some finicky dogs, finding an appealing food may be a problem. Other dogs eat well for a while and then seem to stop eating for no apparent reason. Obesity is also a common problem, and despite their best efforts, caregivers seem to have little success in reducing the animal's weight. These are the problems discussed in this chapter after first taking up the topic of normal canine feeding behavior.

Normal Feeding Behavior

Many people believe that a natural diet for canids is almost solely meat. However, the diet of wild canids consists of the entire carcass of rodents and larger mammals, and occasionally vegetative matter such as fruits and seeds. Like their wild ancestors, most dogs tend to eat rapidly. When wolves bring down prey, there is often competition for food from packmates, and the animals that eat rapidly receive the most food. Wolves have a remarkable ability to gorge themselves, and it has been reported that they can consume up to one-fifth of their own body weight at one time. Even dogs fed commercial food have been reported to consume 10% of their body weight in canned food at one time.[1] Dogs also prefer canned food over semi-moist food, and both are preferred over dry kibble. They also usually prefer cooked meat over raw meat probably because of the production of attractive odors.

Social Facilitation

Having other dogs around can increase eating, particularly in puppies. This effect is temporary, however, and over time, group-fed puppies probably eat no more than those fed alone. The effects of social facilitation are less apparent when food is readily available all day.[1] If food is restricted, dominance interactions, especially among puppies, occur during feeding. The dominant animals may get such a large proportion of the food that the more subordinate ones are undernourished. Feeding puppies with several pans of food is a way of preventing this problem.

Burying Bones

An interesting behavior related to the wild ancestors of dogs is the tendency of some dogs to bury bones. Even when some dogs are in plastic or metal cages, they may attempt to cover a bone by using papers or blankets on the cage floor. Wild canids, including wolves and some species of fox, bury small prey and may go back to the source of the cache during lean months of the year. Some dog owners claim to have seen their animals bury small animals and later uncover them after the tough skin had decomposed. However, it is common for dogs to bury bones but fail to dig them up later, suggesting the maintenance of the full behavioral sequence, from burying to recovering the food, may have been lost in domestication.

Hospital Environment

Familiarity with the environment plays a role in determining a dog's appetite. An animal hospital is not a particularly good place in which to evaluate a dog's eating behavior because the strange environment may suppress eating. The hospital diet is likely to be different from the dog's customary diet, and the time at which the dog is fed may also be different.

Most dogs adapt to a new feeding regimen surprisingly well. One study of eating behavior in hospitalized dogs found that within 3 days most dogs adapted to the hospital regimen, as indicated by how rapidly they consumed their meal after being fed.[2] Although healthy dogs may adapt to a hospital environment, there is evidence that several factors affect a dog's appetite, and sick or convalescing dogs could suffer if the hospital staff rigidly adhere to the principle that a dog will eat if hungry enough.

Conditioned Food Aversions

A canine's likes and dislikes can reflect acquired aversions as well as acquired tastes. Animals may develop an aversion to a food that has made them sick or nauseous. Foods that produce an allergic response in the gastrointestinal system, or that are contaminated with bacterial toxins, can produce an aversion to that specific food. The food itself may be perfectly safe, but one constituent of it causes an aversion. The aversion-producing substance can be removed and the ability to associate a food with gastrointestinal illness will diminish when the animal makes the association that the food is now safe. Although the actual occurrence of acquired food aversions has yet to be demonstrated in animals in nature, the presumed function is to protect animals from repeated ingestion of food with toxic constituents. Foods associated with allergic reactions and gastrointestinal distress leading to the development of an aversion would lead dogs to avoid the food that produces illness.

Learned or conditioned food aversions have been studied in the laboratory by using lithium chloride, which is a substance that causes ingestive nausea and sickness. The taste or smell of the food takes on aversive properties after one or more pairings with the illness-producing treatment.[3] A striking example of aversion conditioning involving predation in canids is the attempt to produce an aversion in coyotes to killing and eating sheep as a possible approach to control predation.[4] The investigators wrapped lamb meat laced with lithium chloride in a lamb's wool covering and allowed captive coyotes access to it. After one or two pairings, the coyotes, who were known sheep attackers, no longer chased sheep in the experimental enclosure. The laced meat approach to reducing coyote predation on lambs has not worked out, however.[5]

Eating Grass

Almost every dog owner wonders about the reason their dogs occasionally eat grass or other plants. Plants, especially grass, are seen in about 5–10% of scat and stomach content samples of wolves and cougars.[6–8] An Internet survey of about 1,600 dog owners whose dogs were observed eating plants at least 10 times, and who spent at least 6 hours daily with their dogs, revealed some insights into plant eating.[9] About 80% of dogs were reported to eat primarily grass, mostly long-bladed grasses. Among dogs, the average frequency of plant eating is daily to weekly. Although sex, gonadal status, and breed group membership seemed to play no role, dogs less than a year in age engaged in grass eating more frequently than adults.

Although a common perspective associates grass eating with a dog feeling ill and vomiting afterward, only about 10% of dogs were reported commonly to show signs of illness prior to grass eating and only 20% regularly vomited after eating grass. Although dogs reported to show signs of illness were more likely to vomit than normal dogs after eating grass, the vomiting may be correlated with, rather than caused by, plant eating.

The picture emerges that grass eating occurs mostly in normal dogs and is not usually followed by vomiting. One perspective gained from studies on whole-leaf swallowing by wild chimpanzees is that plant eating plays a role in expelling intestinal parasites.[10] One must remember that although most family dogs carry few or no intestinal parasites, plant eating may be a predisposition inherited from wolf ancestors that were exposed to parasites. The increased tendency for puppies to eat grass more frequently than adults may be explained by the fact that in nature puppies have little immunity to intestinal parasites and are more vulnerable to blood loss; hence, the prophylactic removal of intestinal parasites by grass eating would be relatively more beneficial. If grass eating is eventually shown by experimental studies to help expel intestinal parasites, grass eating would be the first documented example of herbal medicine including domestic dogs and their wild relatives.[11]

Ingestion of Inappropriate Materials: Pica

Dogs are not necessarily careful about what they chew and swallow. A mouthful of dirt now and then causes no problem. However, for no apparent reason they sometimes consume larger quantities of dirt, gravel, pieces of wood, or rubber objects, even to the extent of causing stomach or intestinal impaction. Because of its prevalence, the ingestion of feces is discussed as a separate section following this section.

Typical History

The necessity to deal with this problem may come about because of surgery on the stomach to remove pebbles or other objects. The owner may have tried correcting the dog directly for consuming inappropriate material, and by the time the dog is presented for the problem behavior, the behavior may occur only when the owners are not around to deliver corrections.

Diagnosis

Although there is usually no distinctive aspect of behavioral or medical history suggesting a specific nutritional deficiency cause for the behavior, a physical examination, hematology, blood chemistry, and other indicated diagnostic tests, as appropriate, may be needed to rule out pathophysiological causes. A possible contributing factor is understimulation when a dog is left alone in an uninteresting environment. On the other hand, the behavior may be related to anxiety-producing situations. Another differential diagnostic possibility is attention-seeking behavior, which could be diagnosed by the owner noting that the behavior does not occur when the dog believes it is alone (Chapter 15). Compulsive behavior is another possibility if the behavior occurs in the same form repeatedly and the dog appears to be driven to consume certain objects, whether or not the owners are present (Chapter 18).

Treatment Guidelines

The first concern is restricting access to the substrate the dog consumes. If boredom is felt to be related to the problem, steps should be taken to enrich the environment, including instituting consistent human interactions with the dog, such as playing fetch or walking. If the behavior fits the attention-seeking model, Chapter 15 should be consulted. If the behavior is due to separation anxiety, this problem should be addressed as outlined in Chapter 10.

If the behavior seems to be compulsive or of undetermined etiology, and the behavior is threatening to the dog's health, this is an area where remote punishment in the way of a citronella spray or shock collar may offer an expeditious resolution. Guidelines for the use of remote punishment with a citronella spray or even a shock collar are given in Chapter 18 under treatment for acral lick dermatitis. Remember that the dog must have ample opportunity to engage in acceptable behaviors. This approach most certainly will necessitate staging the dog's access to objects inappropriately eaten and arranging the treatment sessions so the dog is likely to believe that the correction came from the objects.

Coprophagy

There are two aspects to this problem. One is a dog eating its own feces or that of other dogs, such as canine housemates. The other is of dogs eating cat feces or, less commonly, horse feces. Eating cat feces is usually more easily managed than eating dog feces.

There is no widely recognized explanation of this behavior but some possibilities have been suggested. In ancestral wolves both males and females were innately programmed to consume fecal droppings of puppies in the nest or den until puppies were able to eliminate on their own. Given this innate predisposition in one context, engaging in the behavior in another, albeit inappropriate, context may be viewed as a reaction to extreme boredom or understimulation. Dogs that habitually consume their own feces are often confined dogs and receive little human interaction. In other instances, eating their own feces can be a type of attention-seeking behavior. Owners may react emotionally to the sight of their dogs eating feces, and a dog may acquire this behavior as a means to garner additional attention.

The severity of this problem ranges from the dog occasionally eating a bit of feces to consuming a large proportion of their own and/or other dog's feces regularly. Coprophagy in nature would be maladaptive because an animal could acquire bacteria or viruses to which it is not immune. Whether in nature or on the domestic scene, the behavior is maladaptive if for no other reason than little nutritional material is taken in. Although in most instances coprophagy is of fresh feces, if the feces are old and contain parasite larvae hatched from parasite eggs, the behavior would infect or reinfect dogs with parasites.

Typical History

Some owners may contact the clinician after one or two episodes of a dog consuming its own feces, and others will seek help only after it has persisted for months, figuring that the behavior was temporary. Because the behavior seems to be intensified in dogs that are closely confined, it is important to understand the environment of the dog and whether the housing situation has changed from being rather free-ranging to a more confined environment at the time the behavior started. The owner may have to do some additional observations, such as determining whether fecal consumption continues when the dog is given a more free-ranging or enriched environment. It is also necessary to determine whether the fecal consumption is of the dog's own feces, that of another dog, or that of cats. Given the difference in makeup of dog and cat feces, consumption of cat feces would appear to constitute a different problem than a dog eating its own or another dog's feces.

Diagnosis

Coprophagy can theoretically be explained as attention-seeking behavior or (rarely) as a compulsive disorder. Another explanation is that the behavior reflects an inappropriate manifestation of an innate predisposition toward consuming feces of pups in the ancestral wolfpack.

Treatment Guidelines

Treatment guidelines are discussed under the topic of consuming dog feces or cat feces.

Consuming dog feces

As with consuming other inappropriate objects, the first approach should be to address the environmental issues related to confinement, lack of stimulation, or attention-seeking aspects that contribute to the behavior. Particular attention should be paid to enriching the environment and increasing social interactions. Giving the dog long-lasting food treats, such as food-stuffed rubber toys or hard plastic flavored toys, may help increase the dog's mental stimulation and decrease the dog's propensity to eat feces. One can also scatter food treats around the yard or set it up so that the dog has to forage for food. Perhaps allowing a dog access to a window facing the street may also help counteract boredom while human family members are gone.

After as much as possible is done to reduce the factors that maintain the behavior, remote punishment of the behavior can be used if needed. Following the principles of effective punishment, lacing fecal droppings with an aversive substance such as hot cayenne pepper sauce is perhaps the most frequently used approach. So as to prevent any unpunished ingestion of unlaced feces, the environment accessible to the dog should be kept clear of all fecal droppings except those used in the conditioning trials. As a last resort, an alternative form of remote punishment is the use of a citronella spray or shock collar, in staged sessions, described for acral lick dermatitis in Chapter 18.

Consuming cat feces

This problem can best be managed by restricting the dog's access to cat feces, assuming that the problem stems from an attraction to the feces rather than as a reflection of boredom or close confinement. Enclosed litter boxes that are cleaned very frequently to prevent odors or isolation of the litter box to a space inaccessible to the dog are possibilities. The use of remote punishment as mentioned above may have to be considered.

Anorexia

We are accustomed to dogs being relatively undiscriminating and rapid eaters, so when they do go off food, it is often quite noticeable. There are several pathophysiological possibilities ranging from the onset of acute infectious disease to intestinal obstruction, as well as behavioral causes. These can usually be differentiated by a thorough medical workup.

Typical History

Dog owners are aware of their dog's individualistic eating behavior. Most dogs can go a day or so without eating, which can be due to hot weather or a change in daily routine, such as the owners going on vacation. Dog owners will generally seek a clinician's advice when there is a major deviation from this pattern for a prolonged period of time. A loss of appetite may be absolute, with the dog refusing all food, or it may be specific to the diet being offered or with the dog eating only food proffered by the owner. In the history it will be necessary to obtain as much information about the past occurrence of the behavior, its onset, and times of the day or week when the anorexia is most prominent, as well as under what circumstances the anorexia occurs. The history should delve into whether the dog's reluctance to eat may occur only if it is cared for by a certain person.

Diagnosis

If the anorexia is an aspect of onset of acute illness in the dog, other signs including fever, lethargy, and depression are likely to be present. Anorexia is a common aspect of illness and is discussed in Chapter 7. Other possibilities of a medical nature are a conditioned food aversion perhaps caused by food allergy, anosmia due to upper respiratory conditions, gastrointestinal obstruction, and food poisoning. Some drugs, particularly those used for cancer chemotherapy, result in an intestinal upset and nausea and may produce an aversion to the food that the dog eats during its treatment. One behavioral cause is attention seeking, which might be suspected for dogs accustomed to lavish attention focused on them when they eat. This syndrome is discussed in Chapter 15. Some dogs have a close bond with a human family member or another dog; when that bonded individual leaves the family or dies, dogs may go off food as a manifestation of depression.

Treatment Guidelines

If an allergy is suspected, eliminating the allergen may not restore an appetite if the food still has the same general olfactory and taste characteristics. It may be necessary to change the olfactory and taste characteristics of the food to sidestep the aversion.

When the loss of appetite is due to loss of the sense of smell, such as secondary to a severe upper respiratory disease, placing salted meat, baby food, or warmed canned dog or cat food into a dog's mouth may stimulate taste receptors and interest the animal in eating again.

As mentioned, anorexia is an adaptive response to febrile illness in general. By losing its appetite, an animal in the wild will stay in its den conserving heat to facilitate acquiring a febrile body temperature to combat a bacterial or viral infection. In this situation it is best to not force-feed the dog at the height of the illness, but to provide optimal nutrition when appetite is recovered in the convalescent stage (Chapter 7). If necessary to maintain body condition in a debilitated animal, internal or parenteral nutrition must be provided to the animal.

Attention-seeking anorexia might have started with a transient illness or even as an aspect of loss of interest in eating stemming from the loss of a canine family member or departure of a close human attachment figure. The approach for attention-seeking anorexia is covered in Chapter 15. With regard to anorexia brought on by the departure of a family member, it may be helpful to point out that extra attention given to the dog, although a reflection of good intentions, prolongs not only the depressionlike behavior but also prolongs the accompanying anorexia.

Obesity

Most people recognize that obesity is primarily a problem of eating too much food for the caloric output, and is the most common nutritional disorder in dogs and cats.

In addition to the overall disadvantages of excessive body weight, some dogs are especially vulnerable. Bulldogs and other breeds that have a brachycephalic head structure may have difficulty exercising if overweight, and they benefit from weight control. In addition to the adverse effects on health, excessive weight can be a real detriment when dogs reach an advanced age and have to be lifted or otherwise handled by their caregivers. The issue of a possible hormonal imbalance commonly comes up, and it is generally believed that castrated or spayed dogs have a higher tendency to become fat than animals with intact gonads. From experimental work there is no question that ovariectomy leads to at least a modest tendency toward increased body weight, increased food intake, and higher fat levels.[12] In female dogs, ovariectomy appears to lead to a minor gain in body weight and food intake. However, the gain is around only 2 to 3 pounds.[13] Experimental findings pertaining to the effect of castration and food intake in males are equivocal. Males that are castrated undergo a moderate reduction in both food intake and body weight, and some muscle mass is replaced by fat tissue.[14]

In both female and male dogs, one could conclude that the effects of gonadectomy on weight gain are probably minor, and that the occurrence of obesity is most appropriately attributed to the owner's behavior in simply feeding the animal more than it needs for its energy output.

In addition to owner-inspired obesity, the possibility of a genetic predisposition toward obesity should be given consideration. Some animals may have an inherited tendency to be fat and may have an appreciably larger number of fat cells than other dogs. The number of fat cells an animal has tends to persist throughout life, and the number of fat cells tends to set the level for total volume of body fat.

Typical History

Obesity may be brought up by the clinician to the owner as an aspect of a dog's general overall health. This is a problem that can exacerbate multiple medical problems such as arthritis, cardiac disease, and diabetes. It is important for the clinician to recognize that it is inherent in people's love and affection for animals that they wish to nurture them. One of the main ways of nurturing a dog is by giving it food that it seems to really enjoy. Thus the history might focus on aspects of the owners' behavior and how they express interaction with the dog rather than on the dog's eating behavior.

Diagnosis

Certain disease conditions may lead to obesity and should be ruled out by history and/or clinical tests. These are hypothyroidism, hyperadrenocorticalism, and tumors of insulin-producing cells. A genetic predisposition may be evident from reviewing the weight of the dog's parents and siblings. Aside from the pathophysiological causes or a genetic predisposition toward obesity, the main reason dogs overeat is because they are offered an excessive amount of highly palatable food, and they lead a rather inactive existence. Like wolves, dogs are capable of consuming considerably more than they need on a daily basis.

Treatment Guidelines

For the dog that has only recently become overweight, a general medical workup is in order to rule out or rule in pathophysiological causes of the excessive appetite or tendency to gain weight on the same amount of food. After medical conditions are ruled out or resolved, attention is focused on the owner's behavior, because the owners control what the dog eats. A number of strategies have been proposed to help dog owners deal with obesity.[15,16] In general, you should counsel a client to look for other ways of showing love and nurture for a dog, such as playing its favorite game, teaching it commands or tricks, grooming it, or taking it for walks. It may be useful to point out that when a dog's diet is changed to being less palatable, this may be the time to switch the nurturing role away from the food bowl to other types of interaction. Establishing a routine with a diet that the dog will eat to maintain an appropriate weight and good health will be easier on the dog and the owner in the long run and be of immeasurable value as the dog gets older. Increasing the dog's exercise output may also help reduce the obesity as long as the diet is not also increased. Vigorous exercise, such as playing fetch or running alongside the owner who is jogging, might be suggested if these changes in exercise can be maintained on a regular basis.

References

1. Mugford RA. External influences on the feeding of carnivores. In: Kare MR, Maller O, eds. The Chemical Senses and Nutrition. New York: Academic Press, Inc., 1977.
2. Boulcott SR. Feeding behaviour of adult dogs under conditions of hospitalization. British Veterinary Journal 1967;123:498-507.
3. Garcia J, Hankins WG, Rusiniak KW. Behavioral regulation of the milieu interne in man and rat. Science 1974;185:824-831.
4. Gustavson CR, Garcia J, Hankins WG, Rusiniak KW. Coyote predation control by aversive conditioning. Science 1974;184:581-583.
5. Forthman Quick DL, Gustavson CR, Rusiniak KW. Coyote control and taste aversion. Appetite 1985;6:253–264.
6. Andersone Z. Summer nutrition of wolf (*Canis lupus*) in the Slitere Nature Reserve. Proceedings of the Latvian Academy of Sciences 1998;52:79–80.
7. Mech LD. The timber wolf and its ecology. In: Fauna of the National Parks of the United States: The Wolves of the Isle Royale. Washington: United States Government Printing Office, 1966.
8. Robinette WL, Gashwiler JS, Morris OW. Food habits of the cougar in Utah and Nevada. Journal of Wildlife Management 1959;23:261–273.
9. Sueda KL, Hart BL, Cliff KD. Plant eating in dogs: Characteristics and determination of underlying causes. Unpublished observations.
10. Huffman MA, Canton JM. Self-induced increase of gut motility and the control of parasitic infections in wild chimpanzees. International Journal of Primatology 2001;22:329–346.
11. Hart BL. The evolution of herbal medicine: Behavioural perspectives. Animal Behavior 2005, 70:975-989.
12. Wade GN. Sex hormones, regulatory behaviors, and body weight. In: Rosenblatt JS, Hinde RA, Shaw E, Beer C, eds. Advances in the Study of Behavior. Vol. 6. New York: Academic Press, Inc., 1976;201–279.

13. Houpt KA, Coren B, Hintz HF. Effect of sex and reproductive status on sucrose preference, food intake, and body weight of dogs. Journal of the American Veterinary Medical Association 1979;174:1083-1085.
14. Gentry R, Wade GN. Androgenic control of food intake and body weight in male rats. Journal of Comparative Physiology and Psychology 1976;90:18-25.
15. Houpt KA. Feeding and drinking behavior problems. Veterinary Clinics of North America Small Animal Practice 1991;21:281–298.
16. Norris MP, Beaver BV. Application of behavior therapy techniques to the treatment of obesity in companion animals. Journal of the Veterinary Medical Association 1993;202:728–730.

Chapter 17

Problems with Sexual and Maternal Behavior of Dogs

Concerns about various aspects of reproductive behavior may range from inappropriate sexual behavior by companion dogs to difficulty in breeding animals maintained by commercial breeders or family breeders having their first litter. Under the topics of sexual behavior, this chapter deals first with sexual inadequacy and lack of interest on the part of designated breeding males or females; then it explores objectionable sexual behavior, such as mounting of people, inanimate objects, and other dogs by male dogs. An understanding of normal behavior is needed to deal with both types of problems, so this section includes a brief description of normal sexual behavior of males and females before going into problem areas. Under the topic of maternal behavior, the problems of maternal neglect of puppies and attacking or cannibalism of the young are covered. Again, a discussion of normal behavior is essential to establish a reference point for problem behavior.

Normal Sexual Behavior

Male puppies typically exhibit sexual mounting as a normal part of play behavior. As puppies approach adulthood they have less interest in mounting as part of play and channel their sexual responses toward females in estrus. Prior to puberty, females display scarcely any sexual responses, and their sexual behavior develops normally without early sexual play. The ovaries of females reaching puberty secrete estrogen twice a year. Estrogen has the effect in most animals of increasing general activity. Thus, a female dog usually moves about more, vocalizes more frequently, and may act nervous during estrus. Urine and vaginal secretions of female dogs in proestrus and estrus are attractive to males. Dog owners report that male dogs are attracted from some distance away to the vicinity of an estrous female, presumably by one or more chemical attractants in the urine. Because they communicate the message of sexual receptivity, these sexual attractants are sometimes termed sex pheromones. These pheromones are probably not so potent as to be detected in the air by males from miles away, but they could certainly be noticed by males on their neighborhood treks. The nature of the pheromone of female dogs is not known. Female dogs that are in estrus may mount other females. Dog owners with two female dogs may occasionally even observe a spayed or an estrous female mounting an estrous female, or vice versa.

Adult mating behavior generally begins with anogenital investigation of the female, some attempts at playing with her, and a few mounts with pelvic thrusting (Fig. 17-1). A female may mount the male, especially if the male's sexual advances are rather slow. When genital intromission occurs, it is somewhat a result of trial and error thrusting. Thus, a male may mount and thrust several times before achieving intromission. The female aids in intromission with her receptive responses, such as the lateral curvature of the rear quarters, deviation of the tail, and movement of the external genitalia. Male dogs differ individually in the extent of their courtship patterns, with some attempting copulation almost as soon as they are placed with females, and others taking longer.

At the time of genital intromission, a marked change occurs in the behavior of the male. As the front legs are pulled caudally, the tail is deflected downward, and stepping activity of the rear legs occurs (Fig. 17-1). Some animals show alternate stepping of the back legs so high that they are thrown off balance. This initial part of copulation lasts for usually 15–30 seconds. At this time the sperm-dense fraction of semen is expelled. Also at this time the penis engorges within the vagina and the male and female are effectively locked together (Fig. 17-1). The bulb of the penis is so engorged that it must remain in the vagina until erection subsides.

During this phase of copulation the female usually stands rigidly, but toward the end of this reaction the female often starts twisting and turning. The male is likely to dismount, but if not, she is likely to throw the male off. The male then turns and lifts one leg over the penis so that the two animals end up in the tail-to-tail, genital-lock position. The genital lock generally lasts from 10–30 minutes, although a lock as short as 5 minutes or as long as 60 minutes is within the normal range. Prostatic fluid, but little sperm, is ejaculated during the genital lock. A lock is not necessary

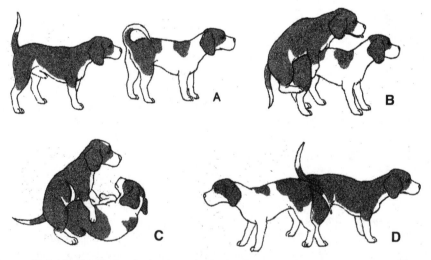

Figure 17-1   Mating behavior in dogs. In A, the female is shown in the receptive posture with tail deviation as the male investigates the female. In B, intromission occurs and the female is motionless during the intense thrusting of the male. In C, the dogs are locked and the female engages in twisting and turning, often throwing off the male. In D, the dogs remain quiet in the genital lock, lasting 10–30 minutes.

for fertilization to occur because litters can be produced by artificial insemination. Although it was once believed that contraction of the female's vaginal constrictor muscles maintained the male's erection during the genital lock, it is now known that erection of the penis is from penile muscles contracting and occluding the venous return, while the arterial blood to the erectile tissues is increased. If the penis becomes engorged prior to intromission, or if it is pulled from the vagina prematurely, detumescence can be facilitated by touching the distal end of the penis. After the genital lock breaks apart the male invariably spends a good deal of time licking the penis and adjacent genital areas.

An interesting aspect of breeding in dogs is that they seem to be not nearly as beset by sexually transmitted diseases as domesticated hoofstock such as cattle and horses. The answer, at least partially, reflects characteristics of canine sexual behavior. In nature the monogamous behavior of the wolf kept females from being exposed to many other males; the less exposure, the less the opportunity to pick up a genital disease. Another important preventative behavior is the almost compulsive manner in which the male licks the penis immediately after the termination of the genital lock. If a female happened to be harboring a genital pathogen that might have infected a male and impaired his future fertility, the male's thorough licking would physically remove much of the contamination. Furthermore, canine saliva has antibacterial substances. Thus genital licking is helpful in preventing a male from picking up a pathogen from a female.[1,2]

Problems with Inadequate Sexual Behavior in Breeding Animals

Problems may be transient or of long duration. One type of temporary problem relates to the need some males have for familiarity with the environment before engaging in sexual interactions with the female. For this reason, females are usually brought to the male's environment for breeding. However, if a male dog readily adapts to new environments, there is no reason that he could not be brought to the female's home. Lack of correct orientation of mounting by the male may reflect some social isolation as a puppy and too little sexual play and contact with other puppies during early life. This could be a relatively permanent problem and not necessarily be amenable to correction through behavior modification.

Females may show a preference for certain males even when they are in full estrus. A less-frequent occurrence is that some male dogs prefer to mate with certain females and tend to reject other females that are fully receptive. In modern breeding operations we expect male dogs to be promiscuous breeders and not choosy as to the sexual partner. Keep in mind, however, that the ancestor of the dog was basically monogamous and predisposed to be selective with regard to mates. The term silent estrus refers to the condition in which a female shows the physiological, but not the behavioral, signs of estrus. Presumably the brain is not responding to estrogen secretion the same as the genital system. However, because some female dogs have been observed to have definite preferences for certain males, they may not appear to be in estrus when in fact in the presence of a different male they would show some sexual interest.

When problems with breeding dogs become too difficult to handle behaviorally, artificial insemination is frequently employed. If it is necessary to obtain semen from male dogs for artificial insemination, that breeder should keep in mind that the ejaculatory response is susceptible to inhibition. In some instances, one may need to place a receptive female near the male to provide some sexual stimulation. To evoke ejaculation, the body of the penis proximal to the glans should be stimulated until rhythmic contractions begin. If this process does not produce ejaculation, then placing mild pressure on the tip of the urethral process at the same time may evoke ejaculation.

Objectionable Mounting Behavior

Male puppies may mount people as part of play behavior and, as long as it is not discouraged, it will continue. Most puppies will outgrow this behavior. Until then a correction is usually sufficient to stop the behavior. If there was little opportunity for the dog to interact with other dogs when it was young, it is possible that in some dogs the mounting of people is a reflection of overattachment to people during early life. The main point to keep in mind in correcting persistent mounting is to correct every act and avoid any reward of mounting by attention or social interaction.

The mounting of people or dogs by adult dogs is most common in males and, if seen in gonadally intact males entering adulthood, castration is indicated. One can expect a resolution of this problem in about 25% of problem dogs and improvement of at least 50% reduction in about 70% (Fig. 17-2).[3]

For the neutered male dog that continues to engage repeatedly in highly objectionable mounting despite correction, the owner should discourage this behavior by completely ignoring the dog, even to the point of walking out of the room every time the dog mounts. As a last resort, the owner can use some sort of remote punishment, such as an ultrasonic noisemaker or squirt gun triggered without the dog seeing it (Chapter 3). Basically every act of mounting must be punished, which means that the opportunity to engage in the behavior must be physically prevented until one is prepared to administer the punishment. With a remote punishment it is important that the correcting stimulus be associated with the mounting and not with the person delivering the punishment.

Normal Maternal Behavior

Maternal behavior is an area in which the behavior of the dam is so important to the survival of the offspring that evolutionary forces have programmed the neural circuitry for this behavior into the brains of dogs. Even a mother that has had no previous opportunity to observe or engage in the care of a newborn suddenly, at the time of parturition, performs a relatively complex sequence of maternal tasks, which continues and changes until her offspring are able to survive on their own. The specific elements of maternal behavior are performed with perfect timing and precision.

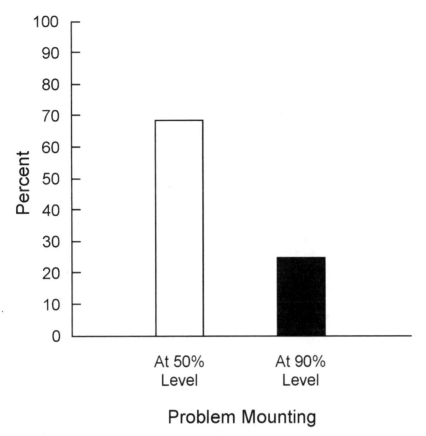

Problem Mounting

Figure 17-2 Effects of castration in improving mounting behavior in males. Shown is improvement at the 50% level, representing at least 50% improvement, and at the 90% level, representing virtual resolution. Shown are percent of dogs responding at each level.

The mother has an emotional attachment to her young that represents the strongest interindividual bond in nature. She is even willing to risk her life for these new animals which she hardly knows yet. Although maternal care is essential for the welfare of newborn, social interactions with the mother and littermates also prepare the young for later social behavioral patterns and temperament. These interactions are crucial for shaping the behavior of pups to be desirable as pets; deprivation of this interaction, by early weaning or orphanage, may be behaviorally costly.

Many professional dog breeders and family breeders are anxious to step in and help canine mothers when any aspect of maternal behavior appears insufficient or the lives or comfort of the pups are threatened. For example, supplemental bottle feeding and assistance in weaning pups onto solid food are often provided, as well as help in the birth processes by cleaning and grooming the pups, cleaning the mouth, stimulating respiration, and inducing the first defecation. Although the innate aspects of these maternal behaviors are programmed into the brain, this programming is not immutable, and our intervention through centuries of dog domestication has facilitated survival and reproduction of mothers with potential deficits in this behavioral programming.

In nature, offspring from mothers who have poor mothering behaviors would not survive. Thus, poor mothering reaches a dead end. Contrast this with the domestic dog where, with some mothers, few or no pups would survive if assistance were not provided to bitches in giving birth and raising young. Under our care bitches who have poor mothering skills may produce as many offspring as those bitches who have complete and effective maternal behavior from birth through weaning. The result is that the gene pool of most domesticated breeds includes a great deal of variability in elements controlling maternal behavior among individual dogs. The problems of maternal neglect and infanticide, covered later, probably reflect some relaxed natural selection coupled with confronting a bitch with an urban birthing environment for which she has little evolutionary preparation. Perhaps it is amazing that mother dogs do as well as they do.

Because relatively few of the basic behavioral patterns of mothering are learned, it is erroneous to assume that major deficiencies in maternal care stem from a bitch's inexperience, or to think that a bitch will necessarily learn the required behavior with subsequent litters. Some habituation, however, may play a role in making experienced bitches less nervous or anxious than naive ones. To the degree that nervousness interferes with the behavior of growing pups, or leads to infanticide, the experienced bitch may be a better mother. Dog owners occasionally ask whether having a litter of puppies will have a lasting calming effect on the mother. Although this effect may occur occasionally, perhaps by chance, there is no documentation to support this notion. It is certainly not advisable for a client to have a bitch bred to try to solve a behavior problem involving excitability or excessive activity.

There are two aspects of canine maternal behavior that differ from other domestic animals. One is that their wild ancestors were monogamous, with both parents available for caring for the newborn. Sires stayed around and customarily played a role in the care of the litter. Secondly, females of the ancestral wolf pack that did not conceive often went through mammary gland development, produced milk, and displayed maternal behavior at the same time of year as their packmates with offspring. When this occurs in a domestic dog it is referred to as pseudopregnancy. The extended family of the wolf includes aunts who serve as nursemaids, the sire, and other male wolves of the pack who, along with the mother, often help at the time of weaning with feeding of the young by regurgitating food for their consumption. All members of the pack play a role in teaching wolf pups to hunt. Because pack members are usually related, they are contributing toward the survival of offspring with which they share some genes. The following is a summary of stages in the changes in maternal behavior as a function of age of the offspring.

Behavior Before and During Parturition

Licking of the mammary gland area and genital areas increases just before parturition. A mother frequently licks and cleans the nipples that the pups will eventually latch onto for suckling. Maternal saliva has antibacterial properties,[1] which further removes potentially harmful bacteria from the nipples. Given that the newborn pup has not yet received any antibody-rich colostrum, and has a gut that is easily penetrated by bacteria, licking the mammary area is an important disease protection behavior of the mother. In addition, newborn pups may not attach to a nipple that does not smell or taste like maternal saliva. This keeps the pup from latching onto some non-nipple area that might be contaminated with coliform or other potentially pathogenic bacteria.

A pregnant bitch often becomes somewhat restless and nervous a few days prior to parturition. The dog may follow the owners around excessively and may also tend to lie down for only a short while, get up, move, and then lie down again. The birth process can begin almost any time after this restlessness is evident (assuming the estimated time of gestation has elapsed). Pups are delivered in four phases: 1) contraction, 2) delivery of fetuses, 3) delivery of the placentas, and 4) the interval between deliveries. Uterine contractions begin in the first stage, and there is a good deal of straining. Most bitches lie down during contractions, and they may frequently move and change positions. Uterine and abdominal contractions become more intense in the second stage as the fetus moves rapidly through the birth canal. The female often breaks and tugs at the fetal membranes with her teeth as the head or buttocks of the fetus appears at the vulva. This tugging on the membranes may actually pull the fetus through the birth canal.

After the newborn passes through the birth canal, the bitch consumes the fetal membranes and licks the newborn vigorously, which usually causes the first respiratory movements. The mother continues to lick and groom the newborn, and when the placenta is delivered, it is usually eaten also. The mother generally bites off the umbilical cord while she is eating the placenta. The mother's eating of the placenta and umbilical cord, with the associated pulling and stretching, seems to cause constriction of the blood vessels in the cord so that little or no blood loss occurs. A neonate pup may sometimes be accidentally wounded by a bitch puncturing the abdominal wall after chewing off the cord. If the umbilical cord is not broken soon after birth, it may be necessary for a person to intervene at this point. During licking and grooming of the newborn the mother concentrates more on the anogenital region of the newborn, stimulating defecation and the expulsion of meconium.

Between deliveries the mother continues to lick and groom the newborn animals as well as her own genital region and also cleans the bedding that has been soiled with amniotic fluids. The stages of labor vary widely in duration, with some puppies born just a few minutes apart and others an hour or so apart, but the total duration of parturition usually does not exceed 12 hours. Following the birth of the last pup, the female lies almost continuously with her young for a period of about 12 hours.

Nursing and Other Aspects of Maternal Care

Nursing is the focus of much of the interaction between a bitch and her puppies. This interaction begins as soon as the young begin to suckle, which can occur before the delivery of the last newborn. Although finding a teat might appear to be a random process, it is more systematic than that. Moving toward the warmth of the mother's body, neonates crawl slowly and irregularly with paddlelike movements of the front legs while pushing with the hind legs. They "scan" the area ahead by moving their heads from side to side, and eventually they come into contact with the mother's ventral wall. The young then climb onto the mother's body and nuzzle into the mother's fur until they locate a nipple, using chemosensory cues from the mother's saliva.

A problem somewhat related to the use of odor cues of nipples is the occasional reluctance of pups that are delivered by cesarean section to attach to a nipple. Because the nipples may have been scrubbed as part of the surgical preparation, there may be no odor of maternal saliva on the nipples. A remedy is to rub maternal saliva on the nipples, which had previously been washed and disinfected in preparation for the operation.

The first stage of nursing lasts for 3 weeks after parturition, and through this phase the mother initiates essentially all nursing sessions. The bitch approaches the pups and lies near them and then arouses them by licking. With time the newborn become very adept at finding teats and responding to the mother's solicitous behavior. Apparently puppies do not take specific nipple positions.

In the second phase of nursing, beginning in about the third week and extending to the fourth week, the young are able to leave the bed. With their eyes and ears functioning well, they are able to recognize and interact with the mother outside the bed. Nursing sessions may occur inside the bed or outside and are now mostly initiated by the young. Usually the mother cooperates by immediately lying down or by exposing her teats if she is already lying down.

The period from about the thirtieth day after birth and extending into weaning constitutes the third phase, when practically all nursing sessions are initiated by the young. Increasingly, the young follow the mother, and as time progresses, the mother begins to avoid nursing attempts of the young. She may lie with her mammary region against the floor or go to where the young cannot reach her. Near the end of this phase, when the mother is increasingly less accessible to the young, the young become capable of taking adult food.

In wild carnivores, where young must eventually learn to kill prey, the transition from nursing to solid food is gradual. Various strategies to facilitate the transition in the wild are used in different species. In wolves, the pack members, including the dam and sire, feed their pups by regurgitating a freshly consumed meal. Wolf pups eagerly "beg" for the partially processed food by pawing and biting at the lips of an adult who has just returned to the nest. In time the pups are also introduced to freshly killed small game, or parts of a carcass of a larger prey, which are brought to the den. The prey dragged to the den undoubtedly pick up bacteria from the ground which should act as a sensitizing dose of common environmental bacteria for development of the infant immune sysytem.[4]

It is only when pups have acquired hunting skills by traveling with the older members of the pack that the pups are capable of living on their own. Under domestication, modern lactating female dogs only infrequently regurgitate food to their young in the manner of wolves. When this does occur dog owners should not be overly concerned or assume the bitch is ill. They should understand this is a normal aspect of canids in nature. The absence of regurgitation does profile the need for caregivers to provision puppies at the time of weaning with food that is palatable and easily chewed.

A lactating bitch will usually accept puppies from another litter, a behavior common in polytocous, or litter-bearing, species. The adopted puppies may even be a couple of weeks older than her own, or even of another species, such as young cats, skunks, or squirrels. This open-arms adoption policy stands in contrast to that of monotocous species, which normally produce just one offspring—such as cattle, sheep, and goats—and where rejection of alien young is so prominent. In the dog's ancestry, there was apparently no natural selection for a wolf mother to reject another's young. In all likelihood, the only young that would show up in the nest in nature would be those related to her. Ungulates, on the other hand, give birth in a group where accepting an alien young would squander the mother's resources on nonrelated offspring.

Interactions Between a Mother and Her Young

Newborn puppies are in contact with their mother around the clock. Puppies also spend a great amount of time interacting with littermates. Thus, the interaction with the mother is not only important for the survival of the offspring, but it also provides the foundation for the subsequent social behavior of dogs. Although basic social responses are innate, the early experience of a puppy with its mother and littermates refines and develops basic responses, including the appropriate use of submissive gestures. A pup's aggressive behavior is also shaped by interacting with other puppies.

If puppies are exposed only to their littermates and have little contact with people, they tend to develop strong attachments to dogs and only with great difficulty form close attachments to people. They may even exhibit fear and escape responses toward people. If a puppy is removed at about 3 weeks of age from its littermates and then exposed only to people, it may be primarily attached to people and show abnormal social responses toward other dogs. Rather than resolving conflicts by threat and submission, for example, they may readily fight with other dogs. Ideally, puppies should be exposed to dogs and people during the socialization period.

The best age for adoption of a puppy into the new home is dependent on opportunities for socialization of the puppy. If socialization opportunities are inadequate at the breeder, it may be wise to take the puppy home at 6 weeks of age. If the breeder has the time and ability to socialize the puppy adequately to new stimuli, people, and environments, it may be better to keep the puppy in that environment until 8–10 weeks of age if the environment at the new home is not as richly endowed with social opportunities.

Problems with Maternal Behavior

There are two general potential problems with maternal behavior: maternal indifference, and infanticide and cannibalism. On the domestic scene these behaviors may reflect relaxation of natural selection of optimal maternal care in some individuals coupled with unnatural stimuli for which the mother dog has little evolutionary preparation.

Maternal Indifference

Although maternal indifference may be a result of domestication and relaxation of natural selection, it might also reflect a hormonal defect in the endocrine changes that help bring about maternal behavior. It is known that the strong attachment of a bitch for newborn puppies, as well as specific behavioral "housekeeping" tasks, such as cleaning up the puppies and nest, are facilitated by hormonal changes at the time of birth. An alteration from normal hormonal secretions could underlie a deficiency in the induction of optimal maternal care, especially if the stimuli at the particular time are inadequate. For some polytocous species a single newborn may not provide enough stimulation to the mother to maintain satisfactory maternal behavior and lactation, even for the one newborn.[5] If this applies to dogs, the work suggests that the bitch with a litter of only one pup should be carefully observed so that compensatory measures can be taken if she does not provide adequate maternal care.

Infanticide and Cannibalism

Despite the physiological buffering from stressful stimuli, mothers can become activated and engage in behaviors that seem horrifying to dog owners and certainly not in keeping with being an attentive and loving mother. At the top of the list of savage acts is maternal cannibalism of one or more newborn pups. It should be noted that killing and cannibalism of newborn has been observed not only in dogs and cats, but in laboratory rodents and various species of wild animals as well. The thing about this seemingly horrendous behavior is that in nature it may often be viewed as normal. Postparturient female hamsters, for example, almost invariably kill and consume one or more of their offspring as the mother adjusts her litter size in accordance with prevailing environmental conditions and food supply.[6] At other times cannibalism may be brought on by nutritional stress of the mother. In squirrel monkeys, for example, cannibalism may occur with females on a low-protein diet.[7]

Another circumstance when maternal cannibalism can be considered normal relates to detection and removal of sick newborns to save the rest of the litter.[4] Sickly newborns might harbor disease organisms that could be transmitted to littermates. If a mother attacks and consumes the sickly animal, she loses the affected offspring but saves the rest of the litter. The trigger for such cannibalism may be cold or inactive pups. To make this system work, the mother's cannibalism must be triggered by any slight abnormality in the newborn, such that the sick animal is disposed of before opportunistic pathogens multiply in the dying newborn to the extent that the infected newborn threatens the rest of the litter. In nature, the mother, who is relatively immune to environmental bacteria, not only removes the source of threatening bacteria, but obtains a meal by eating the sick pup, thus precluding one more trip away from the den.

The mother cannot, of course, actually diagnose a disease, but must operate on signs that are correlated with disease, such as an inactive, nonresponsive, or cold newborn. Deformed young that would probably not survive in nature could also trigger infanticide and cannibalism, and veterinarians and breeders are familiar with mothers that have killed and eaten physically deformed pups.[8] An explanation as to why a mother dog on the domestic scene would kill and consume pups that are not sick or deformed is that some environmental stimulus may be upsetting and incidentally trigger the cannibalism syndrome. This may happen with a new mother that is not habituated to the birthing environment or some environmental stimuli of which a breeder may not be aware.

In the way of resolution, one could examine the environment of the whelping area for disturbances that might serve as triggers of the behavior so that the rest of the litter, or future litters, are less likely to be affected. A mother that repeatedly engages in infanticide is more likely to continue this behavior, and clients should be advised accordingly.

Pseudopregnancy

Before this behavioral syndrome was understood, pseudopregnancy in dogs was considered an abnormality. This is probably because, of all domestic female animals, only the bitch has been observed to show behavioral signs of pseudopregnancy. At one time the dog was considered a possible animal model of the classic human behavioral disorder characterized by a barren woman whose obsession with wanting a child caused her to experience the physiological and behavioral changes associated with normal pregnancy. It is now known that pseudopregnancy in barren female wolves whose sibling packmate is pregnant is functional, because in a wolf pack there is usually pairing between just the dominant male and one female. Nonpregnant or nonlactating females who are aunts of the pups can serve as nursemaids, and in this way they contribute to the survival of offspring related to them and indirectly enhance their reproductive fitness. Female dogs retain this capacity to varying degrees, so the behavior we see should be considered normal, albeit usually undesirable, on the domestic scene.

In dogs the syndrome starts prior to parturition with the bitch showing enlargement of the mammary area and abdomen. The mammary glands may develop to the point of secreting milk. Many dog owners, not knowing whether the dog was mated or not, might suspect that the bitch is pregnant. Pseudopregnancy usually subsides within the last 2 weeks of the expected parturition. In some bitches, however, the pseudopregnancy continues into parturition with the female displaying behavioral signs of impending parturition, including abdominal contractions and straining. Soon afterward the dog may collect a few stuffed toys and treat them as newborn puppies, licking and hovering over them as if to nurse them (Fig. 17-3). This variant of maternal behavior may continue for as long as a normal lactation, ending at the expected time of weaning, when the bitch abandons the adopted toys and her behavior returns to normal.

Pseudopregnancy does not occur in spayed bitches. The syndrome appears to be brought on by the secretion of prolactin and progesterone, the latter secreted by the ovarian corpus luteum, which forms after ovulation occurs. Spaying a dog in the postparturient stage does not immediately eliminate the behavior, suggesting that prolactin is the hormone responsible for maintaining maternal behavior. Differences in dogs in the predisposition to show behavioral signs of pseudopregnancy would seem to lie in the sensitivity of neural elements in the brain rather than the hormones.

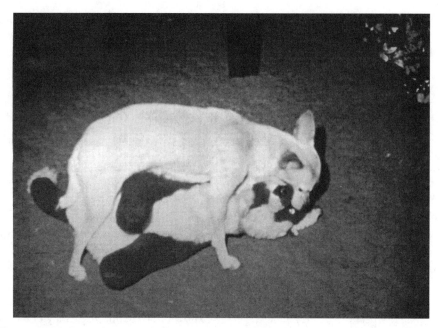

Figure 17-3 Behavioral aspect of pseudopregnancy in a dog. Shown is a Chihuahua attempting to nurse a stuffed teddy bear. The female dog lost interest in the stuffed toy at the approximate time of weaning in mother dogs.

References

1. Hart BL, Powell KL. Antibacterial properties of saliva: Role of maternal periparturient grooming and in licking wounds. Physiology and Behavior 1990;48:383–386.
2. Hart BL, Korinek E, Brennan P. Postcopulatory genital grooming in male rats. Prevention of sexually transmitted infections. Physiology and Behavior 1987;41:321–325.
3. Neilson JC, Eckstein RA, Hart BL. Effects of castration on behavior of male dogs with reference to the role of age and experience. Journal of the American Veterinary Medical Association 1997;211:180–182.
4. Hart BL. Behavioral adaptations to pathogens and parasites: Five strategies. Neuroscience and Biobehavioral Review 1990;14:273–294.
5. Leigh H, Hofer M. Behavioral and physiological effects of littermate removal on the remaining single pup and mother during the preweaning period on rats. Psychosomatic Medicine 1973;35:497-508.
6. Day C, Galef B. Pup cannibalism: One aspect of maternal behavior in golden hamsters. Journal of Comparative Physiology and Psychology 1977;91:1179-1189.
7. Manocha S. Abortion and cannibalism in squirrel monkeys (*Saimiri sciureus*) associated with experimental protein deficiency during gestation. Laboratory Animal Science 1976;26:649-650.
8. Harkness JE, Wagner JE. The Biology and Medicine of Rabbits and Rodents. Philadelphia: Lea and Feibiger, 1989.

Chapter 18

Repetitive, Compulsive, and Stereotypic Behaviors

Whereas the material presented in the preceding chapters deals with problem behaviors that can usually be considered normal or adaptive from the dog's standpoint, this chapter, and Chapter 19 on cognitive dysfunction, deal with behaviors that are abnormal and appear to have no adaptive or functional value from the standpoint of the dog or its evolutionary ancestor. Examples of behavior problems covered in this chapter are excessive tail chasing, repetitive snapping at imaginary flies, chasing shadows, flank sucking, and excessive licking of the carpus or tarsus (referred to as *acral lick dermatitis*). Of all of these behavioral disorders, acral lick dermatitis has received the most attention from clinicians in trying to understand the etiology and exploring various treatments. Common to all of these behavioral problems is that they show a high degree of constancy from one occasion to the next, both within and between animals. The behaviors have no apparent adaptive value from the animal's standpoint, and the dogs seem to be driven or under a compulsion to engage in the behavior.

There has been some discussion about the etiology and nature of these behavioral disorders, especially in comparison to the repetitive and highly stereotyped behaviors seen in confined farm and zoo animals, where pacing, swaying, mouthing, and biting are common. In livestock and zoo animals the stereotypic behaviors are usually attributed to environmental stress from confinement and boredom, and in some instances, crowding or social isolation. The behaviors may be viewed as coping strategies that are reinforced by the release of morphinelike endorphins. A major problem with this comparison is that companion dogs engaging in repetitive, stereotypic behaviors are usually not subjected to the extremes of confinement, boredom, or crowding seen in some livestock or zoo animals.

The repetitive and stereotypic behaviors of dogs share similarities with human compulsive disorders such as excessive hand washing or hair pulling. Psychiatrists generally attribute these behaviors in humans to an effort to prevent or reduce anxiety or stress; patients often report being compelled or driven to perform the behavioral acts. These human compulsive behaviors are often accompanied by an obsession with ideas, thoughts, impulses, or images that cause anxiety or distress, and the compulsions seem to relieve the anxiety caused by the obsessions. Collectively, these human disorders are referred to as obsessive-compulsive disorders (OCDs), and are often treated by serotonergic drugs with antianxiety and antiobsessional properties, such as fluoxetine and clomipramine. Like dogs, human OCD patients do not generally suffer from the confinement, crowding, isolation, or boredom that seem to underlie farm or zoo animal stereotypies. Although the behavioral disorders of dogs covered in this chapter share the apparent compulsiveness of human OCDs in repeatedly performing an identical act, the term OCD implies a verbal report of the patient's obsessions with ideas, thoughts, impulses, or images, which cannot be addressed in dogs. Thus, the human OCD model, with an emphasis on mental obsessions, does not seem to apply to dogs.

Until more is understood about the underlying mechanisms of these behaviors in dogs, it seems appropriate to use the terms *compulsive* and *stereotypic* behaviors. *Stereotypic* refers to the behavioral topography, that identical acts are performed repeatedly, and *compulsive* refers to an apparent internal drive to engage in the behavior that has no anchor in adaptive innate behavior of the ancestral dog or prior learning. Clearly for some of the behaviors there seems to be a genetically related breed predisposition. Doberman Pinschers have been reported to be particularly prone to a flank sucking disorder that is uncommon in other breeds (Fig. 18-1).[1] Acral lick dermatitis is particularly prevalent in large, sporting breeds, such as the Labrador Retrievers.[2] In those instances where there is a genetically related predisposition, perhaps reflecting some neurotransmitter abnormality, the behavior may occur spontaneously; in other instances, the behavior occurs only when evoked by conflict, boredom, or isolation. Not uncommonly, reinforcing attention from the dog owners may intensify the behavior.

With the exception of acral lick dermatitis, the compulsive and stereotypic disorders can all be handled with the same approach with regard to diagnosis and treatment guidelines. Because more clinical research has been directed to acral lick

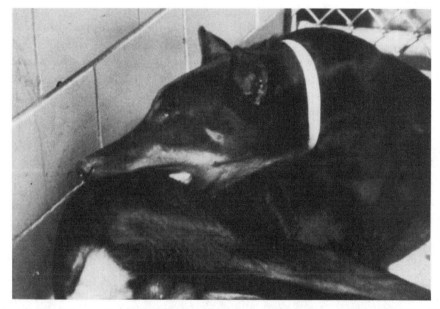

Figure 18-1 Compulsive and highly stereotypic flank sucking in a Doberman Pinscher. This behavior occurred primarily when the dog was alone and undisturbed.

dermatitis than the other compulsive and stereotypic behaviors, this syndrome will be treated as a separate topic.

Compulsive and Stereotypic Tail Chasing, Flank Sucking, and Fly Snapping

Although a large variety of behaviors could come under this heading, the stereotypic behaviors of tail chasing, tail checking (looking at the tail repeatedly), snapping in the air as though to catch imaginary flies, chasing shadows or light flashes, and flank sucking are the most frequently mentioned. All these behaviors appear to be compulsively driven. The onset can sometimes be related to confinement, boredom, conflict, and/or isolation. As often as not, however, no clearly identifiable environmental factor is evident. Given the breed predispositions mentioned earlier, a logical possibility is that an abnormal pattern of neurotransmitter secretion predisposes the animals to engage in the repetitive behaviors in an environmental situation that creates no problem for most dogs but which may evoke the behavior in dogs with the predisposition.

Typical History

Dog owners will often not report these behaviors as soon as they are manifested because they are usually harmless in terms of injury to the dog or inconvenience to the owner. There seems to be a gradual onset, with a dog showing the repetitive pattern on occasion, and which becomes increasingly frequent. When the owner realizes that clearly something is wrong, professional help or advice is sought. Often, the owners will have attempted to distract the dog from the behavior, to calm it down or reassure it. If the owners are pronounced in their comforting or reassurance they may actually be reinforcing the display of the behavior, which then further increases the frequency or intensity. Exploration of the history should deal with possible boredom, confinement, or conflict. It is useful to have the owners bring in a video recording of the behavior, both when they are present and gone from the home, and to take additional notes as to the time and circumstances under which the behavior is most likely or frequent.

Diagnosis

The diagnostic workup to identify possible pathophysiological, environmental, and attention-seeking factors initiating or maintaining the behavior is necessary to order to outline a treatment program. These aspects of diagnosis are profiled in the following sections.

Contributing pathophysiological causes

Some of the stereotypic behaviors may have been initially displayed as the result of a medical problem, such as an irritation of nerves that supply part of the tail, which induced some tail chasing or tail checking. Fly snapping could have been brought on by retinal artery remnants in the aqueous humor or other problems in the visual system. Thus, a general physical examination, with particular attention to any abnormality that could be related to the onset and maintenance of the behavior, is indicated. Keep in mind that the behavioral manifestations of a previous patho-physiologic process that has since resolved may be maintained by reinforcement of the behavior through comfort or attention.

Contributing environmental causes

The main criterion to use in evaluating the degree to which confinement, boredom, conflict, or isolation play a role in initiating or maintaining the compulsive behavior is if the owner can identify the onset of one or more of these factors with the onset of the problem behavior. This role of environmental stress or conflict is emphasized by some authorities as a major contribution to compulsive and stereotypic behavior.[2] If the behavior comes and goes as a result of the occurrence of one or more of these influences, this is strong evidence for a causal link. Environmental factors may contribute to, but not be the sole cause of, the problem.

Attention-seeking behavior

All the behavioral patterns considered under this topic have been, at one time or another, diagnosed as attention seeking. Thus, a primary diagnostic goal should always be to determine whether the behavior is solely or partially maintained by an audience effect (Chapter 15). This may be true even if the behavior looks so driven and compulsive as to not, on the surface, be a credible candidate for an attention-seeking act. Ruling out an attention-seeking cause hinges on determining whether the dog performs the behavior when alone. This task is a little complicated; just watching the dog outside in the yard while in the house will not do. Behaviors such as tail chasing or fly snapping can be observed by having the owners leave the house with a well-placed video camera running when the likelihood of the behavior is high. It may be necessary to confine the dog within the range of the camera, being aware that confinement may increase or decrease the likelihood of the dog displaying the behavior. Alternately, one could quietly sneak back to the house to observe the dog through a window. Sometimes there is physical evidence of the behavior occurring when the owners are away. Flank sucking involves placement of the mouth over the flank area which leaves that area wet with saliva. Thus, when one returns from an absence it is clear that the behavior has been occurring in the owner's absence. Even in such cases, however, a video helps document when the behavior occurs and the role of precipitating stimuli, if any.

If the behavior is greatly reduced but not entirely absent when the owner is gone, one could be dealing with an abnormality that occurs with some basic frequency or tendency, without an audience effect, but which has been exacerbated by the owner's reinforcing attention. If conflict has been implicated as a contributing factor, the animal should be left in the same conflict-inducing environment when left alone for diagnostic observations.

Treatment Guidelines

Treatments discussed in the next sections, ranging from correcting environmental causes to remote punishment, represent a logical series of steps for approach to treatment. The steps are designed first to remove or reduce stimuli or situations that may cause or contribute to the stereotypic behaviors, and second to stop the repetitive problem behaviors directly. After reviewing the following treatment approaches, some dog owners may want to just correct the obvious factors that may be contributing to the behavior and live with the problem rather than deal with remote punishment or drugs to achieve a complete resolution. If a problem behavior seems to be displayed as the result of a medical problem such as an irritation of nerves that supply part of the tail, these pathophysiologic causes should be resolved, if possible. Keep in mind that the behavioral manifestations of a previous pathophysiologic process may continue, even after the medical problem is resolved.

Dealing with boredom, isolation, and conflict

If there is any indication that the onset or maintenance of the behavior is related to confinement, conflict, or boredom, these circumstances should be identified and alleviated if at all possible. A dog kept in a room with four blank walls, for example, could be given access to more of the home, including a window with a sill close to the floor from which it can watch goings-on outdoors. If the dog is receiving conflicting signals from different members of the family in terms of punishment for some misbehavior, the dog's interactions with family members should be structured so that all members of the family are giving the dog the same clear and consistent signals. An understanding of the necessity of using positive reinforcement for guiding behavior should be stressed and attempts to use interactive punishment should be completely discouraged (Chapter 3). The alleviation of environmental factors that may be related to the problem should not be necessarily expected to resolve the behavior, but behavior modification approaches to stop the behavior directly are less likely to be successful if the causes are not initially addressed.

Attention-seeking behavior

The degree to which the behavior might have been maintained completely or partially by the presence of family members (audience effect) should have been ascertained under diagnosis. If there is any indication that the behavior is displayed less intensely, or less frequently, when alone than when the family members are present, the owners should withdraw any reinforcement of the repetitive behaviors. On the other hand, they should calmly reinforce, through praise, food treats and affection, the appropriate and desirable behavioral alternatives. Further suggestions for this aspect of treatment are available in Chapter 15.

Structuring the dog's daily routine

Whether or not boredom or confinement plays a role, regular periods of physical and mental exercise should be structured for the dog as long as they do not exacerbate the compulsive behaviors. Thus, walks or ball retrieving sessions in the morning and afternoon should be recommended as long as these can be performed on a daily and regular basis. Automobile rides for dogs that love outings may be suggested. Food-dispensing toys could also be recommended for mental exercise. Keep in mind that a main source of conflict for some dogs is plenty of interaction with owners on the weekends and isolation and boredom during the week when the owners are at work. Increasing the interaction, if it only occurs on weekends, could actually exacerbate the problem. Dogs that are kept in outdoor runs may be predisposed to engage in compulsive or stereotypic behaviors because of such confinement combined with inconsistent interaction with the owners.

Preventing the compulsive behavior

When efforts such as reducing stress and boredom and enhancing social interaction reduce the general factors related to the likelihood of the repetitive behavior, it may be necessary to restrict the specific stimuli that evoke the compulsive behavior to the degree that it is feasible. Controlling illumination in the room so as to reduce the intensity of shadows or light flashes that activate chasing shadows or lights are some possibilities. By lowering the tendency for an animal to engage in the compulsive behavior, the stage is set to reinforce alternative behaviors. For example, playing fetch either within or outside the house in the presence of attenuated shadows or light flashes (that previously evoked the chasing behavior) is an example of reinforcing an alternative acceptable behavior. Some problems, such as tail chasing or flank sucking, may be prevented by the use of Elizabethan collars, but these collars undoubtedly add to the stress that an animal may already experience.

When it is determined that the treatment parameters are fully explored or implemented and there is still no major alleviation of the behavior, there are two further treatment possibilities. One approach is to attempt to control the behavior with psychotropic medication (see next section). The other approach is to explore the use of remote punishment such as shock or citronella spray collar. This type of remote punishment, if applied correctly, appears to offer an expedient and time-saving approach when environmental and pathophysiological causes are ruled out as main contributing factors. It is necessary to follow the principles of remote punishment (Chapter 3), which means that every act of the repetitive behavior must be punished,

---

COMPULSIVE BEHAVIOR

Causes
- Conflict, confinement, stress, boredom
- Neurotransmitter abnormality
- Learned behavior from endorphin release

Resolution
- Alleviate stress, conflict, and boredom.
- Structure environment and interaction with owner.
- Consider drug treatment.
- Implement remote punishment with citronella or shock collar.

and the behavior must be punished immediately after its performance. Thus, it is only those behaviors that can be physically prevented, except when the owner can deliver a punishment, that lend themselves to such types of behavior modification. The use of a shock or citronella spray collar combined with restraint to prevent unpunished problem licking is described in detail in the next section. It is absolutely essential that the person delivering the citronella spray or shock through the remote control device be dissociated from the delivery of the punishing stimulus, so that the dog comes to believe that it is the behavior that brings on the punishment, not the owner. Dog owners must understand both the rationale and theoretical basis of this type of therapy, as well as the specific application.

Psychotropic drug treatment

The same antianxiety, serotonergic drugs used in people with OCDs, namely clomipramine[3] and fluoxetine,[4] have been shown to reduce the frequency of compulsive behaviors in dogs. Such treatment generally requires medication for at least 2 or 3 weeks before a change in the behavior can be fully evaluated. Although clomipramine is a drug frequently used with dogs, selective serotonergic reuptake inhibitors (SSRIs) may be effective as well (Chapter 6). Clinical trials reveal that, although the behaviors may be reduced or eliminated, withdrawal of the drug is usually followed by a return of the behavior. Thus, it will usually be necessary to keep the dog on such a drug for several months and only then experiment with gradually reducing the dosage while following the behavior modification principles outlined earlier in this chapter.

Acral Lick Dermatitis

Acral lick dermatitis (ALD) is the name given to a repetitive and seemingly compulsive behavior in which a dog excessively licks an area on the carpus or tarsus (Fig. 18-2). This problem is usually referred to a dermatologist initially for medical workup because of the skin lesion. Although local irritation or itching undoubtedly helps maintain the excessive licking, the licking maintains the dermatological lesion, and in some instances may have been responsible for creating the lesion. Regardless of whether a dermatitis or a licking problem came first, the excessive licking helps maintain a cycle of irritation leading to more licking. When presented with a dog with a carpal lesion the common practice is to prevent licking by the use of a conical Elizabethan collar or other collar while the affected area is treated and allowed to heal. The use of such restraint collars is undoubtedly stressful, and an alternative is a bandage or sleeve on the leg, which should cause less overall stress if the dog will allow the bandage or sleeve to stay in place. Substances that are marketed as licking repellants work only on dogs that have a low predisposition to lick the affected area.

Dermatologists usually conclude that a dog presented with ALD is showing a behavioral problem when the affected area has completely healed with no signs of infection and the dog is still drawn back to licking this area to the point where a

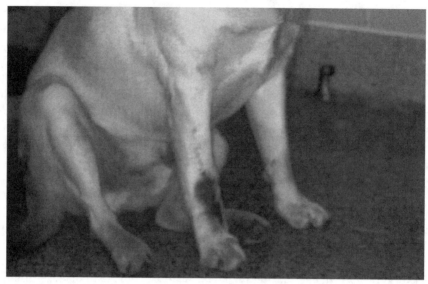

Figure 18-2 A wound resulting from compulsive and stereotypic excessive licking, referred to as acral lick dermatitis. This behavior occurs primarily when the dog is alone and undisturbed. Although psychotropic drug treatment may suppress or reduce licking, remote punishment has been shown to result in more permanent resolutions.

wound is likely to be created again. Currently it does not seem to be possible to determine whether an ALD lesion began as a behavioral problem or dermatological problem, or what proportion of excessively licking dogs fall into each etiological category.

It should be emphasized that licking is a normal type of grooming in dogs important for the maintenance of hair coat and removal of ectoparasites. Licking of wounds (aside from ALD or surgical sites) has an adaptive, cleansing function because saliva has antibacterial substances and epithelial growth factors that enhance the rate of wound healing.[5] The absence of grooming would be as abnormal as excessive grooming. Acral lick dermatitis is an example of normal behavior with abnormal manifestation. Compulsive licking of the carpus results in the epithelium eventually being eroded, leading to bacterial infection in the deep tissue, which then produces irritation attracting more licking. Continuous irritation over the carpus can result in a buildup of connective tissue as a cutaneous granuloma, commonly called a *lick granuloma*.

One explanation of the occurrence of ALD stemming from an ethological explanation is that ALD reflects abnormal activation of a vestigial grooming control center in the brain resulting in a compulsion to lick. There is evidence for an endogenous control mechanism responsible for regular grooming bouts seen in cats[6] and bovids,[7] among other common mammalian species. In dogs, grooming is not very orderly or well organized, and regular grooming bouts do not occur as in cats. When relatively calm and relaxed, a dog in sternal recumbency, with an abnormally activated grooming center producing an urge to groom, might turn and lick a convenient protruding part of the body closest to the mouth, which would be the carpus. For a dog that commonly rests with its head curled to the side and with an abnormal compulsion to lick, the tarsus is a convenient place to lick. The same process of licking irritation and infection over the tarsus would follow as with dogs that especially lick the carpus.

Typical History

This problem is often presented in dogs after there is a cutaneous wound, most frequently in the carpus, but sometimes on the tarsus. Less frequently other body parts are involved, but theoretically there is no reason that a different part of the body could not also be excessively licked. It is important for the clinician to evaluate carefully the circumstances when the excessive licking first started and the current environment for any signs of conflict, confinement, or boredom. There might be a time, being confined in a kennel, for example, when the excessive licking first began. Any measures taken by the owner to stop the behavior should also be evaluated and indications explored as to whether the owners' attempts at dealing with the problem helped or exacerbated the problem.

Diagnosis

There is usually no competing diagnosis with this behavior because of the typical lesion, location, and sign of excessive licking. Enough history should be explored to rule out that the behavior has attention seeking as a contributing cause. This is usually evident from the fact that the dog is prevented from grooming (directly admonished by the owner for licking) when the owners are present and engages in the behavior only when the owners are gone. The owners can see damage to the affected area when the dog is left alone; this finding in the history generally rules out attention seeking as a major contributing cause.

Treatment Guidelines

As with the other compulsive and stereotypic behaviors, the approach to treatment should emphasize first the alleviation of causative factors, including allowing for complete healing of the affected area. Second, measures (covered in the next section) can be taken to directly stop the licking of the affected area.

Complete healing of the skin lesion

Because of the damage to the skin, immediate attention must be given to prevention of further excessive licking by the use of a sleeve, body shirt, and/or bandage. A restraint collar should be used if necessary. Secondary skin infections must receive medical attention, which may require a full medical workup for signs of abnormal thyroid function and exacerbation by skin allergies and a skin biopsy to determine the depth of the involvement. There is a possibility of a secondary bone or periosteal infection if the skin infection has gone into deeper tissues. Prevention of licking the lesion is necessary until there is no indication that irritation is coming from the affected area that would provoke licking again. Appropriate treatment with antibiotics is indicated to treat any infection.

Dealing with boredom, isolation, and conflict

Any evident environmental source of stress, boredom, or conflict should be removed, as discussed earlier for other compulsive and stereotypic disorders. If confinement seems to be related to the problem, the owner should be encouraged to seek an alternative type of housing. Structured, regular outings—in the way of walks, runs, or ball chasing—should be implemented on a daily basis.

Drug treatment

Of the compulsive behaviors, acral lick dermatitis is the most frequently studied with regard to suppression of the behavior. The antianxiety agents clompramine[3,8] and fluoxetine,[4] as well as narcotic antagonists,[9,10] have all been effective in at least reducing the behavior, but after completion of a course of treatment, the behavior appears to return. It could be that eventually additional drugs will be developed that may be more effective in controlling this behavior.

Remote punishment: Citronella spray and shock collars

Although treatment with serotonergic drugs, such as clomipramine or fluoxetine, may suppress the compulsive licking for the duration of treatment, longer-term resolutions have been accomplished only with the use of remote punishment. Such behavior modifications are most readily provided by the use of a citronella spray or mild shock collar. Use of the principles with regard to use of remote punishment should be reviewed in Chapter 3; important aspects are immediately delivering the punishing stimulus as soon as there is any attempt at carpal licking and punishing (stopping) every act of such licking attempts. This means that at the times when the owner is not around and is unable to punish the behavior, the licking must be prevented with a bandage, body suit, or collar. The remote punishment must be strong enough to stop the licking. It is important that the shock or citronella spray not be associated with the person delivering it. Before starting the punishment program, dogs should be habituated to the special collar. Because the collar must be charged regularly or have its batteries charged, it is necessary to trade off between a real and a dummy collar while the dog has a restraint collar or body suit on. When the special collar is used later it will not be associated with its weight.

For the first few training sessions the restraint collar or body suit is removed and the dog observed from a place where the owner can see the dog but not be readily seen by the dog. A recommended procedure is that the person delivering the spray or shock through the remote control device be outdoors and the dog inside where the animal can be watched through a window. The remote punishment is delivered every time the dog turns to lick the affected area. The first trial should be conducted for at least 1 hour, and at the end of the trial the restraint collar or suit should be replaced. After a few such sessions, and when the dog no longer attempts licking the affected area for an hour or so, the training sessions can be conducted in other locations. For this step the owner might carry the remote control device concealed while constantly watching the dog. When the dog turns to start licking the affected area, the punishment should be immediately delivered while the person seemingly

---

ACRAL LICK DERMATITIS

Causes

- Confinement, boredom, and conflict
- Skin disorders
- Neurotransmitter abnormality
- Disorder of grooming control system

Resolution

- Allow wound to heal with licking restraint.
- Alleviate boredom, conflict, and stress.
- Implement remote punishment with citronella spray or shock collar.
- Use serotonergic drug treatment.

---

goes about his or her business so that the dog cannot perceive that there is any connection between the person and the delivery of the punishment.

The clinical trial using a shock collar of the type used for field training found that dogs received an average of only 10 shocks before the problem was resolved, with a range of 7–21 shocks.[11] In this trial the behavior was immediately eliminated and no other abnormal repetitive behavior arose in its place. This suggests that the excessive licking is not necessarily a manifestation of stress or anxiety, because otherwise one would expect another type of stereotypic behavior to occur in its place. In some instances a "refresher" session with the shock collar was necessary a few months later. The citronella spray collar is likely to work as well as a shock collar, but there are no clinical data addressing this aspect.

References

1. Hart BL. Three disturbing behavioral disorders in dogs: Idiopathic viciousness, hyperkinesis and flank sucking. Canine Practice 1977;4(6):10-14.
2. Leuscher UA, McKeown DB, Halip J. Stereotypic and obsessive-compulsive disorders in dogs and cats. Veterinary Clinics of North America Small Animal Practice 1991;21: 401–413.
3. Hewson CJ, Luescher A, Parent JM, Conlon PD, Ball RO. Efficacy of clomipramine in the treatment of canine compulsive disorder. Journal of the American Veterinary Medical Association 1998;213:1760–1766.
4. Rapoport JL, Ryland DH, Kriete M. Drug treatment of canine acral lick. Archives of General Psychiatry 1992;49:517–521.
5. Hart BL, Powell KL. Antibacterial properties of saliva: Role of maternal periparturient grooming and in licking wounds. Physiology and Behavior 1990;48:383–386.
6. Eckstein RA, Hart BL. Grooming and control of fleas in cats. Applied Animal Behaviour Science 2000;68:141–150.
7. Hart BL, Hart LA, Mooring MS, Olubayo R. Biological basis of grooming behaviour in antelope; The body-size, vigilance and habitat principles. Animal Behaviour 1992; 44:615–631.
8. Goldberger E, Rapoport JL. Canine acral lick dermatitis: Response to the antiobsessional drug clomipramine. Journal of the American Animal Hospital Association 1991; 27:179–182.

9. Dodman NH, Shuster L, White SD, Court MH, Parker D, Dixon R. Use of narcotic antagonists to modify stereotypic self-licking, self-chewing, and scratching behavior in dogs. Journal of the American Veterinary Medical Association 1988;193:815–819.
10. White SD. Naltrexone for treatment of acral lick dermatitis in dogs. Journal of the American Veterinary Medical Association 1990;196:1073–1076.
11. Eckstein RA, Hart BL. Treatment of canine acral lick dermatitis by behavior modification using electronic stimulation. Journal of the American Animal Hospital Association 1996;32:225–230.

Chapter 19
Behavioral Aspects of Aging Dogs

Thanks to improvements in nutrition, medical care, and protection from accidental death, our pet animals, like people, are living longer. And, just as with people, old age in pet dogs is accompanied by physical changes, including arthritis, disturbances in endocrinological function, heart problems, visual impairment, and loss of hearing. The geriatric stage of an animal's life is when closer attention must be paid to functioning of the thyroid gland and the pituitary-adrenal axis and to monitoring organ systems for signs of cancer. Old age in dogs is sometimes also accompanied by behavioral changes, which include disorientation, signs of loss of recognition of family members, onset of fear reactions, and signs of irritability. The purpose in this chapter is to help clinicians understand the nature of behavioral problems of aging dogs and to be able to communicate with dog owners the reasons for such behavioral changes. As a special topic, advice gleaned from caregivers of geriatric dogs is provided about how to make life easier for both the dog and the caregivers.

Challenges of Caring for an Elderly Dog

The presence of an aging dog, especially one that has been a family member for most of its life, presents not only challenges to which caregivers must respond, but it also presents emotional challenges. From a study involving an interview with a group of caregivers of older dogs, there are useful perspectives or a philosophy about living with an aging dog, as well as practice tips that make life easier for both the dog and caregiver.[1]

Philosophical Attitudes

The first thing to mention is that old dogs have their positive aspects. Many caregivers feel they are more mellow, less excitable, and even more loving than younger dogs. In compensation for the additional time and expense required, many of the caregivers felt their old dogs were more faithful and grateful for their care than younger dogs. This canine-style gratitude may provide a level of companionship and devotion that one sees only in an older dog.

Managing an Older Dog

Although the loyalty of caregivers to their aging dogs is beyond question, and their willingness to adapt to the extra care and medical expenses laudatory, it is important that dog owners be counseled on the means by which they can make this process as convenient as possible and to understand the biological basis of many of the behavioral changes they observe in their beloved canine family member.

Impairment of hearing and vision

These changes are common in old dogs. In one study about 40% of owners of 11–12-year-old dogs reported visual impairment; this progressed to about 70% in 15–16-year-olds. Hearing loss is more common and was reported for about 50% of 11–12-year-olds and 90% of 15–16-year-olds.[2] Because deaf dogs cannot hear verbal commands, hand signals should be used. For partial deafness, clapping the hands or stomping the floor is a way of gaining their attention. For dogs that are blind, it is a major disturbance when one rearranges the furniture. One should be sure to use more verbal commands for dogs that are blind or that have severe visual impairment. Dogs that are severely impaired in both hearing and vision will require communication through tactile means such as stomping on the floor and teaching the dog to respond to being touched on parts of the body such as the head, meaning to come.

Arthritis

Of the common physical problems of old dogs, arthritis emerges as needing particular attention. Thus, elevated food and water bowls and ramps to the bed (if the dog sleeps on the owners' bed) and the car may become essential. Use of a special sling or towel for lifting may be necessary if the dog has difficulty getting up or walking. The canine form of wheel chair, the cart with a sling to support the dog, is needed in some instances of severe joint or neuromuscular problems. Comfortable bedding seems to be very important, and foam beds and heating pads (even in the summer) are frequently used. It is important to watch for the slipperiness of wood and tile floors in older dogs that have lost some of the control of their gait and to cover such floors with mats or rugs.

Just as we are learning with people, it is beneficial for dogs with arthritis to receive exercise. Some people find that artificial turf is useful for outdoor areas that tend to be muddy, especially for dogs that lie down a lot. It is particularly important to maintain a proper weight for dogs as they age, because it is easier on their joints and it is easier for the caregiver to lift and care for them. Thus, counseling for diet is perhaps more important than with younger dogs.

Dental problems

These problems are as prominent in old dogs as visual and hearing impairment. Because frequent brushing of the teeth is useful, behavior modification in habituating the dog to the brushing in gradual steps with positive reinforcement is recommended (Chapter 3). Keep in mind that many dog treats are hard, and when a dog has dental problems, softer treats may be more appropriate.

Anxieties

Although only some dogs undergo severe cognitive impairment in their elderly years, most will show some impairments of memory and hearing. The possible value of a diet rich in antioxidants will be covered later in this chapter, but caregivers should understand that the impairment of memory and learning can make aging dogs act somewhat like a puppy. Anxieties that emerge in an aging dog may be similar to the initial anxieties in puppies. Separation anxiety, for example, is normal for puppies but is habituated as the puppy gains experience in being left alone repeatedly (Chapter 20). When an elderly dog, previously habituated to being left alone, shows separation anxiety, it may be because the habituation was lost as a function of impairment of learning and memory. The same is true for anxieties related to loud noises or strange people. Utilizing training techniques to rehabituate the separation anxiety and fears of noises by desensitization and counterconditioning may be useful (Chapter 3).

Irritable aggression

In some older dogs the onset of aggression, particularly of an irritable nature, is puzzling, especially if the dog was nonaggressive before. Puppies usually learn to suppress irritable aggressive tendencies by taking a subordinate role. If this learning is impaired in an older dog, the irritable aggression may occur because there is less cerebral modulation of this aggression. One should handle the aggression in an indirect manner, as with dogs of younger age.

House soiling

This problem is frequently due to age-related urinary and/or fecal incontinence. Although medication may help, some management is advisable. Plastic mats and sheets may be useful for areas most likely to be soiled. Enzymatic cleaners are the most useful to clean up urine puddles. It is particularly important that the caregiver pay attention to the dog's subtle requests to go outside. This may be the time when dog doors are a major help for dogs that may need to make trips to the outdoors more frequently than when they were younger, but one may have to use ramps to make the use easier for the arthritic dog. Some people find diapers useful. Baby gates are frequently used to restrict dogs from carpeted areas where house soiling would be a problem or at certain times such as night. If the dog is incontinent, and the skin or hair coat regularly soiled but the dog does not like baths, one can use wash cloths to clean the dog. Experienced caregivers of older dogs say to expect a lot of laundry.

Loss of the learned generalization that the house is a "den" (Chapter 14) may also lead to house soiling. Learning is also involved as dogs signal to owners the need to go out. This signaling behavior is subject to being less reliable with age-related impairment of memory. As one would with house-training a puppy, start with the basics and restrict access to the house until house-training is relearned. Another idea is to place the sleeping bed of the dog near the door to go outdoors, so that less cognitive involvement is required for this important task.

If flies are bad because of urine or fecal leakage, it alleviates the problem if the dog is kept inside. Many older dogs find life easier inside the house. Also, having the dog inside allows for closer supervision and for one to use padded beds. For the inside-outside dog, fly repellants may be useful for dogs that are incontinent and exposed to flies.

Sleep-wake cycle problems

The older dog that used to sleep through the night and now is moving about at night may severely deprive owners of sleep; this problem alone prompts some people to confront whether they can keep the dog any longer. There are no nursing homes for old dogs, but a dog may be given its own sleeping quarters away from the bedroom. Keep in mind that with longer periods of sleeping, older dogs may tend to lie in one position for an excessively long duration and should be checked for decubital ulcers.

Euthanasia and saying good-bye

One can hardly be in the field of companion animal health care for very long without seeing the need to counsel caregivers of old dogs about how to face the death of their dog and address questions about euthanasia and sources for help in loss of a pet (see Chapter 29). Caregivers of old dogs, when asked about the point at which they would elect to have a dog euthanized, most often mentioned when the dog is experiencing pain and suffering. Also mentioned frequently is when the dog is perceived to be experiencing reduced quality of life. Less frequently mentioned is when the dog is no longer able to walk or is showing incontinence.

Cognitive Dysfunction

Owners of older dogs describe a variety of behavioral changes that can generally be grouped into five categories: 1) disorientation in the immediate environment, 2) change in social responsiveness toward human family members, 3) house soiling with concomitant loss of signaling to go outdoors, 4) disturbance of sleep-wake cycle, and 5) a reduction in activity.[3] A reduction in general activity could reflect a limitation of several organ systems and/or cognitive dysfunction.

The signs of dogs with disorientation due to cognitive dysfunction include staring into space, getting lost in the house or yard, getting stuck in corners, and standing at the wrong door or wrong part of the door to go out. The signs associated with dysfunction in social interaction include a perceived loss of recognition of human family members, often indicated by a decrease in greeting owners. Other changes in social interaction are less soliciting of attention from the owners and/or a change (increase or decrease) in following owners around the house. House soiling due to cognitive dysfunction is characterized by the dog urinating and/or defecating in the house, along with reduced signaling to go out or decreased use of a dog door. Of course, medical explanations such as urinary incontinence and diarrhea, and secondary behavioral explanations, such as separation anxiety, should be ruled out. Signs of a disturbance in the sleep-wake cycle are regularly waking up the owner at night by pacing or vocalizing, sleeping less at night, and/or sleeping noticeably more during the day. Interestingly, disorders in all of these categories have their counterparts in Alzheimer's disease of humans.[4]

Because the behavioral changes involve deficits in memory and learning, the terms *cognitive dysfunction, cognitive impairment,* and *cognitive dysfunction syndrome (CDS)* have been used in discussing these behavioral changes in aging dogs.[5] In a strict sense cognition refers to learned associations where an animal makes new responses that appear to reflect abstractions from previously learned material.[6] Thus, reference to cognitive dysfunction for dogs who get lost in the house or seem to no longer recognize family members is not necessarily accurate. Nonetheless, loss of orientation in the home or yard and impaired recognition of family members reflect impairment of memory and learning and would be logically correlated with impairment of cognitive function.

It is assumed that some sort of neuronal, neurotransmitter, metabolic, cerebrovascular, and/or biochemical degenerative changes in the brain underlie the behavioral changes. A noteworthy aspect of impairment of memory and learning in dogs is the accumulation of beta-amyloid deposits in the frontal cortex and hippocampus, areas of the brain especially involved in cognitive behavior. Research shows the amyloid deposits are similar to the early stage amyloid plaques seen in the brains of humans with Alzheimer's disease (AD).[7,8] Laboratory research on aging dogs has shown that the degree of beta-amyloid deposition in the brain corresponds to the degree of impairment in learning complex tasks.[8,9] The neuropathological and behavioral changes seen in some aging dogs are, in fact, similar enough to humans with dementia to suggest to investigators that dogs are a useful model for human dementia.[10]

Prevalence and Predictability of Cognitive Impairment in Dogs

Research has found that there is a progressive, age-related prevalence of dogs showing signs of cognitive dysfunction, and in the number of signs related to one or more of the behavioral categories of dysfunction (Fig. 19-1). The percentage of 11–12-year-old dogs classified as mildly affected (impairment in one behavioral category based on having two signs of dysfunction related to that category) is about 20%; another 10% are severely affected (impairment in two categories). Among 15–16-year-olds, 30% are mildly affected and 35% severely affected (Fig 19-2). This study also showed that despite the fact that dogs of large body size die at a younger age than smaller dogs, presumably as a function of more rapid aging in the cardiovascular, musculoskeletal, and endocrine systems, the brain does not seem to age more rapidly in larger dogs. Small-bodied dogs are as likely to be severely impaired in cognitive function, at any given age, as large dogs.[3]

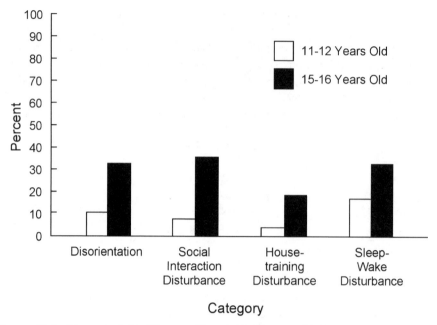

Figure 19-1   Percent of 11–12-year-old and 15–16-year-old dogs with impairment in various behavioral categories. There is a significant progression of impairment as a function of age. (Data from Neilson et al. 2001.[3])

Experienced clinicians know that the behavioral signs of cognitive dysfunction could be a reflection of an organ system abnormality other than, or in addition to, brain degeneration. Quite likely is the possibility that other neurological diseases, hypothyroidism, arthritis, and cardiovascular disease will intensify some signs that also reflect the loss of memory and learning. In fact, it would be unusual to find a 15–16-year-old dog severely impaired in cognitive function without any substantial impairment in nonbrain organ systems. Although some disorientation within the house or yard can be attributed to complete or partial loss of vision, the onset of visual impairment accounts for only a small proportion of dogs developing disorientation during the same time period.[2] In most instances, disorientation seems to be independent of visual impairment.

Some work has addressed the question of the predictability of dogs developing severe cognitive dysfunction by prospectively monitoring changes in dogs 11–14 years of age for 6–18 months. As in Alzheimer's disease,[4] dogs initially observed with one, or a few, signs of cognitive impairment and considered mildly impaired were much more likely to be severely affected later than dogs without any initial signs of cognitive impairment.[2]

Effects of Gonadectomy

An issue of some importance is the degree to which gonadectomy in dogs might predispose them to age-related behavioral changes associated with cognitive impairment. Research over the past decade revealed that estrogen for women and testosterone for men may be protective of AD; laboratory research showed benefi-

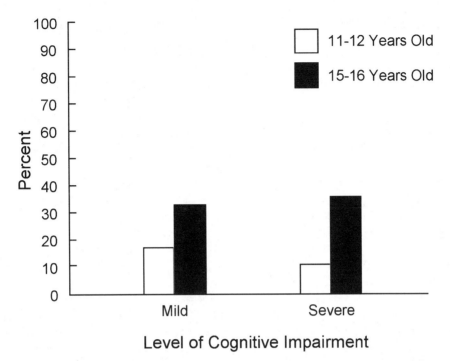

Figure 19-2   Percent of 11–12-year-old and 15–16-year-old dogs with mild cognitive impairment (one category of dysfunction) and with severe impairment (two or more categories of dysfunction) (Data from Neilson et al. 2001.[3])

cial effects of estrogen and testosterone for neuron survival and adaptive growth in vitro. Removal of estrogen by ovariectomy, or postmenopausal fall in estrogen, may predispose women to AD.[11,12] In elderly men the diagnosis of AD is associated with low levels of free testosterone, even after adjustments for age, education, smoking status, body mass index, diabetes, and any cancer diagnosis.[13]

In a study of aging dogs that had signs of mild cognitive impairment, gonadally intact males did not progress to a more severe stage of impairment compared with neutered dogs, of which about 50% progressed to the severe stage.[14] The most logical conclusion of this small study is that the presence of circulating testosterone appears to slow the progression of impairment in cognitive function in dogs already showing some signs of impairment. This finding is in line with current research on the neuroprotective role of testosterone and estrogen, as studied at the cellular level, and the role of estrogen in preventing Alzheimer's disease in humans. One would expect gonadal estrogens would have a protective role in female dogs just as testosterone seems to have for male dogs. When one considers the conventional procedure of spaying or neutering dogs at an early age, it is almost surprising that the effects of early gonadectomy are not more noticeable. Although one should not question the value of spaying and neutering as important to the control of unwanted pets, the possible increased likelihood of some predisposition toward severe age-related cognitive impairment in gonadectomized dogs profiles the importance of learning about preventing and treating the problem.

Prevention and Treatment of Age-Related Cognitive Dysfunction

Caloric restriction is the only known regimen of life-style change that increases the life span of animals—ranging from rats to primates[15] and now including dogs[16]—and also allows them to stay young longer in terms of overall health, memory, and learning. Because a spartan, low-calorie diet is too unappealing for people (or their companion animals), there is currently a major research interest in attempting to find alternative dietary regimens to lengthen life span, prolong overall health, and preserve cognitive function. One of the hallmarks of caloric restriction is the maintenance of mitochondrial function and control of oxidant production. There are a myriad of studies on various possible dietary supplements on brain function in animals and humans. In one of the more noteworthy of such studies, feeding old rats the mitochondrial metabolite, carnitine, and the antioxidant, lipoic acid, reversed age-related mitochondrial degenerative change and lowered oxidative damage in liver cells,[17–18] while at the same time increasing the binding affinity of brain- and memory-related enzymes.[19] In essence the old rats, especially those with impaired cognitive performance, became more like young rats.

The work on rats has led other investigators to study the performance of old dogs under laboratory conditions on tests involving difficult discrimination tasks. Short-term studies of 1 year revealed that dietary supplementation with carnitine and lipoic acid, along with vitamins E and C, significantly reduced the impairment that aged dogs showed on difficult discrimination tasks.[20,21] Knowing that behavioral enrichment of laboratory beagles would probably help prevent age-related declines in learning ability as well as dietary supplementation with mitochondrial cofactors and antioxidants, investigators tested laboratory beagles with behavioral enrichment and dietary supplementation alone and combined compared with control husbandry and diet. Both interventions reduced age-related decline, but the combination of the two had the greater protective effect on learning ability.[22]

Dogs that would be logical candidates for treatment with dietary supplements to protect against a cognitive decline are those advancing in age. One does not have to wait for signs of disorientation in the home or yard, reduced social responsiveness, or loss of house-training. Although dog foods formulated with these supplements are increasing available, the addition of mitochondrial support supplements and antioxidants to a standard or therapeutic diet is also an option. Behavioral enrichment, especially that involving some problem solving and cognitive function, can be started much sooner and is likely to be useful in preventing cognitive decline. It is important in evaluating a dog that shows behavioral signs related to cognitive dysfunction to rule out, and treat as appropriate, deterioration in organ systems that might be involved in the behavioral changes or impacting overall health. Treatment of signs of cognitive dysfunction is just one aspect of the care needed for maintaining the health and welfare of aging dogs.

A drug that may be useful in alleviating the behavioral signs associated with cognitive dysfunction is L-deprenyl (selegiline HCL). This drug appears to ameliorate the signs of cognitive impairment in some dogs by possibly reducing the depletion of the neurotransmitter dopamine and providing for some neuroprotective and antioxidant support.[23]

Conclusion

The role of the clinician is to advise the caregivers of elderly dogs about the importance of medically monitoring the dogs and offering suggestions to make life easier for themselves as well as the dog. Intervention in the way of dietary supplementation with antioxidants is a step most dog owners can easily take by supplementing the food themselves or using a specially formulated diet for older dogs. Treatment with dopaminergic and neuroprotective drugs may be indicated for dogs showing clear signs of cognitive impairment. Caregivers should enjoy the extra love and devotion that an aging dog can offer in response to the sympathetic care given to them in their declining years. When the time comes to say good-bye, caregivers can rest assured that they have done their part.

References

1. Hart LA, Dorairaj K, Camacho S, Hart BL. Nurturing older dogs: Attitudes and experiences of caregivers. Journal of the American Veterinary Medical Association 2001; 37:307–310.
2. Bain MJ, Hart BL, Cliff KD, Ruehl WW. Predicting behavioral changes associated with age-related cognitive impairment in dogs: A longitudinal study. Journal of the American Veterinary Medical Association 2001;218:1792–1795.
3. Neilson JC, Hart BL, Cliff KD, Ruehl WW. Prevalence of behavioral changes associated with age-related cognitive impairment in dogs. Journal of the American Veterinary Medical Association 2001;218:1787–1791.
4. Ashford JW, Schmitt F, Kumar V. Diagnosis of Alzheimer's disease. In: Kumar V, Eisdorfer C, eds. Advances in the Diagnosis and Treatment of Alzheimer's Disease. New York: Springer Publishing Co., 1998:111–151.
5. Ruehl WW, Hart BL. Canine cognitive dysfunction: Understanding the syndrome and treatment. In: Dodman NH, Shuster L, eds. Psychopharmacology of Animal Behavior disorders. Malden: Blackwell Science, 1998;283–304.
6. Shettleworth SJ. Cognition, Evolution and Behavior. New York: Oxford University Press, 1998;3–48.
7. Cummings BJ, Su JH, Cotman CW, et al. b-Amyloid accumulation in aged canine brain. A model of early plaque formation in Alzheimer's disease. Neurobiology of Aging 1993;14:547–560.
8. Cummings BJ, Head E, Afagh AJ, et al. b-Amyloid accumulation correlates with cognitive dysfunction in the aged canine. Neurobiology of Learning and Memory 1996;66: 11–23.
9. Head E, Callahan H, Huggenburg BA, et al. Visual-discrimination learning ability and b-amyloid accumulation in the dog. Neurobiology of Aging 1998;19:415–425.
10. Cummings BJ, Head E, Ruehl WW, et al. The canine as an animal model of human aging and dementia. Neurobiology of Aging 1996;209:259–268.
11. Haskell SG, Richardson ED, Horowitz RI. The effects of estrogen replacement therapy on cognitive function in women: A critical review of the literature. Journal of Clinical Epidemiology 1997;11:2149–2164.
12. Yaffe K, Sawaya G, Lieberburg I, et al. Estrogen therapy in postmenopausal women: Effects on cognitive function and dementia. Journal of the American Medical Association 1998;215:1288–1291.

13. Moffat SD, Zonderman AB, Metter EJ, et al. Free testosterone and risk for Alzheimer disease in older men. Neurology 2004;62:188–193.

14. Hart BL. Effects of gonadectomy on subsequent development of age-related cognitive impairment in dogs. Journal of the American Veterinary Medical Association 2001; 219:51–56.

15. Beckman KB, Ames BN. The free radical theory of aging matures. Physiological Review 1998;78:547–581.

16. Kealy RD, Lawler DF, Ballam JM, Mantz SL, Biery DN, Greeley EH, Lust G, Segre M, Smith GK, Stowe HD. Effects of diet restriction on life span and age-related changes in dogs. Journal of the American Veterinary Medical Association 2002;220:1315–1320.

17. Hagen TM, Ingersoll RT, Wehr CM, Lykkesfeldt J, Vinarsky V, Bartholomew JC, et al. Acetyl-L-carnitine fed to old rats partially restores mitochondrial function and ambulatory activity. Proceedings of the National Academy of Science USA 1998;95:9562–9566.

18. Liu J, Head E, Gharib AM, et al. Memory loss in old rats is associated with brain mitochondrial decay and RNA/DNA oxidative: Partial reversal by feeding acetyl-L-carnitine and/or R-alpha-lipoic acid. Proceedings of the National Academy of Science USA 2002;99:2356–2361.

19. Liu J, Killilea DW, Ames BN. Age associated mitochondrial oxidative decay: Improvement of carnitine acetyltransferase substrate-binding affinity and activity in brain by feeding old rats acetyl-L-carnitine and/or R-alpha-lipoic acid. Proceedings of the National Academy of Science USA 2002;99:1876–1881.

20. Milligram NW, Head E, Muggenburg B, et al. Landmark discrimination learning in the dog: Effects of age on antioxidant fortified food, and cognitive strategy. Neuroscience and Biobehavioral Reviews 2002;26:679–695.

21. Milligram NW, Zicker SC, Head E, et al. Dietary enrichment counteracts age-associated cognitive dysfunction in canines. Neurobiology of Aging 2002;23:737–745.

22. Milgram NW, Head E, Zicker SC, Ikeda-Douglas CJ, Murphey H, Muggenburg B, Siwak C, Tapp D, Cotman CW. Learning ability in aged beagle dogs is preserved by behavioral enrichment and dietary fortification: A two-year longitudinal study. Neurobiology of Aging 2005;26:77–90.

23. FDA Freedom of Information Summary, Selegiline. Exton, Pa: Pfizer Animal Health, 1998.

Chapter 20
Selecting and Raising Puppies

The primary concerns under this topic are giving advice to clients regarding the source of a puppy, methods for raising it to avoid behavior problems as an adult, and how to make the dog an enjoyable member of the family. Although advice in raising puppies may be given to clients with young animals when they come in for routine vaccinations or examinations. the ideal time for advice in selecting a dog is before the pet is obtained. Sometimes a client's behavioral concerns may stem from an unfortunate or adverse experience with a previous pet, and the client desires help in obtaining a new dog with the hope of avoiding similar problems in the future. This chapter covers the background information that may be useful in presenting to a client different options with regard to selection of breed, selection of sex, neutering, and rearing practices.

In the selection of a companion animal, the role of the clinician boils down to suggestions about matching the most appropriate companion animal to the person or family seeking advice. A number of parameters are considered in recommending particular pets for particular environments. One decision may be whether to adopt a dog or a cat. Within a species there are questions about size, hair length, coat color, potential for allergies to the pet, and whether the animal should have a purebred or mixed-breed background. Size and color are important, but the parameter that will have the most effect, and contribute most to the richness of the relationship the pet will have with the family, is its behavior. Both dogs and cats offer affection and companionship. The particular advantages of cats are mentioned in Chapter 27, "Selecting and Raising Kittens." If the person seeking advice wants an active playmate, a companion for car trips or animal-oriented social outings, or as a home-security alarm system, cats cannot compete with dogs. On the other hand, if the prospective owners are physically or emotionally limited in the time or energy they can devote to active interaction with the pet, a cat is likely to be a better mate. Occasionally clients with one dog ask about adopting a new dog in an attempt to help correct a behavior problem, such as separation anxiety, with the resident dog. Although such adoptions sometimes do help with problems in the resident dog, they frequently do not work. The best advice is to adopt an additional dog only if the client wants a new dog, not to solve a problem with the current dog.

Some people have an opportunity to adopt an adult dog and want to avoid the hassles of puppyhood. This may lead to unexpected behavior problems, so in these instances potential adopters should learn about the background of the dog. Adult dogs put up for adoption may have barked incessantly, been difficult to house-train, fought with resident pets, or been fear-biters with regard to children. They may also have been wonderfully behaved pets for which the owners are seeking a new home because of constraints on keeping pets in a new home. In adopting an adult from a shelter one should find out as much as possible about the animal's background and behavior. A behavioral profile of the dog's behavior before relinquishment to a shelter may not always be available, but animal shelters are increasingly providing profiles based at least on temperament evaluation at the shelters. Although these temperament evaluations have not proven to be predictive of future behavior in a new home, they may be of some value in selecting a pet.

Source and Age of Adoption

For the client who is interested in obtaining an 8-week-old puppy from a healthy litter, raised by an attentive mother, in a household where good nutrition and kind treatment are evident, the main preadoption advice you can offer would be to point out the most appropriate breeds and gender to be considered. Other sources of puppies are shelters and breeding kennels. The section later in this chapter on early experience covers the main concerns one would have in looking into the environment of the source of adoption. At family and kennel breeders one also has an opportunity to obtain information about individual genetic background. Genetic background as a function of breed membership is covered in a subsequent section.

The Dam, Sire, and Progeny

Although some behavioral predispositions can be obtained from information about breed identification, there is a good chance the behavior of the puppy as an adult will resemble that of the mother. In normal circumstances one is free to observe the interaction of the dam with members of the family, strangers such as the person considering adoption, and other dogs. It is also helpful to learn about the behavior of the sire, either by means of telephoning the owner of the sire or observing the sire directly. One can, in some situations, even go to the extent of "progeny testing" by inquiring as to the behavior of puppies from previous litters. This will involve some effort, but it could lead to some practical results. For example, if a client has had unfortunate experiences with a flank-sucking Doberman or an aggressive Australian Shepherd, it would be a good idea to talk to the owners of the dam, sire, and siblings from previous litters to confirm the absence of problem behaviors of particular importance.

The Age for Adoption

Many dog handlers and breeders point to a body of experimental and practical evidence to support the notion that puppies should be adopted between the ages of 6 and 8 weeks for optimal socialization with both dogs and people. There is, theoretically, a window extending from about 3–12 weeks of age in which socialization of puppies to people and other dogs is most easily made. Adoption before 6 weeks may interfere with the socialization to other dogs, especially if the puppy is adopted into an environment without contact with other dogs. Adoption after 8 weeks may curtail the period of easiest socialization to people in the new home.

Puppy Temperament Testing

A great deal of information is written in the popular dog literature about puppy temperament tests, with about as many different temperament tests as there are authors of the papers or books. The truth is that no puppy temperament test has been found to predict adult behavior reliably. Clearly puppies within a litter can differ markedly with regard to docility upon being handled by people, tendency to approach or avoid people, and ease with which signs of aggression or dominance are evoked. But these differences do not reliably carry into adulthood. Behavioral predispositions with a genetic basis theoretically could be evaluated in puppies, but differences among puppies are probably masked by a preponderance of puppy behavior. Furthermore, developmental stages are greatly influenced by the new home environment interacting with genetic predispositions.

In selecting a puppy, one really cannot avoid interacting with the litter, and one puppy is likely to appeal more than others. It would be hard to avoid basing part of the selection on the behavior of the puppy. However, one should realize that impressions about a puppy are not a predictor of behavior as an adult. There is simply too much development, both behavioral and physiological, yet to occur during maturation that influences behavior. Undoubtedly the day will arrive when some genetic markers will be available through genetic analysis that may be associated with traits to be avoided, such as aggressiveness or excessive fearfulness.

What about the runt of the litter? Admittedly, most runts turn out all right, but there is a greater chance of future problems involving its emotional behavior. If the runt was not able to receive sufficient food there is a possibility of undernutrition early in life. The runt is also more likely to be harassed by its littermates, and this may have enduring effects on its behavior. It is true that stunting of body size may not involve the brain. However, when one sees marked somatic stunting there is no way of knowing how severely the central nervous system, and hence behavior, may have been affected.

Behavioral Characteristics of Dog Breeds

The more we know about the specific behavioral attributes or disadvantages of various breeds of dogs, the more success we will have in recommending the best match of dog breed for specific families or households. The idea of matching certain breeds of dogs with certain types of people or households requires a reliable, unbiased approach to determine typical breed characteristics. People who want dogs live in a variety of environments, ranging from small apartments to houses with lots of open space. The human environment may range from that of a single man or woman to a large family with young children. Some people who want a dog as a watchdog may be relatively unconcerned about the dog's behavior toward children.

A family with young children, and who already have a watchdog, may have the opposite concern. With some people, the ease of training may be of paramount importance.

The current popular literature contains statements about breed differences in behavior, such as aggressive temperament, trainability, loyalty, and mellowness with children. However, the perspectives obtained are from breeders and breed associations and are likely to reflect personal biases. Often the selection is approached on the basis of size and coat color or hair type. Information about specific behavioral attributes of various breeds of dogs is essential for the selection of a dog as a family or personal pet. A general guideline of basic behavioral characteristics of breeds is needed to help prospective pet owners narrow their choices. With a general guideline in hand, one can then go to local dog authorities, such as breeders and trainers, for information about behavioral characteristics of particular genetic lines within breeds to decide on an individual dog. Of course, to make a meaningful recommendation, one must learn something about the environment in which the dog will be living and the personalities and lifestyle of the people involved. Most people have some idea about the type of dog they want. Clients should be cautioned to reduce their emphasis on size, head shape, and coloration, or whether the puppy is cute or not, and place emphasis on the behavioral characteristics of the prospective adult dog most appropriate for them.

The information on breed rankings, with respect to problem behaviors mentioned in various chapters in Section II, is from a data-based set of breed profiles of frequently registered breeds.[1] The information was obtained by interviewing a large number of small animal veterinarians. They were randomly selected so as to represent male and female authorities equally and to represent eastern, central, and western regions of the U.S. about equally. The behavioral traits are deemed those of most interest to prospective dog adopters. The idea of asking a large number of authorities to provide data for breed profiles is predicated on three principles: 1) breed differences in behavior actually exist, 2) the behavioral differences are known in general by authorities such as small animal veterinarians who have extensive experience with dogs of many breeds, and 3) the information about behavioral differences that exists in the minds of such authorities can be obtained by interviewing a large number of authorities with an interview format that minimizes the opportunity for them to rank breeds with which they have a personal connection.

The guidelines presented for breeds high and low in particular behaviors are just general guidelines as to the suitability of certain breeds for various environments or human-animal interactions. Early experience and behavioral interactions with human family members play an equivalent role in the behavioral characteristics of any particular dog. This said, if the selection of a puppy can be narrowed to a single breed or two, one can go to dog breeders or trainers for more information about behavioral characteristics of particular blood lines within a breed to decide on the source of the puppy.

What about mongrels versus purebred dogs? Many or most mongrels turn out to be very acceptable pets. The advantage of selecting a purebred over a mixed breed is that with the purebred one has more success in predicting what the dog will be like as an adult. One can have some success in judging the future behavior of a puppy of mixed breed on the basis of the characteristics of the likely breed contributions to a particular dog.

Gender Considerations and Effects of Neutering

Some of the same behavioral traits that vary from breed to breed also vary significantly between sexes. In Figure 20-1, traits in which males rank higher than females and in which females rank higher than males are presented. Because these are the same traits for which breeds were ranked, one can see the interactions here. If one wishes to obtain a dog from a breed that ranks moderate with regard to aggressive dominance over the owner, for example, but wants to minimize this aggressive tendency, a female would make a good choice. On the other hand, if one were choosing a dog from a breed ranking low in aggressiveness, the choice of a female over a male would not be such an important consideration.

Because male dogs are increasingly castrated as puppies or juveniles in the interest of pet population control, the question may arise as to the degree to which behavior is altered by castration. Too many times people feel that castrating a male dog early in life will make it calmer, less destructive, less aggressive toward the owner, or better with children. The objectionable behaviors altered in males, to a major degree by neutering (but not necessarily totally prevented), are mounting of other dogs or people, urine marking in the house, aggression directed toward other male dogs in the family and aggression directed toward human family members.[2]

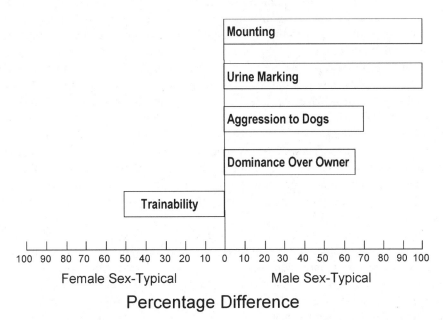

Figure 20-1 Behavioral predispositions that are female sex-typical and male sex-typical. The data are portrayed for neutered males and females. Note that behavioral differences are expressed quantitatively with some characteristics more strongly sexually dimorphic than others. (Data from Hart and Hart 1988[1] and Hart and Eckstein 1997.[3])

Castration before puberty seems to have no greater effect on the likelihood of these objectionable behaviors than does castration as an adult.[3]

With female puppies there is no indication that spaying at 6–8 months of age will have any lasting influences that are different than the same procedure performed in adulthood. The experience of one or more estrus periods, or even raising a litter of puppies, has not been shown to have any lasting influences.[3]

Influence of Early Experience

Of all the domestic animals kept by man, our relationship with dogs and cats is unique. We inevitably play some role in their early experience because they are raised within a family setting from the day they are born. Studies on the effects of early experience translate into a number of useful working principles with regard to raising puppies.

Prenatal and Neonatal Life

In the first 2 weeks after birth, and even extending back into the late prenatal period, the brain undergoes rapid development. Neurons are still multiplying and there is extensive growth of axons and dendritic branches. Eventually, neuronal growth and development are largely curtailed. Corresponding events that influence the brain just after birth can have influences that are difficult to reverse in the adult dog. In the neonatal period, for example, severe protein deficiency can impair normal brain development. Such malnutrition would be unusual in normally raised litters of puppies, but it is a possibility with excessively large litters and where there is a little runt that could, theoretically, suffer from impairment of brain development.

Sometimes there are concerns about the risks of handling the newborn puppies, and some breeders may feel that puppies should not be handled for the first couple of weeks. In families where children are present this can be an almost impossible assignment. What kind of advice should one offer about the effects of such early handling? From work with rats, mice, and cats, it is clear that the handling of neonatal animals for a few minutes each day may result in more rapid development of some organ systems, such as earlier eye opening, earlier development of motor coordination, and slightly accelerated growth. In light of these effects of early handling, clients could be advised that some handling of puppies is permissible as long as it does not become excessive.

Maternal and littermate interactions are another area of concern during early development. A mother spends almost all her time with the infants—nursing, grooming, retrieving, and sleeping. A fairly extensive body of literature on laboratory animals indicates that the severe disruption of this relationship can have important consequences on the behavior of the young as juveniles or adults. Understanding the effects of maternal deprivation is important because practitioners are frequently called on to give nutritional and medical advice to individuals who want to raise animals that have either been weaned very early or raised as orphans. It is unfortunate that in the literature available to pet owners so little is mentioned about the possible adverse effects of raising orphans without contact with mothers or lit-termates and how such effects can be minimized. It is impossible for a person to substitute for the round-the-clock care that a mother dog is able to offer, but human comfort, handling, and petting can partially substitute. Puppies that are orphaned and hand raised should, if possible, be kept together rather than be separated in an incubation box or among several households.

Period of Socialization

The period between 3 and 12 weeks of age is one that has been billed as particu-larly important for social responses. If a dog is deprived canine contact from about 3 weeks of age, it is likely to be socially inept around dogs. The puppy may not dis-play appropriate signals indicating submission when threatened by a dominant indi-vidual, or it may not correctly read submissive gestures of another. Some dogs that persistently get into fights with other dogs, injuring themselves or others, may fall into this latter category. In other instances a dog may act extremely fearful or exces-sively submissive as a function of inadequate exposure to other dogs. If people do not interact much with a dog during this period, especially after adoption, the dog may be either excessively fearful or inappropriately aggressive toward people.

When a family or single person is going to adopt a puppy, and there are no other dogs or puppies around, it is wise not to adopt the dog until at least 8 weeks of age so as to let the puppy develop social responses toward other dogs as long as the breeder is providing for other aspects of appropriate socialization. This is the time to consider puppy socialization classes, which are becoming increasingly popular. One study revealed a correlation between puppies attending puppy socialization classes and long-term retention in the home.[4] In the case of dogs raised where there is not frequent human contact, they should be adopted a week or so earlier than 8 weeks so that there is more time for optimal socialization with people. Of critical importance here is that the dog learns to take a subordinate role to people it inter-acts with, including children. Although early enrollment in an obedience class is valuable, this is no substitute for frequent and appropriate social interaction each day.

If a potential adopter desires to have a dog that will respond favorably around children, but they have no children at the present time, one might recommend that they look for a puppy that is born to a family breeder that has children with which the dogs frequently appropriately interact. They also should consider adopting the dog perhaps as late as 10 weeks of age, so as to allow more favorable behavior toward children. Following adoption, the owners should regularly have the dog exposed to children.

Avoiding Problem Behaviors

Some of the problems that may be avoided by early attention to various aspects of canine ethology and learning principles are house soiling, separation anxiety, bit-ing, fear of strange noises, obnoxious begging, barking, scratching at doors, fear related aggression, canine sibling rivalry (toward new babies), dominance-related aggression toward human family members and aggression toward other dogs in the same family or away from the home. The resolution of each of these problem behaviors in adult dogs is dealt with in Section II and the principles for preventing these problem behaviors are generally a modification of the treatment guidelines for resolution of the problem behavior.

House-Training

House-training is probably the most frequently discussed topic in puppy-raising advice covered in books on raising and training dogs. The fact is, as a reflection of an evolved adaptation to guard against accidentally reinfesting themselves with intestinal parasite larvae, dogs have an innate predisposition to keep the den and rest areas clean of feces and urine.[5] This predisposition allows dogs to be relatively easily house-trained, and one might say that sometimes dogs are house-trained in spite of the owners' attempts. If dogs did not have the basic inherent predisposition to keep the nest and rest areas clean, house soiling in dogs would be much more prevalent than it is and house-training much more challenging.

The house-training process is basically that of facilitating the acquisition of the behavioral orientation for the puppy that the house represents a "den" and adjacent "rest" areas. In addition, house-training helps the puppy develop signals to indicate when it wants to go outdoors to eliminate. However, there is one caveat; the den sanitation predisposition was maintained in the wolf ancestor by natural selection because the behavior reduced reinfestation with fecal-borne endoparasites and pathogens. Under domestic conditions, where dogs are treated for endoparasites, den sanitation is no longer under natural selection. This relaxed selection has led to more variability in the strength of this den sanitation predisposition among dogs than would be characteristic of the wolf ancestors. Thus, some dogs may be easier to house-train than others simply as a reflection of a weakened den sanitation predisposition.

It is easiest for a puppy to express its den sanitation behavior in the house if it is first maintained in a small space by use of fences or gates. If left in a small space for a relatively short period the puppy will usually control its elimination until it is taken outdoors to eliminate. After this routine becomes reliable—and the dog no longer soils the confined area and defecates or urinates soon after being taken outdoors—it can gradually be allowed greater access to the house while the routine of toilet outings is continued.

Puppies that are adopted during the winter and cannot be taken outdoors might need to be initially paper trained. This is begun by placing papers at a place in the confined area farthest away from the bed, food and water. To provide cues that will eventually be associated with use of the outdoors, a small amount of dirt and leaves may be placed on the papers. The soiled papers should be regularly cleaned up, except one layer of slightly soiled papers should be placed on top to provide an olfactory signal of the toilet area. After the puppy regularly uses the paper, the amount of paper spread could be gradually decreased and the puppy allowed greater access to the rest of the house. When tolerable weather arrives the next step will be to shift the dog's behavior from use of the newspapers to the outdoors. Usually one can just walk the dog to the appropriate place. Some trainers suggest placing the papers outside initially in the area in which they want the puppy to elim- inate. During house-training, areas of the house that are soiled should be cleaned up immediately with an enzymatic cleaner and covered with plastic or made tem- porarily unavailable to the dog.

Some puppy owners may want to train their puppy to eliminate in certain areas of the yard or on certain substrates. For example, in training a puppy to avoid the lawn, it is useful to go out with the puppy on most outings and walk it to the appro- priate areas until the dog relieves itself in the intended area. This desirable behav- ior should be acknowledged with praise. Whenever feces are left on an inappropri- ate substrate they should be picked up and a little fecal material placed in the in- tended toilet area to reinforce the olfactory signal for that area.

Separation Anxiety

Separation anxiety can usually be understood as a normal behavior of puppies upon being deserted. In nature, wolf puppies would rarely be abandoned, and even adult wolves would usually be in contact with their pack. Thus, when a puppy's family walks out and leaves it alone, the puppy may have an emotional reaction ranging from mild anxiety to panic.

One of the common manifestations of separation anxiety occurs when puppies are left alone at night. Imagine the distress of a puppy removed from the around- the-clock company of its mother and littermates and brought into a strange home where the only companionship is from human family members and these "pack" members abandon it at night. From this standpoint whining and yelping is under- standable. This puppy form of separation anxiety may be prevented by placing the puppy in an airline shipping crate on a chair near the side of the bed of the owners, so that the puppy can see and hear the owners throughout the night. This also gives the human family members, as well as the puppy, a better night's sleep. The habit- uation to being more separated begins by gradually moving the puppy's sleeping bed, an inch or so per day, away from the owner's bed. Eventually the puppy's bed can be across the room on the floor. If the goal is to have a dog sleep in another part of the house, the habituation process for nighttime sleeping can be continued, in gradual steps, until that goal is achieved.

A more difficult task is the habituation of separation anxiety when owners leave the house. The only way to habituate a dog to being left alone during the day is to schedule departures. Such habituation is much more easily accomplished with pup- pies and young dogs than it is with older dogs who have a history of anxiety or panic- like reactions when abandoned. The prevention of separation anxiety, by leaving the puppy alone frequently during the day for no reason other than habituation, may strike some dog owners as not sympathetic to the puppy's distress upon being left alone. In fact, there may be a tendency not to leave the puppy alone unless neces- sary to avoid this anxiety. However, puppies should be left alone frequently, if pos- sible, with staged short-term departures starting at an early age. When these depar- tures become somewhat routine, food treats should be paired with the departures so that the puppy learns to associate a food treat with being left alone. When the dog readily eats the food treat upon being left alone, this is usually a sign that at least anxiety is at a low level. Departures should be varied in duration, although it is certainly easiest to begin the habituation process with short departures that are repeated.

Fear of Loud Noises

It is natural for puppies to be fearful of strange noises; in nature strange noises might be a clue of harmful events to follow, such as a predator or unfriendly conspecific. However, strange noises that are repeated and never followed by an adverse consequence result in habituation to that particular noise. As with separation anxiety, puppies are usually more easily habituated to strange noises than adult dogs. They are commonly habituated to the sounds of vacuum cleaners, lawn mowers, fireworks, and thunderstorms without the owners even being aware of the process. On the other hand, unhabituated fear of loud, but harmless, sounds is common. One thing that makes fear reactions in dogs somewhat worse than they would normally be is that owners often try to comfort their puppies when they notice some fear or anxiety, apparently wishing to assure the puppies that nothing is wrong. This reinforcement of fearful behavior can exacerbate rather than improve the reaction.

Habituation of puppies to certain loud noises by intentional exposure to the fear- or anxiety-evoking noise is important if the puppy would not be exposed to these sounds until later in life. Although not the best idea, the stimuli can be presented at full strength. In adult dogs such habituation would usually involve exposure to a graded stimulus. The louder and more frightening the noise, the more necessary it is to present the stimulus in a modified or dampened form for the first exposures and then gradually increase the intensity. Habituating dogs to gunshots or firecrackers, for example, proceeds most easily with the use of muffled gunshots (use blankets over a starter pistol, cap gun, or gunshot recording) at the beginning of the training sessions.

When intentionally exposing dogs to anxiety-evoking stimuli one should offer a food treat to countercondition the emotional response; theoretically, the noise becomes associated with the positive effects brought on by food treats. When the dog is readily taking a food treat upon presentation of the noise, this is an indication that there is only weak fear or anxiety. The habituation process is continued as the sound is presented more intensely in graded steps. For the muffled shot, layers of blankets can be removed. The habituation is completed when the loud sound can be presented with no muffling.

Fear-Related Aggression

Just as with fear of strange sound acoustics, it is natural for young dogs to be fearful of strangers, whether they are other dogs or people. When they have a fear, a natural response is to escape, or if this is not possible, to threaten in some way so as to drive away the fear-inducing person or other animal. If the threatening behavior, such as a growl, drives away the fear-evoking individual, that behavior pays off because the aversive aspects of fear are relieved. If the growl does not induce people to withdraw, the dog may escalate its level of threat behavior by snapping; if this level of threatening behavior is effective, this new level is reinforced and replaces the milder threat behavior. Fear-related aggression directed toward children is not uncommon because dogs are frequently not properly habituated to children as puppies.

Preventing this problem requires an understanding that the behavior stems from a fear and not an offensive type of aggression. The prevention is to assure that a puppy has exposure to all of the types of possible fear-evoking individuals it will encounter as an adult. The dog needs repeated exposures to strangers and children when it is a puppy, and these exposures should be filled with fun, including petting, playing, and dispensing of food treats.

Obnoxious Begging, Barking, and Scratching

Behaviors such as scratching a door or barking to get inside the house are not manifestations of emotional reactions, but natural responses of dogs in a family setting. If barking or door scratching never results in any payoff in terms of being allowed in the house, the behavior will not increase in frequency. These behaviors may not completely go away because scratching and barking at the door probably exist at some natural level. The rule is never to reward the objectionable behavior. As to reinforcing acceptable behavior, one might require a period of quiet behavior for 10 minutes before allowing a puppy inside or simply reward the puppy for sitting by the door. In Chapter 3, a way of training a dog to ring a bell, or use some other acceptable behavior to indicate it wishes to come in the house, is outlined.

Clients have sometimes shaped objectionable behavior to the most offensive form by deciding not to give into a relatively mild form of an objectionable behavior, such as scratching at the door. However, when the behavior becomes very intense, the owners may then give in, reinforcing the more objectionable form of the behavior. The results in the case of scratching is that an intense and persistent form of the behavior replaces the milder form.

Canine Sibling Rivalry

One of the types of strange stimuli that can make a puppy or adult dog anxious and defensive is a new baby. Although dogs may be habituated to adults, juveniles, and young children, a new baby is clearly a different type of stimulus. Dogs, of course, can habituate to babies as easily or even more easily than to children because babies generally do not pursue them and poke them or pull their hair.

The problem of sibling rivalry arises when the young dog finds itself neglected whenever the baby is around. The dog may develop a dislike of the baby because the appearance of a baby is often accompanied by a reduction in pleasant and rewarding interactions with human family members. To make matters worse, people will often try to assure the dog they still love it by giving plenty of affection and treats to the dog when the baby is not around; this increases the contrast in social interactions with the dog when the baby is present and when the baby is not present.

There are several tips that can be followed to avoid this problem. If the soon-to-be parents intend to make other changes when the baby arrives, such as using a crate or moving the dog's sleeping place, they should do it early so the dog does not associate this change with the arrival of the baby. The owners should also start exposing the dog to new sights and sounds of a baby. Perhaps they might walk around carrying a doll or pushing a stroller. They could bring home baby clothes from friends and introduce these novel odors to the dog to incorporate the scent of a newborn. When the baby comes home from the hospital one parent who is more bonded with the pet could greet the dog while the other person carries the baby into the house. This keeps the dog from being ignored if its favorite person is holding the baby. In gradually introducing the baby to the dog, one should make it fun and rewarding for the dog to have the baby around. The only time the dog should get any attention or treats is while the owner is holding or working with the baby.

Dominance-Related Aggression

There is a natural tendency for dogs, as with their wolf ancestors, to aspire to a position of dominance over other pack members. Generally, expressions of aggressiveness are limited by the assertion of control by the human pack members. As long as any attempts at aggressive dominance by the puppy or young dog are appropriately corrected there is little problem. In the ancestral wolf such corrections would take the form of threats or snaps directed toward the unruly young pup. Instead of growls and snaps, human pack members use other forms of expression of control, such as a loud, low voice or restraint to accomplish the same end. A reluctance by people to control adequately the social interactions of a puppy that tests them may lead to future problems with related aggression.

The likelihood of this problem is related to the inherent predisposition of a dog to attempt to exert dominance over the owner. Such a predisposition is influenced by gender, breed membership, and individual genetic makeup within the breed. Regardless of a puppy's genetic or experiential background, family members should assert themselves when any signs of testing of the owner occurs. The degree to which this expression of human family control needs to be maintained depends on the temperament of the dog. Some dogs readily accept a subordinate role; other puppies will need a more structured environment. All puppies should frequently be given commands—such as "sit," "lie down," and "stay"—and food and praise should be used to reinforce obedience. Obedience classes are generally useful to help reinforce the control of human family members over their dogs.

Conclusions

This chapter deals with the selection of a puppy from the standpoint of the source, breed, gender, and individual genetic makeup. The effects of early experience are profiled with regard to socialization to people and other dogs. Habituation to separation and frightening environmental stimuli are most easily managed in puppies. Clinicians should be in a position to counsel prospective and new puppy owners about not only the selection of a dog but the importance of attention to early experience and training, especially for the avoidance of some of the common problem behaviors that are seen in adult dogs.

References

1. Hart BL, Hart LA. The Perfect Puppy: How to Choose Your Dog by Its Behavior. San Francisco: Freeman Press, 1988.
2. Neilson JC, Eckstein RA, Hart BL. Effects of castration on behavior of male dogs with reference to the role of age and experience. Journal of the American Veterinary Medical Association 1997;211:180–182.
3. Hart BL, Eckstein RA. The role of gonadal hormones in the occurrence of objectionable behaviours in dogs and cats. Applied Animal Behavior Science 1997;52:331–344.
4. Duxbury MM, Jackson JA, Line SW, Anderson RK. Evaluation of association between retention in the home and attendance at puppy socialization classes. Journal of the American Veterinary Medical Association 2003;223:61–66.
5. Hart BL. Behavioral adaptations to pathogens and parasites: Five strategies. Neuroscience and Biobehavioral Reviews 1990;14:273–294.

Section III
Behavior and Behavior Problems of Cats

Cats endear themselves to us in many ways. For one thing they are, without question, the cleanest and most fastidious in personal care of all domestic animals. Their grooming behavior, driven by an internal, clocklike generator, regularly evokes bouts of grooming, which tend to progress over the body in a posterior direction.[1] Such programmed grooming, which is effective in controlling ectoparasites,[2] was important for the ancestral cat and is genetically retained in the domestic cat. Grooming not only is useful in controlling fleas and other surface parasites, but it also removes stale oil and dirt. This aspect of grooming helps maintain the insulating value of the *pelage,* a property that is vital for optimum insulation so important to small mammals with a heat-losing body surface to mass ratio. Another endearing behavior of cats is their fastidious toilet behavior; just place a litter box in a corner and clean it regularly, and they are automatically toilet trained. Would that dogs, or even human counterparts, be so easily trained. Of course, this behavior was also important to the welfare of ancestral cats that were exposed to potential reinfection by intestinal parasites. Defecating in the den or nest areas invites reinfestation. Both grooming and toilet behavior can and do deviate from normal. In subsequent chapters we deal with the resolution of problems related to too much grooming and too little fastidious toilet behavior (Chapters 21 and 26).

An intriguing, and still poorly understood, behavior of several felids is purring. The behavior is reported for civets, genets, cheetahs, and even mountain lions. The physiological mechanism of purring is a brain-coordinated laryngeal modulation of respiratory air flow.[3] The various stimuli that evoke purring and the value to the ancestral cat are still not understood.

The old adage that cats have nine lives is another special feline topic worthy of mention. The adage probably stems from the ability of cats to survive falls from heights that would be fatal to almost any other mammal. In one study of cats falling from apartments in New York City, 90% of 115 cats falling from an average of 5–6 stories high survived.[4] Doing the math, one can see that on average, a cat could fall from a 5-story apartment onto pavement nine times before its number was up. Keep in mind a human's chance of surviving a fall of only 50 feet is about 50:50. Admittedly, cats are small with considerable wind resistance, and their maximum velocity from falling is half that of humans. But the flying squirrel posture, gyroscopelike righting reflex landing them on their feet, and their impact-absorbing flexed limbs, which spread out the shock, are unique to cats. Because the ancestral cat, like the domestic cat, undoubtedly climbed trees, and for millions of years cats have been falling out of trees, natural selection has shaped the strategy of surviving falls from heights.

One other unique aspect of cat behavior related to the feline ancestor is its social behavior. Mammalian species found in nature may be classified social or asocial and as territorial or nonterritorial. Social species are drawn together and often interact in some sort of social network. Asocial species, which comprise most species in nature, generally live in a solitary fashion, and if territorial, do not share a territorial space and do not have a social network with conspecifics aside from breeding and raising young. Asocial species often live in territories adjacent to conspecifics and are aware of the coming and going of their neighbors.

Cats, which are territorial, are the only domestic species in which the wild ancestor is considered asocial. Modern cats, however, have the ability to thrive in a wide range of social and asocial living environments, ranging from an environment where there is a despot with all others being subordinate[5] to an environment where social interactions are largely amicable with a recognizable social hierarchy.[6] Nonetheless, even in relatively amicable situations, the asocial background from the ancestral wild cat seems to surface from time-to-time as a component of intercat aggression (Chapter 22). One aspect of aggression between cats is that the density of cats within a neighborhood, and certainly within some households, is higher than one would find in the environment of the ancestor. This may contribute to the occurrence of aggressiveness in cats because they cannot conveniently leave an environment where altercations with other cats occur.

To be sure, conflicts are reduced by neutering males and spaying females. In a sense the practice of gonadectomy renders cats somewhat abnormal compared with the ancestor, but it contributes in a major way to the relatively peaceful coexistence of cats with each other in our environment.

Territorial species often have territorial marking behavior by which they leave strategically placed physical marks and substances that give off volatiles, or scents, on one or more prominent objects in the environment. Often urine is used, and at other times special scent glands are used, to deposit scent-producing substances on target objects. For animals in nature the territory is the area that is actively defended. A home range is the area the animal may occupy from time to time but is not necessarily defended. Because so many cats range freely outside the home, aspects of territoriality are important to understand.

For all domestic cats kept inside a home the territory includes all or part of the house. For indoor-outdoor cats the territory may also include the yard or even adjacent properties. Sometimes the limits of the cat's territory are difficult to determine. Cats may have a home range spanning over adjacent yards and wooded areas that are roamed through during normal day-to-day activities. Indoor-only cats, of course, do not have a home range beyond the territory of the house.

There are three types of important territory marking in domestic cats; cheek gland rubbing, scratching vertical objects and urine scent marking (see Chapter 21, Figure 21-1). All these types of markings involve leaving a chemical scent or odor. A characteristic of territorial marking is that the mark must be periodically renewed to maintain freshness, thus serving as a reminder to conspecific intruders that the territory is currently occupied. Most cat owners are familiar with the rubbing of the cheeks on vertical or prominent objects in the territory. Common targets are door thresholds, other cats in the household and/or the caregiver's legs. One interpretation of this behavior is that the cat is attempting to maintain a communal scent among the inhabitants in the household. One of the commercially available feline facial pheromones (Feliway®) claims to mimic this cheek gland pheromone and predispose a cat to feeling calm in an unfamiliar environment.

The types of marking in cats that can lead to problems for their owners are urine spraying and scratching. Marking associated with a cat scratching the surface of a corner of a couch can lead to serious damage. Scratching creates a visual mark and at the same time rubbing secretions from the front feet onto the object. After a cat starts scratching a target, be it a tree trunk or a piece of furniture, the odor attracts the cat back to the roughed-up area for repeated scratching to freshen up the scent. The resolution of objectionable scratching of furniture is discussed in Chapter 23.

The third type of marking is urine marking or urine spraying, typically on vertical surfaces. Urine marking, along with other types of house soiling, constitutes the most frequent group of feline problem behaviors for which veterinarians are consulted and is dealt with in Chapter 21.

The free-ranging manner of many cats brings up the issue of territoriality. A common occurrence is where a cat's attachment to its territory is so strong that when the owners move to a new home, not far away, the cat repeatedly leaves the new home and returns to its old territory. This is not the only explanation for returning to the old home; a cat may be escaping something aversive in the new home. For example, at the time of moving the neighbor near the new home may have a harassing dog or bully cat. At the old home the cat may not have shared a territory or home range with a dog or another cat.

As a resolution of this problem, if there is evidence that there is a situation in the new home that is aversive to the cat, consideration should be given to alleviating this situation. Ideally, cat owners should be aware that the introduction of a new cat or a new dog carries with it special problems and techniques for adapting a cat to the new household resident. Owners should wait until the cat is settled into the new home to bring in new canine or feline housemates.

For the cat that is strongly attached to the old home, it might be restricted to the house for several months before it is allowed to have access to the outdoors. The indoor-outdoor cat could be put outdoors on regular occasions using a leash and harness so that it develops an attachment to the area surrounding the house without having the freedom to leave. It is hard to say how long it will take for a cat to develop an attachment to a new territory when it is restricted. It is better to err on the side of restricting the cat too long than to risk having it wander off.

References

1. Eckstein RA, Hart BL. The organization and control of grooming in cats. Applied Animal Behaviour Science 2000;68:131–140.
2. ———. Grooming and control of fleas in cats. Applied Animal Behaviour Science 2000;68:141–150.

3. Frazer Sissom DE, Rice DA, Peters G. How cats purr. Journal of Zoology, London 1991;223:67–78.
4. Diamond J. How cats survive falls from New York skyscrapers. Natural History 1989;8:20–26.
5. DeBoer JN. Dominance relations in pairs of domestic cats. Behavioural Processes 1977;2:227-242.
6. Macdonald DW, Apps PJ, Carr GM, Kerby G. Social dynamics, nursing coalitions and infanticide among farm cats, *Felis catus*. Advances in Ethology Supplement 1987;28: 1–64.

Chapter 21

Feline House Soiling: Urine Marking, Inappropriate Urination, and Inappropriate Defecation

Cats are famous for their fastidious personal hygiene and, in fact, are usually so reliable in this behavior that one hardly needs to give a second thought to house-training them.

No other domesticated mammalian species discreetly digs a hole for elimination and then nicely covers it. It is not that cats "know" this is the right thing to do; clearly natural selection has played a role in shaping an innate predisposition toward this behavior. However, despite the fact that cats are known for their fastidious eliminative behavior, house soiling is the most frequent feline behavior for which veterinary consultation is sought.[1-3] Aside from the possibility of medically related causes of house soiling, this problem may reflect the choice of an inside toilet area separate from or in addition to the litter box, urine spraying of household objects, or a combination of behaviors. Understanding the way in which natural selection has shaped eliminative behavior is critical in solving problems associated with elimination.

Normal Eliminative Behavior

Because of an aversion to close contact with feces and urine, cats, like other denning or nesting species, have an inherent predisposition to keep the nest area free of fecal contamination. This is an evolved trait that protects them from exposure to fecal-borne parasites and pathogens. Cats go one step further, however, with their strong predisposition to bury fecal and urine deposits. Behaviorists have speculated from time to time about the evolution of the burying aspects of feline toilet behavior. One likely explanation is that this behavior helps cats avoid parasites or pathogens in nature.[4] By burying feces, cats avoid parasite larvae or intestinal pathogens that they could acquire through contact with uncovered feces. Burying the feces may also help keep fecal-borne tapeworm segments out of the reach of rodents who are intermediate hosts of a tapeworm species; cats who eat rodents with the encysted tapeworms acquire the tapeworms. The same is true for keeping feces away from cat fleas that ingest tapeworm eggs and are the intermediate host of a tapeworm species that infects cats when the flea is consumed after being groomed off. Another possible advantage of burying feces and urine is that in nature cats rely on small rodents for a food supply, and by burying freshly deposited feces and urine they are reducing cues of their proximity, which might otherwise induce rodents to avoid the area or at least be much more vigilant for a feline predator.

The burying behavior so characteristic of domestic cats, and presumably their evolutionary ancestors, makes them particularly nice house pets; fortunately, this burying behavior can be expressed in places as farfetched from the evolutionary environment as high-rise apartments. A cat owner need only provide a suitable litter and a container. Some people have even gotten away with hiding the litter container under a cabinet. The commercial version is the litter box dome enclosure which also prevents the access of canine housemates to the litter box. Modern technology has even provided mechanical, self-cleaning litter boxes. The problem with these innovations is that they may be pushing the limits of what some cats would consider even remotely "natural," and they commonly react by choosing an alternative toileting area in the house.

The aversion to feces and urine deposits, which plays a role in den sanitation, seems paradoxical with regard to the tendency for house cats to be attracted to the smell of residual urine and feces in selecting a place for elimination. In nature, urine and feces are not deposited randomly but in certain toilet areas.

Although cats may identify toilet areas by the mild residual odor from past use, they are turned off by the accumulation of too much urine and feces. As mentioned, the adaptive value of this behavior is that, in nature, they would be otherwise walking through a parasite minefield from the accumulation of feces kept moist from urine. A little fecal and urine odor, perhaps not unlike a restroom sign, is fine, but an accumulation is definitely aversive. Understanding this aspect of normal feline behavior can aid in realizing the importance of litter box management.

General Aspects of Problem Elimination

Lack of litter box use may be a sign of a pathophysiologic problem in the urinary system (e.g., urinary cystitis) or the gastrointestinal system (e.g., diarrhea), making it difficult for the cat to get to the litter box conveniently or to go outdoors for every elimination. In some instances a painful process in the joints, particularly arthritis, may make going into and out of a litter box difficult and lead to house soiling. Although the behaviorist must rule out, or rule in, a pathophysiological cause of the house soiling, in this chapter only problem elimination with a primary behavioral cause will be covered in reference to treatment guidelines. However, it must be remembered that a cat that has recovered from a medical condition leading to problem house soiling can continue to display the problem house soiling after resolution of the medical problem.

Aside from lower urinary tract disorders or other pathophysiologic problems, there are two behavioral reasons for problem urination: (1) a change in toilet area, referred to as *inappropriate urination*; and (2) *urine marking* (spraying). House soiling with feces may be due to a pathophysiological problem or change in toilet area, referred to as *inappropriate defecation*. Sometimes there is more than one etiology leading to house soiling. Urine marking appears to involve no urinary abnormality and, thus, is basically a behavioral problem.[5]

Diagnostic Issues

Generally with inappropriate elimination the cat changes its toilet area to another part, or parts, of the house and the litter box is no longer used. If a cat is urinating inappropriately, it still may use the litter box for defecation. Urine marking often occurs in circumstances arousing anxiety, such as agonistic encounters, social interactions, and/or territorial encounters with other cats. Urine marking is typically done with a standing posture, hind legs straight, tail up and quivering, while the cat alternately steps with the back legs and sprays urine on a vertical surface (Fig. 21-1). Frequent targets can include walls, windows, stereo speakers, and kitchen appliances. Spraying may also hit horizontal surfaces. Less frequently, objects may be marked using the squatting posture but still in the context of spraying a target, such as the owner's clothing.

It may be difficult to determine whether urine deposits on horizontal surfaces are a reflection of inappropriate urination or urine marking. Urine marking cats that deposit urine on horizontal surfaces usually spray urine on vertical surfaces at other times. Thus, the deposition of urine on vertical surfaces, at least on some occasions, is a clear diagnostic indication of urine marking. With urine marking the litter box is usually still used for urination and defecation. Problem urination may involve both urine marking and inappropriate urination, but the occurrence of both at the same time in the same cat is probably infrequent. Table 21-1 outlines some of these features in differentiating inappropriate urination from urine marking.

In dealing with both inappropriate urination and urine marking it is important to obtain a careful history about the location of soiled areas, management of litter box hygiene, and environmental events or social interactions with other cats that might be related to the onset of the problem. This is best done without expressing any judgment as to what is the best type of management or blaming the cat owner for less than the best management, so as not to bias the response of the owners. Having the client draw a rough map of the house floor plan with soiling locations, litter box locations, and areas of interaction with other outside or inside cats can be very useful. Because the treatment of inappropriate urination differs from that of urine marking, it is important that the clinician correctly diagnose the problem behavior. A study of diagnostic approaches to urine marking by veterinarians revealed that about 30% did not seem to recognize the critical element of deposition of urine on vertical targets as a key diagnostic feature in differentiating urine marking from inappropriate urination.[6]

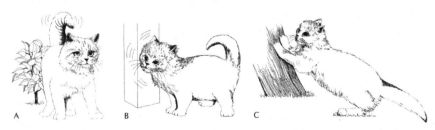

Figure 21-1   Three types of scent marking by cats. In addition to urine spraying (A), this illustration shows scent marking by a cat rubbing secretions from glands at the corners of the lips (B) and from glands located in the feet when the cat scratches something (C).

Table 21-1   Guidelines in differentiating problem urination reflecting inappropriate urination from urine marking (spraying).

Behavioral Signs	Inappropriate Urination	Urine Marking
Posture	Squatting	Usually standing
Amount of urine	Emptying bladder	Small amounts
Litter box usage	Usually stops using box	Continues to use litter box
Target area	Attractive horizontal substrate	Usually vertical
Precipitating factors	Aversion to litter box	Agonistic intercat interactions
Inappropriate defecation	Common	Usually not a problem

Individual Differences

One of the issues about inappropriate elimination that is overlooked is the genetic variability among cats in the degree to which they show fastidious toilet behavior. As mentioned, sanitary toilet behavior was undoubtedly present in the ancestral cat and is still retained by most cats in modern urban environments. In nature, the behavior of burying feces and urine in an appropriate substrate was acquired and maintained through natural selection. Assuming this eliminative behavior had a health-related function such as protecting offspring along with adults from exposure to parasites or pathogens, mother cats that deviated in nature from this sanitary behavior would leave fewer offspring than the more fastidious felines. Hence, the genetic programming of the behavior in nature was maintained with relatively little variability.

As cats have been domesticated and fecal-transmitted parasites and diseases controlled with medical intervention, natural selection that maintained the innate basis of the behavior has been relaxed. Now, cats that are not very sanitary live and reproduce about as well as the fastidious ones; when a behavioral pattern is almost irrelevant to reproductive success there is increased variability in the genetic elements controlling the behavior.[7] This is one reason that optimal litter box behavior may be easily thrown off in some cats by strange litter material or the addition of a new cat, and yet other cats are barely fazed.

There is no simple way of determining the exact role of genetic components of the sanitary toilet behavior of any particular cat as opposed to all of the environmental and medically related factors underlying problem elimination. Understanding the genetic aspects does help, however, in approaching each situation on a case-by-case basis, with the knowledge that genetics, as well as early kittenhood experience and current circumstances, all play a role. That said, if a family breeder or cattery has a cat with consistent and notoriously poor litter box habits one might think twice about breeding this cat.

Because house soiling may involve pathophysiological considerations for inappropriate elimination, as well as a potential need for psychotropic medications, cat owners should immediately think of consulting their veterinarian about this problem behavior. Interviews with a large number of owners of cats with problem urination revealed that 70% had contacted their veterinarians; friends and the Internet were other frequently consulted sources.[6] Those not consulting their veterinarians usually expressed that they did not believe their veterinarian could help with the problem. There is clearly room for veterinarians and feline advocacy organizations to let cat owners know that this is a problem that can be resolved and that they should involve the family veterinarian. Finally, although the comments of this chapter are intended to help clinicians in resolving problem elimination in a client's home, the same principles apply to boarding cats away from their home. The last thing a client wants is to have a cat thrown off in elimination behavior stemming from being boarded inside a cage with a tiny litter box lined with newspaper.

Inappropriate Urination and Defecation

There are several possible medical causes for inappropriate urination, including lower urinary tract disorder, age-related cognitive dysfunction, weakened urinary bladder sphincter control, mild arthritis, and neurological problems. Weakened anal sphincter control, uncontrollable diarrhea, and colitis may be involved in inappropriate defecation. After these causes are excluded or resolved, the problem is considered primarily behavioral. In some instances problem elimination could reflect more than one cause.

Typical History

The cat presented for this problem is usually one that was previously consistent and reliable in using a litter box and/or outdoor toilet area and for some reason is now defecating and/or urinating on the floor or on another horizontal substrate. With regard to house soiling just with urine, the cat owner may not have distinguished between urine marking and inappropriate urination, although if urine is deposited on vertical objects a good number of cat owners are aware that this is different than their cat finding a new toilet location. Sometimes just one or two carpeted areas are used exclusively, and other times several areas are used, almost as if by random. A carpet, because of the texture and possibly the odor, may share enough properties with soil or sand to be an attractive toilet alternative for the litter box. Some cats are drawn to a bathtub or sink for elimination; perhaps a small bit of water associated with these areas is an attractive influence. The soil in large planters is also logically attractive as a toilet area to cats. Some clinicians have noted that urinating in bathtubs or sinks may involve a urinary tract disease rather than urine marking.

Aspects of the history that are important to gather are changes that might have occurred in the household at the time the problem began. For example, there may have been an introduction of another cat, puppy, or adult dog that has changed the social dynamics in the home or even the cat's access to a litter box. With the addition of new cats the owner may not have added the appropriate number of litter boxes or may not be changing litter boxes more frequently to accommodate more frequent use of the boxes. In multicat households, different cats may prefer different types of litter material and a new cat may not like the litter material that is used for the resident cat. An owner may have moved a litter box to a part of the house where it is inconvenient or unappealing for the cat. There may have been changes in the house, such as installation of new carpet (new odor and texture) or introduction of new furniture, that became appealing to a cat if its attraction to the litter box was rather marginal. With regard to a cat that uses outdoor areas for urination and defecation, a change in weather may be involved. The history should focus on whether the problem stems from aversion to the litter box (or outdoor areas) or attraction to the household target or location. Aversion to the litter box may be indicated by a cat not covering the feces, straddling the box to avoid touching the litter, shaking its paws after touching the litter, digging outside the box on the floor of the room, and running from the box after elimination. Such aversion-related behavior may have been noticed prior to the onset of house soiling and could have been a behavioral marker that the cat would later be house soiling.[3]

Probably the most common cause of aversion to a litter box is infrequent cleaning of the litter box and changing of the litter. Aversions are also sometimes related to the introduction of new litter material that may have differently sized granules or deodorizing chemicals. If the caregiver introduced a new plastic litter box without thoroughly washing it, strong volatiles characteristic of new plastic may be driving the cat away. The size of the litter box may be too small for the cat to be able to move around appropriately. If an owner uses plastic liners, the cat may develop an aversion if, while covering urine or feces, the cat's claws catch the liner. The use of liners has been associated with an increase in inappropriate elimination.[8] Cats that are brought into the home from an animal shelter or from a different home may be introduced to a type of litter different from that to which they were accustomed or with which they were raised. One should inquire about the type of litter and litter box previously used by a cat in its previous home or shelter and whether there were any problems in the cat using the other litter box. Another reason is that the cat may associate pain or trauma with litter box use, such as with arthritis making climbing into the litter box painful.

An aversion to the location of a litter box can develop for a number of reasons. The litter box may be situated in a very busy area or in an area where another pet that the cat does not get along with, such as a new puppy, spends a good amount of time. It may be located near something that may have startled it, such as a washing machine or dryer. It may be too close to where the cat is fed; cats prefer to eliminate away from the feeding area.

Diagnosis

Initially, the clinician should determine whether the problem is inappropriate urination or urine marking, according to the criteria discussed previously and listed in Table 21-1. Assuming that urine marking is ruled out, the next step is to rule out a pathophysiologic cause by history and clinical tests. Interstitial cystitis, which has been reported to be related to the onset of problem urination, is not diagnosed by urinalysis and generally requires endoscopic examination of the urinary bladder.[9] The history should have clarified the possible aspects of the household management and interactions with the family causing aversion to the litter box or attraction to other areas.

Treatment Guidelines

The recommended treatment for inappropriate elimination usually follows along four lines. One is to deal with identifiable aversive aspects of the litter box or outdoor area (for indoor-outdoor cats). The second is to increase the appeal and accessibility of the litter box or outdoor toilet area. The third is to discourage the use of inappropriate areas or to make them unavailable. The fourth, as a last resort, is the use of confinement to reinstate litter box usage. Although there is a tendency for cat owners to want first to try discouraging use of inappropriate areas by some sort of punishment or making the soiled area unavailable, it is important that attention first be given to eliminating aversive aspects of the litter box and attempting to increase its appeal.

Dealing with aversive aspects of the litter box

Litter box aversion is probably more common than most cat owners believe. Understanding the cause of a litter box aversion may be as simple as noticing that the litter box is not being cleaned frequently enough. Daily cleaning of the litter box may be sufficient for a single cat, but a client may not realize that with two additional cats, there should be more litter boxes and the boxes should be cleaned more often. Accommodations should be made because different cats may have preferences for different types of litter. With regard to number of litter boxes, it is best to err on the side of too many. At least one litter box per cat is recommended in multiple cat households; some authorities suggest one litter box per cat plus an additional one for good measure. These litter boxes also have to be separated by distance in the house. If they are next to each other, it is like having one large litter box.

Covered litter boxes, although appealing to cat owners, may result in concentration of urine and fecal odors that are aversive to cats. If the litter box is covered, the owners may not be aware of how dirty it is. Another modern invention, the automated litter box cleaner, may also repel some cats because of the loud noise. Cat owners may have to give up these amenities if they seem to produce an aversion. An aversion may also stem from the client introducing a new litter with a deodorizing additive or a litter box liner that gives off aversive odors or is caught in the cat's claws. Apparently some cats find deodorizing additives objectionable. The problem may be solved by the owners shifting back to the old litter. A new litter box will have an odor associated with new plastic that may be aversive; therefore, a thorough soapy cleansing and rinsing is important. A plastic litter box should be replaced periodically, because the urine soaks into it over time, creating a constant source of odor.

The recommended procedure for management of the litter box is that solids and wet litter or clumped litter should be cleaned at least daily. The clumping, small-granulated clay litter is efficient at localizing the spread of fluid so that the box is easily cleaned and the rest of the litter material remains dry. Even with using a clumping litter, the litter box needs to be dumped and cleaned regularly. If the older litter material of large granules is used, the feces need to be scooped daily, and the entire litter material should be discarded at least weekly and the litter box washed.

There are occasions when use of the litter box presents an opportunity for harassment by a puppy or a child. Most adults know not to bother a cat using a litter box, even if the squatting cat represents an easy target to catch for medication. Any harassment of a cat at the litter box can lead to avoidance of the litter box, and cat owners should be counseled accordingly.

Finally, under the topic of cleaning litter boxes, cat owners should be reminded of new research showing that cat fecal-borne parasites may have adverse effects on wildlife and soiled cat litter should not be flushed down the toilet but rather bagged and dispensed of with garbage. Cat owners may not be aware of the fact that most clumping litter may block sewer lines if flushed down the toilet.

Increasing the appeal of the litter box

After the aversive aspects are dealt with there should be consideration of increasing the appeal and accessibility of the litter box. Given individual differences among cats, it could be that some cats would use any litter material put before them, even newspapers, but others would be easily thrown off by something other than what they used while they grew up. A useful type of experiment to conduct with cats is to offer to them a litter box choice experiment in which the conventional clay litter and sandlike clumping litter are among the selections. If tray liners have been used, some choices should be given without the liners. The litter box experiment might include as many as five to eight appropriately sized temporary litter boxes (cut down from cardboard boxes) to determine a cat's preference for litter (Fig. 21-2). Wood chips and treated newspaper plugs are rarely preferred but could be among the options. Because cats can differ with their choice of litter material, or even the preferred location of the litter box, in multicat households it is important to determine whether there are individual cat differences and to accommodate the cats accordingly. Some cats may not even like the usually popular clumping clay litter, and it may be necessary to use plain sand. Sand offers easy digging and it drains well and this may be why it remains an all-time favorite substrate of outdoor cats. For indoor cats, the preferred litter is fine unscented clumping litter.[3]

Some cats prefer different depths of litter. One could determine the appropriate depth of litter for a particular cat in the litter box lineup mentioned above, where one box has litter 1 inch deep and another box has litter 2 inches deep, and so forth. Another possibility is shaking the litter in the box so that the litter is shallow at one end (1/2-inch deep) and deeper at the other end (2 inches deep) and recording the part the cat uses. In the general case, the deeper, the better.

A special situation may arise if a cat is attracted to a particular throw rug for urinating to the point where the rug is ruined. A litter box size piece could be cut from the now ruined rug, placed in the bottom of the litter box, and sprinkled lightly with litter. The cat may then be drawn to this previously soiled rug remnant in the litter box and start using the box regularly. Gradually, over time, more litter material is added, a spoonful at a time starting around the edges, while pieces of the carpet are cut away until the cat is using the box with only litter material.

The appeal of outdoor toilet areas may be increased by eliminating aversive elements such as harassing dogs or the effects of inclement weather and providing a

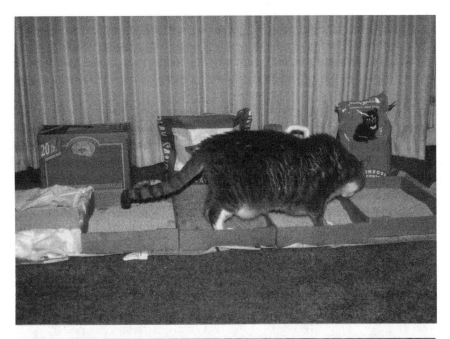

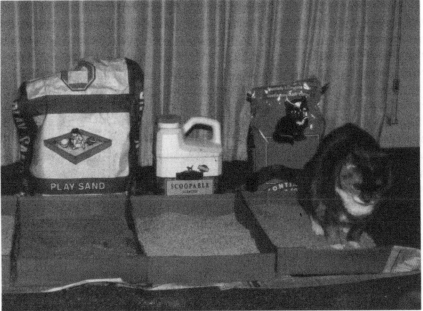

Figure 21-2   Lineup of litter boxes to determine a cat's preference for litter. The array consists of fine clay with liner and without liner, playpen sand, another brand of fine clay, and course clay. This cat seems to prefer the coarse clay.

shelter over one or more designated areas. Taking note of the widespread appeal of children's sandboxes for cats, caretakers could create an outdoor, toilet-area sandbox for the cat at ground level with commercial sand that can be cleaned as frequently as one would clean a litter box.

Discouraging use of inappropriate areas

A paradox regarding urine and fecal odors can affect the problem: Some mild residual odor signals a toilet area to a cat, but strong odors signal excessive buildup of feces and are avoided by a cat. Hence, frequent cleaning of the litter box is recommended to avoid the odor of excessive accumulation of feces and urine; the mild residual odors remaining after cleaning remain as a marker of a toilet area.

The areas affected by feline house soiling in most homes are invariably cleaned soon after they are soiled; there is no accumulation of feces or urine, but some residual odor undoubtedly often remains, serving as a marker of a toilet area. For inappropriate targets, vigorous cleaning of previously soiled areas with an enzymatic cleaner is necessary to remove all residual odor cues so that these areas do not retain the slightest hint of odor of a toilet area. To this end the cleaner should not contain ammonia. A number of cleaning products will usually work, although published data reveal that enzymatic cleaners result in the most effective removal of urine odors.[10,11] Residual urine odors on a carpet may make it attractive when coupled with the soillike texture of the carpet. Initial attraction to a newly installed carpet may be related to new carpet odors with enough shared characteristics with residual fecal or urine odors that the cat is attracted to use the new carpet.

One may also take advantage of the fact that, for reasons of protection from pathogens and parasites, cats will generally not defecate or urinate in areas that are customarily used for feeding or watering. Thus, feeding, watering, and playing with a cat in previously soiled areas may discourage the subsequent use of that particular area for toileting. Remote punishment, such as upside-down plastic carpet runners, duct tape, or contact paper placed sticky-side up, room deodorizer, aluminum, heavy plastic, or motion- or light-beam–triggered alarms, may be placed near the target area(s) to discourage the cat's approach (Chapter 3).

Remote punishment to keep a cat away from an inappropriate toilet area works only if the punishment is delivered immediately after the cat enters the off-limits area, and if the punishment is delivered every time the cat approaches the area. Punishment is always more effective if the likelihood of the cat engaging in the

---

INAPPROPRIATE ELIMINATION IN CATS

Causes

- Litter box or outside toilet area aversion
- Attraction to inappropriate toilet areas

Resolution

- Implement litter box hygiene.
- Increase attractiveness of litter using selection experiment.
- Add additional litter boxes.
- Prepare appealing outside toilet area.
- Use enzymatic cleaner for soiled areas.
- Feed or water cat near inappropriate toileting areas.
- Use remote punishment for inappropriate area.
- Confine cat, and then allow gradual access to house.

Case Study: Inappropriate Urination

History

Toby, a 4-year-old male castrated domestic shorthair cat with two feline house-mates, was presented for urinating out of his litter box. He used the litter box consistently until 1 month ago. There is one litter box in the house on the second floor for all cats. The owners use scented clumping litter that is scooped every 3 days and changed every 6–8 months. When Toby uses the litter box he does not cover the urine or feces and rushes to leave the litter box. He primarily urinates on the carpeting behind the couch on the first floor. Medical examination, with urinalysis and complete blood count and serum chemistry panel, were within reference limits.

Diagnosis

Inappropriate urination stemming from too few litter boxes, aversive litter, and inadequate cleaning schedule.

Treatment Plan

1. Increase the number of litter boxes to four, spread throughout the house.
2. Switch to a nonscented, scoopable litter.
3. Clean the litter boxes daily.
4. Change the litter and wash the litter box once every 2 weeks.
5. Clean the soiled carpeting with an enzymatic cleaner.
6. Make the area behind the sofa, previously a target, aversive to approach with the use of upside-down plastic carpet tread.
7. If measures 1–7 do not solve the problem, conduct a litter choice trial to determine whether there is another type of litter that Toby prefers.

Progress Report

The owners followed all instructions, and at 2 months, Toby was consistently using the litter boxes for both urination and defecation. He urinated out of the litter box only once, when the owners were out of town for a weekend and the pet sitter had not cleaned the litter boxes.

---

behavior is reduced first by making the litter box as appealing as possible. It is also easier if there are just a few spots that the cat targets.

Retraining through temporary confinement

If the previously mentioned procedures do not resolve the problem, there is the option of confining the cat in a small space, such as a bathroom or utility room with a tile or vinyl floor, so that the cat has a higher probability of using a litter box. After the cat is regularly using the litter box it may be gradually allowed access to the rest of the house under close supervision. Such confinement is, in itself, somewhat aversive and may produce some anxiety or aversion to the room where the cat is confined. Thus, this approach is recommended as a last resort.

Urine Marking and Spraying

As explained earlier, urine marking is a type of territorial marking that is mostly performed by tomcats. Urine for cats represents a fingerprint and cats can identify the smell of individual cats. In nature, by urine marking prominent objects in its territory, a cat familiarizes itself with its own territory and home range. The pervasive, but mild, urine odor probably makes a cat more self-assured and comfortable and also communicates the cat's presence to other cats in the surrounding areas. Cats probably do not "intentionally" mark the boundaries of their territories as one would put up a fence, but rather mark prominent objects within the territory.[12] Urine marking by females is also undoubtedly useful during the breeding season in attracting breeding males as they wander through the territories of various females.

Recall that urine marking is typically expressed by urine spraying, whereby a cat approaches a vertical target, briefly smells it, and then turns, lifts the tail, and sprays a bit of urine on the vertical target. The urinary bladder is usually not emptied. Frequent targets are walls, windows, stereo speakers, and kitchen appliances. As mentioned, the behavior is normal for tomcats and presumably reflects an aspect of territoriality related to repelling other males or gaining access to breeding females. The behavior is under hormonal control and is usually prevented when males are castrated (Chapters 4 and 27).

Spraying may also be deposited on horizontal surfaces either by squatting or standing while emitting a jet of urine that falls on a horizontal surface. Because some urine deposition on horizontal surfaces (e.g., owner's clothes) is deposited in the same context as spraying urine on a vertical surface, the term *urine marking* is used interchangeably with urine spraying to include marking on both vertical and horizontal surfaces. No studies have reported differences in the frequency with which females and males may distribute vertical versus horizontal marking. It is assumed that if cats engage in horizontal marking, most urine marks are still deposited on vertical surfaces.

Androgen Control of Urine Marking

Although urine marking in males is strongly influenced by gonadal androgen secretion and is much more prevalent in tomcats than neutered males or females, castrated males make up the large majority of cats presented to clinicians for urine marking. A survey of over 100 owners of male cats castrated between 6 and 10 months of age estimated that urine marking in the cats as adults occurred on an occasional basis in about 30%; in about 10% of cats the problem became serious. The same study, which included a survey of over 100 owners of female cats spayed between 6 and 10 months of age, suggested that 5% of females became serious urine markers.[13] Probably a more accurate estimation of the disparity between males and females in the tendency to engage in urine marking comes from a clinical trial involving recruiting cats for treatment of urine marking. The trial found that five times as many males were nominated by their owners and enrolled into the study as females.[14]

Androgens produced by the gonads cause the odor of tomcat urine, which is distinctive from that of females or castrated males.[15] Although the odor of male cat urine is virtually always made less offensive by castration, dealing with spraying behavior is another story. Castration is estimated to be effective in markedly reducing or eliminating problem urine marking in about 90% of urine marking adult male cats.[16] The extent of experience an adult male has in engaging in the malelike behavior, such as urine marking, appears to play no role in the persistence of the behavior after castration. Similarly, as summarized in Figure 21-3, castration at the earlier age is evidently no more effective in preventing the problem behavior than castration at the later age is at eliminating an existing urine marking problem.[17] The persistence of urine marking in tomcats after castration is apparently not due to residual amounts of testosterone, because this hormone is metabolized quickly and evidence from work on laboratory animals has shown that maintenance of malelike behavior is not due to compensatory secretion of adrenal androgens.[17]

The persistence of urine marking in some castrated males may be seen as similar to the persistence of sexual behavior in some castrated male cats. The best explanation is that the neural circuitry for the behavior, established before birth, can be activated by appropriate stimuli even without the androgenic hormonal support that is needed by the majority of cats.[18] In the case of sexual behavior, the stimulus is a receptive female; in the case of urine marking, the stimulus may be agonistic interactions with other cats or other territorial disturbances.

Because urine marking is primarily a male sex-typical behavior, the possible role of perinatal hormones in predisposing some females to engage in the behavior has also become a topic of interest. Investigators studying sexual behavior of laboratory

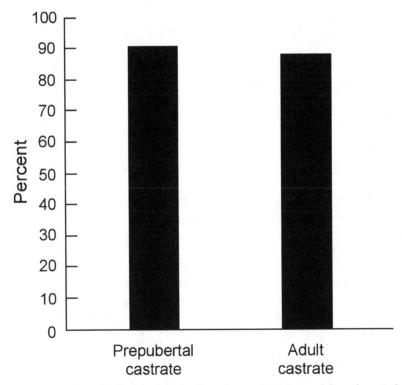

Figure 21-3 Estimated effects of castration of prepubertal or adult male cats in preventing or markedly reducing problem urine marking in the cats in adulthood. (Data from Hart and Cooper 1984[13]; Hart and Barrett 1973[16].)

rodents have found that an intrauterine position of a female fetus between two male fetuses can predispose females to malelike behavior (Chapter 4). This explanation for the occurrence of urine marking in female cats was not supported in a study on cats.[13]

Typical History

Cats will often be presented with complaints by the owner that urine is being deposited on household objects. Frequently the owners are perplexed as to why the problem started and, of course, want to have the problem resolved. When treating urine marking, it is a good idea to explore the reasons why the animal started spraying and continues to spray. Were there antagonistic encounters with other cats in the home or outside the home? Did the owners recently move? Is the cat emotionally upset or especially anxious? Are there new cats in the household? Are there stray cats in the neighborhood coming to the window? Did spraying begin with the onset of the breeding season? Some factors that provoke marking may be transient, such as the onset of the breeding season or the owners moving to a new house, and therefore, after the marking has been reduced or eliminated the problem may be resolved. In other instances, such as the addition of a new cat to the home, the provocative stimuli are more permanent.

In pursuing the history, the who, when, where, and why questions are important to pursue: identifying the culprit (who?); the estimated frequency of the urine deposits and the time that marking occurs (when?); whether the targets are horizontal or vertical surfaces (where?); and the provocative stimuli (why?). Having the owner draw a map of the house identifying the location of litter boxes, feeding areas, resting areas, targets of marking, and places of interaction with cats outside or inside the house may be useful.

As mentioned above, urine marking is primarily a male behavior. The most common owner-identified cause of urine marking is agonistic interactions with cats inside or outside the home. Unfriendly interactions between cats in a home often begin with the introduction of a new cat. Other triggers are a change in home or territory, such as the owners moving to a new home or making an outdoor cat into an indoor cat. It appears that the stress and anxiety from interactions with other cats or a change in daily routine are responsible for initiating and maintaining the spraying in many or most cats. Not surprisingly, therefore, cats from multicat households are overrepresented in cats presented for urine marking.[14]

Considering the role of urine spraying in marking territory and renewing previous marks in nature, thoroughly cleaning deposited urine marks can be expected to eliminate the faint odor cues of a previously marked area that draw a cat back to freshen the marked area. One should obtain information about the way in which old marks have been cleaned when taking the history.

Litter box hygiene is also important and one should inquire about type and frequency of litter box cleaning procedures. Infrequent cleaning and changing of the litter box may be a factor in evoking urine marking, especially in females. Perhaps a chronically soiled litter box raises the level of anxiety or emotional upset in some cats. Inadequate litter box hygiene may be an indication that one should be aware of the possibility of both urine marking and inappropriate urination.

Finally, keep in mind that the owner's estimation of the actual amount of urine marking may differ from that which actually occurs; an owner may initially over-estimate the actual number of marks deposited as opposed to when they subsequently record, on a daily basis, the number of urine marks.

Diagnosis

The main differential diagnostic challenge is to rule out inappropriate urination (see earlier sections and Table 21-1). It is possible in instances where inadequate litter box hygiene is obvious that cats may have both a urine marking and an inappropriate elimination problem. One might expect inadequate litter box hygiene to contribute to urine marking in females more than males because urine and fecal odors may be more upsetting to females than males.

Although a thorough medical evaluation seems advisable, lower urinary tract disorders do not appear to cause urine marking.[5] Urine marking involves finding a target, using a special posture, and spraying only a small amount of urine on a vertical target; this is not the type of behavior that can be readily attributed to a lower urinary tract disorder or systemic disease. Although not likely to be related to the maintenance of the urine marking, any urinary problem that becomes evident during a medical workup should be treated prior to, or concurrent with, treating the urine marking.

Treatment Guidelines

For cats that are spayed or neutered, the treatment approaches emphasize addressing the triggers, managing intercat interactions, maintaining litter box hygiene, cleaning old and newly deposited urine marks, and giving the cat antianxiety medication. Although several approaches, including antianxiety medication, can be used simultaneously, some clients may prefer to attempt to resolve the problem by the measures of environmental hygiene and management of intercat interactions before placing the cat on medication. At the outset the client should record on a daily basis the number of marks that are detected for at least a week before implementing any treatment. By recording urine marks one can assess the improvement when therapeutic measures are instituted. Although the management and hygiene approaches are important, these are therapeutic measures that are not necessarily as easy to profile in the client's mind as the administration of medication.[6]

Castration of gonadally intact males

An estimated 80% of adult males castrated because of a spraying problem can be expected to undergo a rapid decline in the behavior, with an additional 10% or so undergoing a more gradual decline. This leaves approximately 10% that can be expected to persist in the problem behavior if no additional measures are taken to resolve the problem. As mentioned, persistence in spraying following castration is not caused by residual amounts of testosterone, because within 8 to 16 hours after castration testosterone in the blood is reduced to castrate levels. Age or experience in performing the behavior seems to play no role in predicting which cats will respond to castration.[17] Treatment for persistent urine spraying or urine marking in male cats that have been castrated as adults is about the same as for prepubertally castrated male cats.

Management of intercat interactions

As mentioned, unfriendly or agonistic interactions with cats inside the home and outside the home are the most common triggers associated with the onset and maintenance of marking behavior. If cats outside the home are a causative factor, blocking at least the lower parts of windows where a client's cat visually interacts with outside cats, making the yard aversive to outside cats with a motion-sensor sprinkler, removing attractions to strange cats such as bird feeders, or some other way of eliminating the interaction may reduce the urine marking problem.

For agonistic behaviors among cats inside the house, making household arrangements to reduce the opportunity of agonistic interactions, such as parceling out the living space, may prove useful. Separate feeding stations and litter boxes as well as separate rest areas are important to provide. In some instances a physical barrier may be needed to separate warring cats (see also Chapter 22).

Cleaning urine marks

In homes, as well as in nature, cats seem to be attracted to previously marked areas and freshen them with new urine marks, presumably to maintain olfactory prominence. In nature this has an adaptive value on maintaining territorial identification with regard to competing conspecifics. A quick cleanup simply weakens the odors and may encourage more marking. Promptly and thoroughly cleaning all deposited urine marks with an enzymatic cleaner probably removes enough of the residual urine odor to decrease the likelihood of future marking.

Litter box hygiene

Although marked areas should be cleaned because they attract urine marking, litter box hygiene is important for another reason. An infrequently cleaned litter box may discourage use of the box for defecation and urination, and an excessive level of urine and fecal odors may raise the anxiety level of some cats, leading to marking. The best recommendation is to use a scoopable litter and clean it at least once a day (see earlier in this chapter). The box itself should be washed about once a week. Providing plenty of litter boxes, scooping the litter boxes once a day, and washing the litter box weekly, coupled with cleaning of deposited urine marks with an enzymatic cleaner, was found to reduce urine marks significantly. These measures appear to be particularly important in controlling marking behavior of females and may virtually resolve the marking problem in some females.[14]

A recent innovation in the efforts to control urine marking is an aerosol spray containing a feline facial pheromone (Feliway). According to label claims, the pheromone has some similarities to cheek gland secretions, which allegedly induce "friendly" behavior when sprayed on prominent areas in the cat's environment; this in turn is claimed to reduce marking with urine. Clinical trials suggest an effect on urine marking ranging from modest to almost total resolution.[19–22]

Pharmacological approach

Treatment of urine marking with psychoactive drugs has evolved over the past two decades. With the earlier treatments using progestins, diazepam, and buspirone in open-label studies, an estimated 30–75% of cats showed a marked reduction of urine marking.[23] Studies with the selective serotonergic reuptake inhibitor (SSRI) fluoxetine indicate that almost all cats respond with a 90% or greater reduction in marking if treatment is sufficiently prolonged.[24,25] Another serotonergic drug, clomipramine, although tested less extensively, may be as effective as fluoxetine.[25,26]

The medications that have been effective in reducing urine marking have different mechanisms of influences on brain neurotransmitters. The SSRIs increase serotonin primarily by blocking the reuptake of serotonin at the synaptic junction. The tricyclic antidepressant (TCA) clomipramine increases serotonin by direct stimulation as well as by blocking serotonin reuptake. Buspirone has serotonergic effects by presynaptic augmentation of serotonin release. Benzodiazepines, such as diazepam, increase gamma amino butyric acid, a neuroinhibitory transmitter. These medications share the effect of reducing anxiety, suggesting that is the avenue through which problem urine marking is reduced or eliminated.

The only drug for which there are clinical data available for comparison with placebo is fluoxetine. In a double-blind format (1 mg/kg/q24hr), urine marking declined in fluoxetine-treated cats by at least 90% in all cats over 8 weeks of treatment; in placebo-treated cats, marking did not change.[24] A follow-up study,[25] comparing fluoxetine with clomipramine, found that although the mean improvement in urine marking continually improved (Fig. 21-4), it was not until 16 weeks or beyond that some cats responded with a 90% or greater reduction in marking (Fig. 21-5).

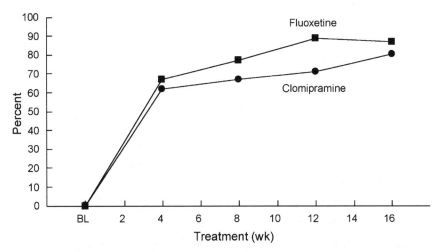

Figure 21-4 Comparative efficacy of fluoxetine and clomipramine in reducing urine marking in cats over a 16-week treatment period. An improvement of 100% is complete resolution. Significant improvement over baseline (BL) was detected for both treatments by 2 weeks, and no significant differences were found between the 2 groups. (Data from Hart et al. 2005[25].) (Reprinted with permission from Hart BL et al. Control of urine marking behavior in cats by long-term treatment with fluoxetine hydrochloride and clomipramine hydrochloride. Journal of the American Veterinary Medical Association 2005,226:378–382.)

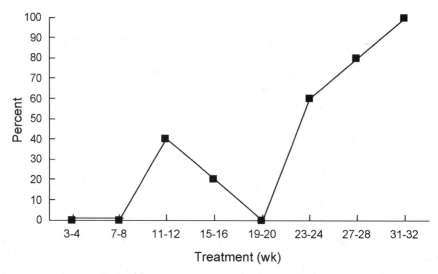

Figure 21-5   Percent of cats reaching at least 90% improvement (reduction in marking) over 32 weeks of treatment with fluoxetine. (Data from Hart et al. 2005[25].) (Reprinted with permission from Hart BL et al. Control of urine marking behavior in cats by long-term treatment with fluoxetine hydrochloride and clomipramine hydrochloride. Journal of the American Veterinary Medical Association 2005,226:378–382.)

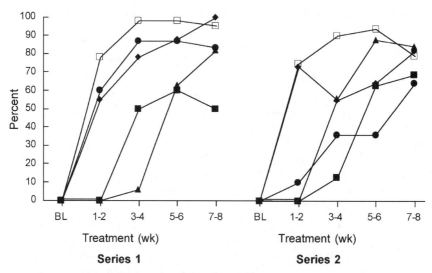

Series 1   Series 2

Figure 21-6   Improvement over baseline (BL) in weekly urine marking rate of five cats during an initial 8 weeks of fluoxetine treatment, which was followed by withdrawal until marking returned to BL rate, followed by a second series of identical treatments for 8 weeks. The graph shows responses of individual cats was about the same over the two series of treatment. (Data from Hart et al. 2005[25].) (Reprinted with permission from Hart BL et al. Control of urine marking behavior in cats by long-term treatment with fluoxetine hydrochloride and clomipramine hydrochloride. Journal of the American Veterinary Medical Association 2005,226:378–382.)

282

In most cats there is a recurrence of urine marking after drug withdrawal, with some often returning to 50% or greater of their original marking rates. There tends to be a correlation between the number of marks at baseline and the level of marking after drug withdrawal. Cats do not necessarily become resistant to the drug or dosage being used, and it is not typically necessary to increase the dosage for cats maintained on long-term drug treatment. When cats are taken off treatment and then treated again after marking resumes, the next course of treatment is apparently as effective as the initial treatment phase (Fig. 21-6).[25] This is useful information for veterinarians when they want to take a cat off treatment to see whether marking returns, knowing that they can expect to control the marking again by putting the cat back on the same regimen. The potential for virtually indefinite treatment in some cats for problem urine marking raises the importance of pretreatment health evaluations with periodic health monitoring during treatment to evaluate any adverse reactions. A general evaluation of health, complete blood count, and serum biochemistry results after 16 and 32 weeks of treatment revealed no major or long-lasting adverse reactions to fluoxetine.

Case Study: Urine Marking

History

Biffy, a healthy, indoor, 4-year-old male castrated Burmese, was presented with an 8-month history of urinating on vertical surfaces in the house. About the time that the problem started, new neighbors had moved in with an outdoor cat that frequently wandered into the client's backyard. Biffy's favorite areas for spraying were next to the sliding glass door in the back of the house, the back of the refrigerator, and the corner of the dresser facing a window opening to the back. The owners have tried verbally scolding him and spraying him with a water bottle when they see him act as if he is about to urine mark, but they very rarely catch him "in the act." The owners prefer to avoid use of drugs for dealing with the problem unless necessary.

Diagnosis

Urine marking, probably evoked by visual interactions with the neighbor's cat

Treatment Plan

1   Discourage visits of the neighbor's cat into backyard by using a motion-activated water sprayer.
2.   Do not punish Biffy for marking-intention behavior, but if caught in the act use remote punishment, such as a handheld water sprayer.
3.   Clean urine deposits with an enzymatic cleaner.
4.   Follow litter box hygiene guidelines.
5.   If these methods do not completely eliminate the marking by the end of 2 weeks, based on daily record keeping, consider administration of an anxiolytic medication.

Progress Report

After 4 weeks of following the treatment plan, Biffy improved and marked only 1 time per week on average. This was, however, still a problem for the owners. Fluoxetine (1 mg/kg once daily) was administered, and after being on the medication for 4 weeks, Biffy had completely stopped the marking behavior.

URINE MARKING IN CATS

Causes

- Territorial or social disturbance: other cats, new house
- Emotional disturbance: anxiety
- Neighborhood cats: breeding season, visual stimulation

Resolution

- Castrate males.
- Implement litter box hygiene.
- Use enzymatic cleaner on urine spots.
- Manage intercat interactions.
- Use serotonergic drugs.

Although in the clinical trials, for the sake of consistency, owners are often told not to attempt to change intercat agonistic interactions, in clinical practice one would recommend managing the household to reduce such aggressive encounters. Along with attending to the cleanup of urine marks and litter box hygiene, reduction of agonistic intercat interactions should reduce the recurrence of urine marking following drug withdrawal. A gradual withdrawal of drug treatment should also reduce the recurrence.

Conclusions

Although the necessity of antianxiety medication is profiled in the treatment of urine marking, there are important environmental and behavioral management issues that can be expected to play a role in the overall success of any treatment plan. In all instances, old and new urine marks should be scrupulously cleaned to remove any odor cues indicating a marking place. The litter box should be maintained with a heightened level of hygiene so as to maintain its appeal as a toilet area and to reduce the buildup of aversive fecal and ammonia odors. Stimuli that may have triggered and that may maintain urine marking, such as agonistic intercat interactions, should be reduced or eliminated to the degree possible. These management procedures, although not necessarily adequate to resolve most urine marking problems, will contribute to the degree the antianxiety medication resolves the problem and may reduce the likelihood of recurrence of marking after drug withdrawal. Drug treatment recommended is a serotonergic medication such as fluoxetine for at least 16 weeks or until no marking occurs over an 8-week period. The drug should be withdrawn by a gradual schedule of every other day if marking does not return. If marking returns, much longer treatment may be necessary.

References

1. Olm DD, Houpt KA. Feline house-soiling problems. Applied Animal Behavior Science 1988;20:335–346.

2. Beaver BV. Housesoiling by cats: A retrospective study of 120 cases. Journal of the American Animal Hospital Association 1989;25:631–637.

3. Borchelt PL. Cat elimination behavior problems. Veterinary Clinics of North American Small Animal Practice 1991;21:257–264.

4. Hart BL. Behavioral adaptations to pathogens and parasites: Five strategies. Neuroscience and Biobehavioral Reviews 1990;14:273–294.

5. Tynes VV, Hart BL, Pryor PA, Bain MJ, Messam LL. Evaluation of the role of lower urinary tract disease in cats with urine-marking behavior. Journal of the American Veterinary Medical Association 2003;223:457–461.

6. Bergman L, Hart BL, Bain MJ. Evaluation of urine marking by cats as a model for veterinary diagnostic and treatment approaches and client attitudes. Journal of the American Veterinary Medical Association 2002;221:1282–1286.

7. Price EO. Behavioral aspects of animal domestication. The Quarterly Review of Biology 1984;59:1–32.

8. Horwitz DF. Behavioral and environmental factors associated with elimination behavior problems in cats: A retrospective study. Applied Animal Behavior Science 1997; 52:129–137.

9. Buffington CA, Chew DJ, DiBartola SP. Interstitial cystitis in cats. Veterinary Clinics of North American Small Animal Practice 1996;26:317–326.

10. Beaver BV, Terry ML, LaSagna CL. Effectiveness of products in eliminating cat urine odors from carpet. Journal of the American Veterinary Medical Association 1989;194: 11,1589–1591.

11. Melese P. Detecting and neutralizing odor sources in dog and cat elimination problems. Applied Animal Behaviour Science 1994;39:188–189.

12. Ewer RF. Ethology of Mammals. New York: Plenum Press, 1968.

13. Hart BL, Cooper L. Factors related to urine spraying and fighting in prepubertally gonadectomized male and female cats. Journal of the American Veterinary Medical Association 1984;184:1255-1258.

14. Pryor PA, Hart BL, Bain MJ, Cliff KD. Causes of urine marking in cats and effects of environmental management on frequency of marking. Journal of the American Veterinary Medical Association 2001;219:1709–1713.

15. Bland KP. Tom-cat odor and other pheromones in feline reproduction. Veterinary Science Communications 1979;3:125-136.

16. Hart BL, Barrett RE. Effects of castration on fighting, roaming, and urine spraying in adult male cats. Journal of the American Veterinary Medical Association 1973;163: 290–292.

17. Hart BL, Eckstein RA. The role of gonadal hormones in the occurrence of objectionable behaviours in dogs and cats. Applied Animal Behaviour Science 1997;52:331–344.

18. Hart BL. Gonadal androgen and socialsexual behavior in male mammals. A comparative analysis. Psychological Bulletin 1974;81:383–400.

19. Frank DF, Erb HN, Houpt KA. Urine spraying in cats: Presence of concurrent disease and effects of a pheromone treatment. Applied Animal Behaviour Science 1999;61: 263–272.

20. Hunthausen W. Evaluating a feline facial pheromone analogue to control urine spraying. Veterinary Medicine 2000;95:151–156.

21. Ogata N, Takeuchi Y. Clinical trail of a feline pheromone analogue for feline urine marking. Journal of Veterinary Medical Science 2001;63:157–161.

22. Mills DS, Mills CB. Evaluation of a novel method for delivering a systematic analogue of feline facial pheromone to control urine marking by cats. Veterinary Record 2001;149:197–199.

23. Hart BL. Behavioral and pharmacologic approaches to problem urination in cats. Veterinary Clinics of North American Small Animal Practice 1996;26:651–658.

24. Pryor PA, Hart BL, Cliff KD, Bain MJ. Effects of a selective serotonin reuptake inhibitor on urine spraying behavior in cats. Journal of the American Veterinary Medical Association 2001;219:1557–1561.

25. Hart BL, Cliff KD, Tynes VV, Bergman L. Control of urine marking behavior in cats by long-term treatment with fluoxetine hydrochloride and clomipramine hydrochloride. Journal of the American Veterinary Medical Association 2005;226:378–382.

26. Dehasse J. Feline urine spraying. Applied Animal Behaviour Science 1997;52:365–371.

Chapter 22

Aggression Toward People and Other Cats

Although aggressive behavior of one type or another is the most common problem in dogs for which professional help is sought, aggression in cats is much less frequently the primary presenting complaint. Some survey information indicates that about 65% of feline cases presented for problem behavior involve house soiling, with various types of aggressive behavior comprising the second most common problem category.[1] Certainly, cats can be aggressive toward people, particularly those in the home, and toward other cats inside or outside the home. The solitary lifestyle of cats that characterized their evolutionary background did not appear to predispose this species toward the dominance-related aggressive behavior in their interaction with human family members that is seen in dogs.

Most types of feline aggression are directed toward people as well as other cats, although petting-evoked aggression is reserved for people and intermale and territorial aggression are mainly directed toward other cats. Of aggressive behaviors directed toward people, the most commonly reported is redirected aggression (about 50%) with play-related and fear-related aggression the next most frequent.[2] Although some cats may fight for a position of dominance within a multicat household, the lack of universal striving by cats to compete for dominant positions precludes devoting a label to this type of intercat aggression. In multicat households there may be a cat that is referred to as a bully and that is offensively aggressive to other cats; but as long as the other cats heed the wishes of this bully there are generally no major adverse consequences. As with urine marking, male cats that are neutered or gonadally intact are overrepresented among cats presented for aggressive behavior.[1,2]

In diagnosing and treating feline aggression it is useful to use body posture and facial expressions in differentiating aggression reflecting an offensive predisposition versus aggression reflecting a fearful predisposition. These expressions and postures are shown in Figure 22-1. There are commonly emotional states that reflect a mixture of offensive and defensive predispositions.

Redirected Aggression

The label for this type of aggression comes from classical ethology where aggression that, in typical instances, would be directed to another animal, is thwarted, and

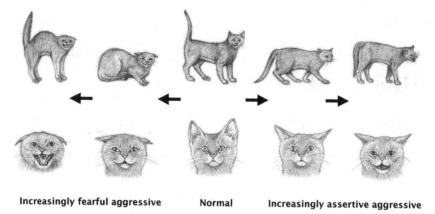

Increasingly fearful aggressive   **Normal**   **Increasingly assertive aggressive**

Figure 22-1 Diagrammatic representation of body postures and facial expressions involved in assertive aggressiveness and fear-related aggressiveness. The change in posture and facial expressions as the cat becomes more assertively aggressive (right profiles) is evident in ear carriage, open mouth, dilated pupils, forward thrust of the body, and tail position. The change in posture and facial expression as the cat becomes more aggressive, but fearful (left profile), is evident in ear carriage, open mouth, pupil dilation, and retreating body posture. The most defined aggressive posture, commonly recognized as the Halloween cat posture, is shown at the far left. These body postures and facial expressions may be useful in diagnosing the type of aggressiveness in a cat described by the client.

the aroused animal then directs its aggression toward another individual. Typically an aggressive response is evoked by the smell of another cat on an owner's or visitor's clothing, the sight of an intruding cat (perhaps through a window), or any fear-inducing stimulus. Because the aroused cat has no access to the appropriate target of its aggressive energy, it then directs the aggression toward a nearby passing object, which is usually the owner or another feline member of the house.

Typical History

Owners may complain that the cat attacked them for no apparent reason and they are rightly worried that a similar event may occur at some time in the future. Careful exploration of the history may reveal that the cat was aggressively worked up through seeing a neighboring cat through a window, or other such stimulus, immediately preceding the attack. In some instances the owner may not be aware of antecedent aggressive arousal. The cat might have been actually fighting with another cat when the owner picked up the cat, and in this highly charged situation, the aroused cat turned and attacked.

Diagnosis

The primary diagnostic possibilities to consider are fear-related aggression and petting-evoked aggression. Fear-related aggression can be ruled out if it is known that the cat is not normally fearful of the person or another cat to which it directed its aggression. The events immediately preceding the aggressive attack are critical

---

REDIRECTED AGGRESSION IN CATS

Causes

- Aroused by aggression encounters with another cat
- Petted by owner soon after arousal

Resolution

- Avoid interacting with aroused cat.
- Wait until cat is eating or grooming to interact.
- Do not break up fight with hands.

---

in firming up the diagnosis and separating this behavior from petting-evoked aggression, which is not preceded by any agonistic encounters with other cats.

Treatment Guidelines

The owners need to identify the triggers, if possible. When their cat is aggressively charged, they need to avoid interacting with the cat. It is necessary to wait until the cat is completely calmed down before petting or picking up the cat, perhaps by noticing when the cat is eating or grooming itself. Above all, owners should be warned not to break up cat fights with their hands even with gloves. If intervention is absolutely needed one should use some sort of object such as a broom to push the cats apart. Alternatively, one could use a heavy blanket to cover the aggressive cat and remove it from the area. If the triggers are able to be identified, but are not easily avoidable, the owner should attempt to desensitize and countercondition the cat to these triggers (Chapter 3).

Play-Related Aggression

This problem relates to the playful stalking, pouncing, biting, and scratching directed toward a moving person by a kitten or juvenile cat that is still at a playful age. Although this problem is covered under the topic of aggression, because of the unpleasant or intolerable biting or scratching of the owner's legs or feet, it is not considered aggression in the ethological sense. Although this behavior may be directed toward other cats as well as people, cats who are targets of another's playful bites or scratches seem to take care of themselves. A clinician's help is needed when there are human targets. This behavior can be reduced or eliminated in cats by following certain recommended practices in raising the cat (Chapter 27).

Typical History

An owner may seek consultation because a young cat is particularly vigorous in its clawing and scratching, and when the owner attempts to push the cat away, this seems to stimulate the cat to return its playful aggressiveness all the more intensely. It may be evident in the history that this behavior is particularly prevalent when there is deprivation in play, such as when an owner is gone during the day and returns from work. On weekends, play-related aggression may be less intense, reflecting less deprivation. Also there may be a predisposition for cats that were orphaned and hand-raised as kittens to engage in this behavior, possibly as a result of early experience with having only people, rather than other cats, as kitten play-mates.

Diagnosis

Usually there is no competing diagnosis because the behavior occurs on a daily or regular basis and is recognized as playful; the cat is not showing any signs of fear toward the owner. The regularity and predictability of the attitude also rule out redirected aggression. Delving into the history may reveal that the owners encouraged aggressive play when the cat was a kitten by rough play.

Treatment Guidelines

Three approaches should be considered and combined as appropriate. The first is to attempt to avoid situations that lead to the cat attacking the person's legs or hands. If playful attacks occur mostly when the owner returns from work, the cat might be placed in a room for an hour or two where it cannot attack. The owners should be counseled not to play roughly with their cat, nor to play with it with their fingers and toes. The owners should consider carrying around small toys, or even wadded up pieces of paper in their pockets, so that when they see their cat approach, they can direct its attention to chase the toy instead of the owner.

The second approach is to establish regular and appropriate play periods using a toy such as a paper ball or feather on a string. Some cat owners have found using a fishing pole with a stuffed stocking tied to the end of the line is an enjoyable play technique because it allows the owner to sit in one place while giving the cat plenty of exercise and play. As a word of caution here, do not use a fine fish line that may tangle the cat; replace the fish line with course cotton thread. Such play periods should be daily or twice daily and at predictable times. This type of play is directed away from the owner's hands and feet.

If play-related aggression continues even after regular play sessions are established, one could employ the third approach, that of using a type of remote punish-

---

PLAY-RELATED AGGRESSION IN CATS
Causes
• Reflects playful behavior
• May be enhanced by play deprivation
Resolution
• Avoid situations that evoke the behavior.
• Redirect cat to appropriate objects.
• Implement remote punishment.

ment such as a water sprayer carried around to spray the cat at the first sign of the playful attack on the legs. An ultrasonic noise deterrent may also work. If possible, the remote punishment device should be used without the cat seeing from where the aversive stimulus is coming. The owners should avoid any attempt to push the cat away with their hands.

Finally, cat owners who want to adopt another cat could conduct an experiment to see whether their cat would get along with another cat of roughly the same age and general temperament by having a friend's cat spend time at their house. This would be an indication that an additional cat might help resolve the problem. Regardless of the success in controlling this problem, the saving grace is that as cats mature the likelihood of this type of aggression becomes much less.

Fear-Related Aggression

This is a type of aggression often shown by cats toward strange people visiting the home, toward owners in certain situations, and toward veterinarians in the examination room or during hospitalization. This type of aggression also occurs between cats. Often the cat indicates that it would like to escape from the fear-evoking situation, but either because of the confined space or owner restraint, this is not possible. The typical Halloween cat posture of a crouched stance, flattened ears, and dilated eyes is the classic threat posture (Fig. 22-1) of a cornered but fearful cat. Most people (and probably other cats) know that an approach beyond a critical distance is likely to evoke an attack. The classical posture is typically seen as an adaptation to look as large and as fierce as possible so as to deter any continued approach by the fear-evoking stimulus. One should also recognize less extreme body language associated with different levels of fear.

Typical History

Cat owners generally understand that the cat is displaying the aggression because it is being forced to remain in a situation from which it would otherwise escape, and that the aggression is a function of fear and a tendency to be protective in the presence of an anxiety- or fear-evoking situation. Owners are sometimes distraught by the fact that they would like their cat to be friendly toward other people or other cats. The fear-related aggression may be the result of the owners attempting forcibly to socialize the cat to fear-inducing stimuli. To the degree the cat's threats and mild forms of aggression keep people away, the behavior is reinforced and becomes more likely in future similar circumstances. In Chapter 27 on selecting and raising kittens, it is mentioned that habituating kittens to children and strangers early in life can often prevent fear-related aggressive behavior being directed toward children and strangers later.

Diagnosis

There is usually no competing behavioral diagnosis when one recognizes the fear-related aspects of body language related to this type of behavior (Fig 22-1) and elements of the history pointing to the cat being fearful. These are the key markers in distinguishing fear-related aggression from play-related aggression, redirected aggression, and petting-evoked aggression.

Treatment Guidelines

In dealing with fear-related aggression directed toward people, the first advice should be to protect people from being bitten or scratched. Cat owners should be advised to avoid picking up or trying to comfort a cat that is aroused and fearful. In an attempt to escape or be defensive, the cat may turn and attack the owner. The treatment in this case involves dealing with the underlying fear of the type of people evoking the aggression. In the ideal situation one would employ some variant of desensitization and counterconditioning approaches in which the cat is exposed to the fear-evoking stimuli but with the distance being great enough that fear is not shown. In the case of fear of children, one might suggest the cat be held comfortably on the owner's lap and then ask a child to come into the room at a distance far enough away from the cat that it does not show any fear response. The owner should call the cat's attention to the child and give the cat a favorite treat. This process is repeated for 10 trials or so through many sessions spread over several days. The owner should look for progress in the cat being habituated to the fear-evoking stimulus. As the cat shows progress in being desensitized, the distance to the fear-evoking stimulus should be decreased to achieve more desensitization.

Dealing with fear-related behavior toward other cats is actually quite complicated because one cannot readily control exposure to other cats as one can with people. If one cat repeatedly attacks another the victim has good reason to be fearful. Given the mobility of cats in a household, and the unpredictability of fear-evoking stimuli, fear-related problem behaviors may be difficult to resolve by staging desensitization and counterconditioning sessions. In some instances just helping a client avoid the fear-evoking circumstances may be a reasonable approach. As a proactive approach one may use fence barriers between the cats involved, so that they can see each other but not interact. The cat with the fear will know it cannot be attacked, so one might employ counterconditioning teaching, such as offering treats in the presence of the other cat.

FEAR-RELATED AGGRESSION

Causes
- Fear of people or cats to whom the cat has not been socialized
- Reinforced by repelling people or cats

Resolution
- Use gradual desensitization to fear-evoking stimulus.
- Countercondition: Pair rewards with people or cats.
- Avoid forcing people on the cat.
- Avoid circumstances where aggression is reinforced.

Case Study: Fear-Related Aggression

History

Ed and Alice, both healthy 8-year-old neutered domestic longhair littermates, were presented for fighting with each other after Ed was brought home from the veterinarian's office for prophylactic teeth cleaning. When they brought Ed back home, Alice growled, hissed, and chased him under the bed. Ed has since become defensively aggressive, which seemed to evoke even more aggressiveness from Alice. The owners have now separated the cats, with Ed kept in the bedroom with the door closed most of the time. When the owners have tried to bring the cats back together Ed tries to get away and Alice chases him.

Diagnosis

Fear-related aggression on the part of Ed in response to aggressive behavior by Alice.

Treatment Plan

1. Continue to keep the cats separated when no one is able to supervise.
2. Systematically desensitize and countercondition the cats to each other by feeding them initially on opposite sides of the bedroom door that separates their spaces.
3. Create multiple hiding places and perches for the cats throughout the house.
4. Rotate the cats between the two designated living spaces.
5. Consider use of an anxiolytic medication for both cats if the problem does not resolve.

Progress Report

At a 2-month follow-up, there was some decrease in fearfulness and aggression displayed by Ed in the bedroom when Alice walked outside of the room. Alice no longer stood outside of the bedroom door or attempted to seek Ed out, but she would display aggression when Ed hissed at her. Ed was then placed on the anxiolytic medication, buspirone. After being on the medication for 5 weeks, the owners reported a significant decrease in the hissing that Ed displayed toward Alice, with resultant decrease in aggression that Alice displayed in return. The owners continued the desensitization and counterconditioning. After an additional 2 months, the owners reported that the cats were now friendly toward each other again. The medication for Ed was gradually discontinued and the problem continued to improve.

The use of a serotonergic drug, such as fluoxetine, to reduce the fear may result in some autonomous desensitization if the cat is allowed exposure to fear-evoking people or other cats at a comfortable pace. There is a precaution to be followed in that the fearful cat, who was inhibited from attacking the fear-evoking person or other cat, may become less inhibited when on an anxiolytic drug and this could exacerbate the problem.

Petting-Evoked Aggression

Petting-evoked aggression is a rather odd behavior wherein a cat, who is being gently petted and nicely held by a person, suddenly turns and scratches or bites the person that has been petting it. By definition this is a type of behavior that is reserved for people and probably has no counterpart in the ethology of the ancestral cat. Nonetheless it is a real phenomenon and one for which there seems to be no cure, although there are guidelines for avoidance of the problem.

Typical History

People who complain about this behavior usually report that they like holding their cat on their lap and petting it. After perhaps as little as 30 seconds, or as long as many minutes, they start to see warning signs of the cat acting restless. A typical sign is the tail switching, a rather uniform marker of an agitated cat, along with its ears rotated back. The cat next digs its claws into a person's leg or bites the nearby arm or leg. One of the problems is that people will see the agitation or restlessness and attempt to pet and comfort the cat all the more, believing they can calm the cat down. If anything, this behavior by the owner tends to escalate the aggression. The best explanation for the behavior is that the cats have a limited tolerance for being petted and are simply reaching their limit.

Diagnosis

After ruling out fear of the owner and any evidence of a trigger causing redirected aggression, the unique circumstances of the cat being petted by the owner prior to the cat turning and attacking generally point to no other competing diagnostic possibilities.

Treatment Guidelines

The most logical treatment is simply to help the owners understand the signals leading to this behavior and to avoid holding and petting the cat for a duration of time that approaches the threshold for attacking. Owners should be vigilant of the warning signs of restlessness and agitation and assume that their cat has a limited tolerance for this type of petting. They simply have to get the cat off of their lap before this tolerance threshold is reached; they should not assume that cats enjoy prolonged petting. If the problem is frequent one might suggest that the owner simply avoid holding the cat in the manner that evokes a response. Alternatively, the least confrontational method of getting the cat off their lap is for the owner to stand up calmly. There are no reports on the effectiveness of anxiolytic drugs on this behavior and probably no reason to involve such drug treatment, provided that the owners are willing and capable of recognizing the signs to avoid triggering the behavior.

Intermale Fighting

Tomcats are known for their predisposition to be drawn into fights with other tomcats in their neighborhood. Tales of tomcats coming home with fight wounds and abscesses are legendary and basically expected by anyone who keeps a tomcat in neighborhood settings where encounters with other cats are frequent. This type of aggression is much more likely between gonadally intact males than between neutered males.

Castration of tomcats is quite effective in changing this behavior, with an estimated 90% of males undergoing a marked reduction or resolution of the behavior.[3]

Although intermale fighting is classically associated with tomcats, castrated males may also be presented for this type of aggressive behavior. Even though the behavior is enhanced by postpubertal secretion of androgen, castrated males (and spayed females for that matter) still have the neural circuitry for this type of behavior. The neural circuitry can be activated by environmental stimuli. For example, a clinical survey indicated that male cats castrated before maturity showed a tendency to fight with other male cats at least on an occasional basis in about 40% of households.[4] Early castration thus carries no assurances that the behavior can be precluded in neutered males.

INTERMALE AGGRESSION IN CATS
Causes
• Natural predisposition of tomcats to fight male cats
Resolution
• Castrate tomcats.
• Separate fighting males if they are in the same house.
• Gradually reintroduce cats in the same house.

Typical History

Clients generally are aware of the strong tendency of tomcats to seek out other tomcats and come home with fight wounds and abscesses. Their cat may be presented after a few such encounters, or when the client desires to make the cat more of an indoor cat. When a neutered male is presented with the problem of roaming and coming home with fight wounds, owners may wonder about whether the castration operation was complete.

Diagnosis

The primary diagnostic feature is the tendency of cats to show tomcatlike fighting, namely seeking out other males and fighting. The tendency to continue to fight, even though the animal is sustaining wounds, results in the cats doing more harm to each other than is customary with more social animals like male dogs, which generally fight until one animal shows submission, generally ending the fight. Within the home it may be difficult to differentiate between intermale aggression between two castrated male cats and territorial aggression (covered later in this chapter).

Treatment Guidelines

For male cats that are gonadally intact, castration is clearly indicated and, as mentioned, the operation has an estimated 90% probability of markedly reducing or eliminating this behavior. For castrated males there are no reports on the efficacy of antianxiety drugs such as those that have proven effective on another tomcatlike behavior, urine marking. Urine marking is related to anxiety, often from aggressive intercat interactions or environmental disturbances. Anxiety would appear to be less important in intermale aggression, so antianxiety medication may have no beneficial effect. There are some case reports of long-acting progestins suppressing this behavior in castrated male cats.[5]

Territorial Aggression

Territorial aggression is perhaps the most common type of aggression occurring between cats. This form of aggression may occur among long-term feline residents of the same household where owners continue to put up with the problem, and it is frequently seen when new cats are introduced to the home. It can also happen where one resident cat returns home from a visit to a veterinary hospital. This type of aggressive behavior was common in the ancestral African wildcat that lived in a solitary state. Among territorial, solitary animals, when an intruding conspecific enters a territory and is detected, it is generally aggressively repelled unless it is an animal of the opposite sex and it is during the breeding season.

In nature this type of aggression is also related to dispersion of the offspring from a natal group. In cats this type of aggression would have been seen between a mother and offspring after they were weaned, taught to hunt, and had reached the age when they could survive on their own. A mother would have repelled the young from her territory and the young dispersed in different directions. Former littermates become intolerant of each other and of the mother in future interactions. Using one's imagination, one sees the emergence of variants of this type of aggression in domestic cats. Cats raised in the same house, where littermates and mother may have gotten along for a year or two, may all of the sudden, for no apparent reason or in response to a relatively insignificant stimulus, develop an aggressive intolerance of each other. Although this type of aggression is not common, one way of looking at this problem is that it may be a manifestation of a behavior that underlies the dispersion process seen in the wild ancestor.

Typical History

Most commonly this type of aggression occurs when a new cat was brought into the home, and despite the owner's best attempts at encouraging the cats to get along fights frequently occur. Perhaps a precipitating stimulus is from an unusual odor on a cat that has returned home from an unfamiliar or unpleasant place, such as a veterinary hospital or boarding facility. Because agonistic interactions between cats in the same house are a leading cause of urine marking,[6] a complicating factor might be that the fighting has led to this even less tolerable behavior.

Diagnosis

Diagnostic possibilities with aggressive behavior between cats, other than territorial, are fear-related, redirected, and intermale. One can generally rule out fear-related

TERRITORIAL AGGRESSION IN CATS
Causes   • Introduction of new cat: territorial defense   • Dispersion effect among resident cats
Resolution   • Gradually expose or reintroduce the new cat.   • Avoid opportunities for the cats to fight.   • Use serotonergic drugs.

aggression if the cats know each other well and have been friendly in the past, although fear can play a role in negative interactions seen when a cat returns home from a veterinary hospital. Redirected aggression can be ruled out by noticing the immediately preceding events leading up to the aggressive encounters. Intermale aggression may contribute to territorial aggression among male cats, and it may not be feasible to attempt to distinguish between these two types of aggression.

Treatment Guidelines

First it is important that owners realize that it is the nature of cats to be less outwardly social as dogs. The owners may have to be satisfied with a simple type of mutual coexistence managed by the owner rather than a friendly resolution. As for addressing serious fighting, keep in mind that fighting between cats tends to evoke more fighting and more fighting could lead to urine marking. The first recommendation, therefore, is to separate the cats into different parts of the household with different feeding stations, litter boxes, and scratching posts but in an arrangement where they can still see each other through a gap of a few feet between fences or gates. If no noticeable aggression is seen for a week or so, gradually the animals can be allowed closer together. The owners should watch to see that the reintroduction does not happen so quickly that the aggression is again evoked.

There are no clinical reports of the results of using antianxiety drugs in these circumstances, but given the efficacy of the serotonergic drugs, such as fluoxetine, on urine marking behavior (Chapter 21), one might be tempted to see whether these drugs would have an effect on facilitating the reintroduction of cats to each other. If there is a reduction of aggressive tendencies, it would probably be best to give both of the cats involved the same treatment. It may be wise, at least at first, to avoid the use of buspirone in the more offensively aggressive cat, because there is some clinical evidence that it can increase aggression.[7]

References

1. Beaver BV. Feline behavioral problems other than housesoiling. Journal of the American Animal Hospital Association 1989;25:465–469.
2. Chapman BL, Voith VL. Cat aggression redirected to people: 14 cases (1981–1987). Journal of the American Veterinary Medical Association 1990;196:947–950.

3. Hart BL, Barrett RE. Effects of castration on fighting, roaming, and urine spraying in adult male cats. Journal of the American Veterinary Medical Association 1973;163: 290–292.

4. Hart BL, Cooper LL. Factors related to urine spraying and fighting in prepubertally gonadectomized male and female cats. Journal of the American Veterinary Medical Association 1984;184:1255-1258.

5. Hart BL, Eckstein RA. The role of gonadal hormones in the occurrence of objectionable behaviours in dogs and cats. Applied Animal Behaviour Science 1997;52:331–344.

6. Pryor PA, Hart BL, Bain MJ, Cliff KD. Causes of urine marking in cats and effects of environmental management on frequency of marking. Journal of the American Veterinary Medical Association 2001;219:1709–1713.

7. Hart BL, Eckstein RA, Powell KL, et al. Effectiveness of busprione on urine spraying and inappropriate urination in cats. Journal of the American Veterinary Medical Association 1993;203:254–258.

Chapter 23
Inappropriate Feline Scratching

Your typical mild-mannered cat can do practically as much damage to a house with its claws as a large dog can with its canine teeth. Scratching trees is an innate behavior of feral cats and presumably the wild ancestor; scratching household objects is the equivalent for the more urbanized feline. Some cats scratch trees or other areas outside the house and the owners are not aware of it, and other cats make their owner's life perfectly miserable by scratching only the most valuable furniture. This inherited behavioral tendency is so strong that even cats declawed still routinely go through scratching motions. Although surgical declawing by removal of the third phalanx (onychectomy) or immobilization of the third phalanx by tendonectomy (or *tenectomy*) may be a last resort to dealing with destructive scratching problems, providing behavioral advice on stopping an old cat from scratching a valuable piece of furniture will impress your clients. In this chapter, background information will be presented on the factors that help attract a cat to scratching certain areas, followed by practical suggestions for inducing kittens to scratch acceptable objects and therapeutic guidelines for older cats with scratching problems.

Natural Scratching Behavior

Observing cats outdoors can teach us a lot about their behavior indoors. Many outdoor cats have a scratching tree that is a prominent object in the environment. Because the cat repeatedly works over the same tree trunk with its claws, it becomes a personal territorial marker because the scratched appearance is readily visible to other cats that might venture by (Fig. 23-1). In the process of scratching trees, cats also rub secretions from glands in their feet onto the tree trunk; this way the scratched tree trunk gains a distinct olfactory character that can probably be recognized by other cats. The chemical mark provides the resident cat with some familiarity with its territory, and the smell appears to attract the cat back to the same tree to restore both the visual and chemical marks. Whether other cats have access to the outdoors or not, many cats have a strong, innate tendency to establish at least one scratching-related territorial mark, preferably on a prominent vertical object of suitable texture. Frequently, the corner of a chair or couch that sticks out into the room is most visible and becomes chosen (Fig. 23-2). As soon as the cat starts

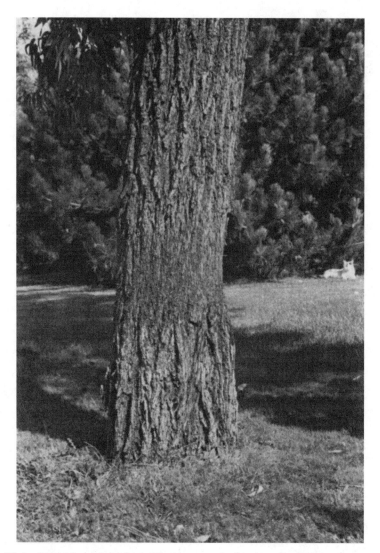

Figure 23-1   Typical scratched tree that is repeatedly scratched and serves as a visual and chemical territorial marker for cats.

scratching a particular corner of a couch, it tends to persist in that place because the spot soon smells like a territorial mark that attracts the cat back again and again.

Scratching also has the function of conditioning the claws. Claws are not sharpened as a knife blade would be sharpened, but are conditioned in that a frayed and worn outer claw is periodically pulled off by scratching, exposing a new and very sharp claw already growing beneath. Worn claws that are removed by scratching may be seen at the base of a scratching post. Cats may also remove these outer claws with their teeth, particularly those on the back feet. Clawing is a natural, healthy behavioral requirement and is not something the animal does to "punish" or displease the owner.

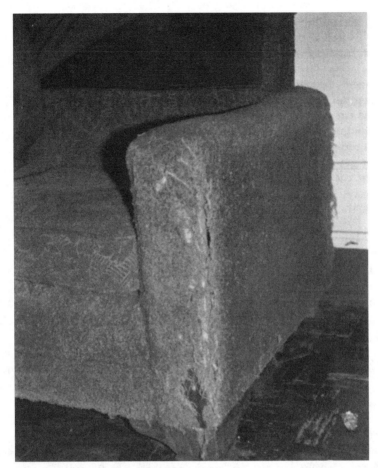

Figure 23-2   Furniture, especially prominent corners of couches or chairs, can become scratched territorial markers for cats inside, just as a scratching tree is outside.

Behavioral Effects of Declawing

Although this chapter focuses on the behavioral approach to resolving problem scratching, something should be said about the surgical operations for dealing with this problem. The common declawing operation, or onchyectomy, involves removal of claws and the third phalanx from the front feet. Another surgical procedure is tendonectomy, which is performed by surgically incising and removing a piece of the deep digital flexor tendon. The third phalanx and claw remains, but the cat can no longer flex the claw, and therefore is unable to dig it into anything. With this procedure, the cat must have its claws trimmed regularly.

Most cats declawed on the front feet can still climb rough-bark trees after the operation using their back claws pushing up. However, coming down from trees may be difficult. The back claws may be used for defense against other cats or dogs if the cat flips over on its back. It would appear that a cat's defense would be weakened, especially if it was accustomed to fending off dogs by scratching with front claws. In general it seems possible that a cat could find its welfare threatened if it were unable to climb smooth-barked trees that it has routinely used for escaping from dogs before it was declawed, and it is also compromised in defense of using the front claws. Therefore, it is highly recommended that declawed cats be kept as indoor cats.

Information from both veterinarians and cat owners indicates that in most instances declawing by onchyectomy does not lead to medical or behavioral problems, and clients are satisfied with the operation.[1,2] After healing, there appears to be little difference between onchyectomy and tendonectomy in adverse effects or client satisfaction.[3,4] One difficulty with tendonectomy is the necessity to continue trimming the nails and an ability by some cats still to scratch—at least to some extent. As mentioned, however, most clients will appreciate coaching on behavioral solutions to problem scratching and prefer the surgical approaches as a last resort.

Training Adults and Kittens for Scratching Posts

To induce a cat to choose an acceptable area to scratch, three principles should be kept in mind.[5,6] First, after a cat starts scratching an object, it tends to return to it. Probably the main reason is to renew the odors apparent to the scratched object. Second, prominent objects and areas are favored. This behavior reflects the predisposition that a territorial marker should be prominent. Finally, the texture of a potential scratching area influences whether it is used. To serve as a scratched object the claws must be able to rough the surface. Typically cat owners have thought of scratching posts for cats, but cardboard scratchers are finding favor.

With regard to the first principle, a kitten should be directed to start on a scratching post or cardboard scratcher before it starts scratching on furniture. The object should be very prominent and kept in an area the kitten frequents until it is being used regularly. One should not wait until the cat is fully grown and capable of serious damage before training it to scratch on a particular object. For a kitten it is useful to place the scratching post or cardboard scratcher horizontally to make it easy for the kitten to develop an attachment to that particular object.

The second principle of scratching comes into play when dealing with the location of the scratching post. Whenever undesirable scratching occurs on furniture, the object should be covered immediately with sheet of plastic to prevent further scratching and kept covered until the cat is regularly scratching an acceptable object. A suitable scratching object covered with appealing material should be put in front of the inappropriately scratched area. Temporarily moving the scratched furniture aside is also a possibility. Another location-related principle is that cats often develop propensities for scratching objects near their sleeping or resting areas, because they tend to scratch just after awakening. Therefore, it is helpful to have at least one scratching post or board adjacent to where the animal sleeps.

The third principle deals with physical characteristics of the scratching object. A flimsy scratching post that is easily tipped over is useless. Many experienced cat owners prefer to use a board attached to the wall rather than a freestanding post. A good dimension for a scratching board is 6–8 inches wide by at least 12–16 inches long. It should be adjustable in height as the cat grows. The best height is usually 12 inches (0.3 meters) off the floor so that the cat may comfortably rest on its back feet while scratching. As mentioned, gaining popularity with cats and cat owners are scratching boards made of corrugated cardboard. The cardboard scratcher may be placed horizontally on the floor or attached to a vertical surface.

Anyone who has lived with a cat scratching problem has probably noticed that cats tend to scratch some types of material more than others. The material on a scratching post should be something a cat likes. Most commercial posts are covered with carpet which, surprisingly, is too durable. As a covering becomes worn out and stringy, the cat likes it better because the post has the odor of the feet and the cat can get a nice drag of the claws. Posts that are made of soft wood such as pine, cedar or redwood are good choices especially if roughened up with a wire brush.

As soon as the kitten is habitually using a scratching post or cardboard scratcher, the scratch object may be moved (a few inches each day) to a spot more preferable to the owner. When it comes time to replace a cardboard scratcher, it would be wise to sprinkle pieces of cardboard with the cat's foot odor from the old scratcher onto the new one. For cats that are adopted into a home, one should, if possible, bring the scratching object with them or at least attempt to imitate the one at the previous home.

Solving a Scratching Problem

In addition to the drive to mark a prominent object in their territory, cats need a substrate upon which they can scratch and remove the outer cuticle and expose the new nail beneath. Although a cat that is allowed at least some access to the outdoors may use a favorite tree or wood post, an indoor-only cat needs a scratching post or cardboard scratcher. Of course, there is no inherent reason why cats should prefer a scratching post to furniture. The following treatment guidelines rely on the information being presented in the first part of this chapter on understanding the principles of scratching and applying these to specific situations.

Typical History

Owners usually contact veterinarians after the destructive scratching has become a major problem and one or more pieces of furniture or draperies are ruined or at least damaged. It is unfortunate when owners wait to get advice until considerable scratching damage has been done, because by then a cat has adopted the scratched object as a territorial landmark, making it more difficult to encourage the cat to switch to another object. Owners may believe that they could simply stop the cat from scratching altogether instead of providing an acceptable scratching alternative. They may have acquired a scratching post or cardboard scratcher at a pet supplier and feel that because the post is labeled as a scratching post or board, cats should automatically be attracted to it. From the cat's standpoint, there is no reason it should prefer a new scratching object to the scratched-up furniture.

Many owners will have attempted some sort of a punishment for the cat, perhaps scolding it when they find it in the scratching mode or even bringing the cat and showing it the scratched area and engaging in some kind of dialogue to convince the cat not to scratch that area. Usually this kind of punishment would encourage the cat to scratch in inappropriate areas mostly when the owner is not around. In general, the sooner a cat owner is supplied with the information needed to understand and redirect a scratching problem, the more easily the problem is solved. The success of the behavioral approach requires a conscientious and consistent effort on the part of the owner to make the program work.

Diagnosis

This behavior problem is fairly evident, so the main diagnostic challenge may be to determine which cat is doing the problem scratching in multicat households. Also it must be determined what objects are being scratched and their locations in the house.

Treatment Guidelines

There are two behavioral aspects to approaching a scratching problem. One is using the natural scratching predisposition to encourage a cat to adopt an appropriate scratching object, such as a scratching post or cardboard scratcher. The second aspect is the use of behavioral modification techniques to discourage a cat from scratching the undesirable object and/or making the inappropriate object unavailable. These techniques are most successful after everything is done first to encourage a cat to express its behavior toward an acceptable object.

The scratched object, such as furniture, should be moved or covered in some way to make it unavailable for scratching. A scratching board or post should be placed as close as possible to where the scratched furniture or object is/was located. A post should be covered with an attractive scratching material, as discussed. After the new object is used by the cat, it may gradually be moved, inch by inch, to an area acceptable to the owners. This needs to be a slow progression so the cat stays oriented to the acceptable scratching object and does not return to the inappropriate object. In some instances it may be useful to have multiple objects throughout the house that all have identical coverings and will all eventually have the same odor of the cat that can be freshened up from time to time. One of these might be near the area where the cat sleeps so that there is an object readily available when the cat awakens

In some instances the old furniture has been so severely damaged that the owner may have the furniture reupholstered. If so, the old covering may be placed on top of the new scratching post. As to the type of material with which to reupholster the chair or couch, the tightly woven nubby materials are probably the safest because the cats typically prefer materials with longitudinally oriented threads.

After a cat is scratching a new acceptable object, the owners may institute some techniques to discourage a cat from going back to the old scratching target by use of remote punishment. One possibility is an electronic device that triggers an alarm when the cat approaches the area. Another would be placing upside-down plastic carpet runners, upside-down sticky tape, or even upside-down mouse traps on the floor near the off limits area. Ambushing a cat by squirting it with a water sprayer when it approaches the off limits area is effective but would require the owner staying around and watching the cat repeatedly until it approaches that area. Keep in mind that remote punishment is most effective if given consistently and immediately after the undesirable behavior.

Cat owners sometimes have questions about the appropriateness of attaching catnip to the scratching post. This is probably counterproductive because cats should be attracted to scratching posts or boards because of the inherent desire to use it as a territorial mark and to condition the claws. Additional motivation such as putting catnip in the post is not needed. There may be a question as to whether there is some value in demonstrating to a cat where to scratch by rubbing his feet on the post. As odd as it seems, this may be beneficial because the cat owner may rub off foot gland secretions on the post, attracting the cat back to the post later.

Some cat owners believe that the redirection of scratching behavior seems too time consuming or involved; these owners may be interested in just reducing the damage done to furniture. An old-fashioned way of doing this is to clip the sharp tip of the claws routinely with a nail clipper; this blunts much of the damage. However, as soon as the old blunted claw is shed, a new sharp one replaces it; owners must be constantly vigilant for the arrival of new claws. Another technique is the use of plastic claw caps which are applied with fast-acting glue to each of the claws of the front feet. On the surface it would appear as though the claw caps may be effective, although the application of a claw cap to each claw is rather labor intensive. There are no clinical studies published on the effects of these products; nor are there surveys done of the opinions of the owners or veterinarians of clients that have used these materials. A possible logical role for claw caps might be temporarily preventing damage while a household is being rearranged and where the owner needs to protect the furniture. If one is actively trying to encourage a cat to scratch acceptable objects, the use of the claw caps would interfere with this new training because the cat is not going to be effective in directing its scratching to another object. Therefore, the claw caps are probably not a long-term solution to a scratching problem.

INAPPROPRIATE SCRATCHING IN CATS

Causes

- Natural tendency for territorial marking
- Renew visual-chemical marks
- Remove worn-out claws
- Preference for suitable texture

Resolution

- Place appealing scratching post in prominent place
- Post should have appropriate covering
- Make scratched furniture unavailable
- Use remote punishment in inappropriate areas
- Gradually move post to side of room

References

1. Morgan M, Houpt KA. Feline behavior problems: The influence of declawing. Anthrozoös 1989;3:50–53.
2. Landsberg GM. Cat owners' attitudes towards declawing. Anthrozoös 1990;4:192–197.
3. Janowski AJ, Brown DC, Duval J, et al. Comparison effects of tenectomy or onychectomy in cats. Journal of the American Veterinary Medical Association 1998;213:370–373.
4. Yeon SC, Flanders JA, Scarlett JM, et al. Attitudes of owners regarding tendonectomy and onychectomy in cats. Journal of the American Veterinary Medical Association 2001;218:43–47.
5. Hart BL. Behavioral aspects of scratching in cats. Feline Practice 1972;2(2):6–8.
6. ———. Starting from scratch: A new perspective on cat scratching. Feline Practice 1980;10(4):8–110.

Chapter 24

Problems with Feeding and Predatory Behavior

Problems with feeding relate to ingestion of inappropriate substances, the loss of appetite, and eating too much (resulting in obesity). Although hunting or predation, is the mainstay of a cat's existence in the wild, concern about cat predation on songbirds has emerged as a major problem; this topic is discussed in terms of selecting and training cats to reduce songbird predation. A discussion of normal feline feeding behavior is relevant to understanding and treating clinical problems in this area, and this topic is discussed first.

Normal Feeding Behavior

In contrast to the "feast or famine" type of existence of big cats, where one large kill may provide enough food to last for several days, the ancestor of the domestic cat preyed on small rodents much as feral cats do today on farms. The caloric value of the typical can of canned cat food is equivalent to that of about one or two mice. Although cat owners tend to feed their cats just once or twice a day, cats will nibble throughout the day if given the opportunity. Adult cats that were given free access to a complete can of cat food were found to distribute feeding across about 12 meals evenly throughout a 24-hour period.[1] The type of food, whether semi-moist or dry, had little effect on the frequency and spacing of meals.

Cats that feed exclusively on a single food, even though nutritionally balanced, may develop a reduced interest in that particular food and favor a more novel diet. Providing animals with increased feeding opportunities and a greater variety in their diet can stimulate an increase in caloric intake.[1] This may be of value in increasing the food intake in an underweight cat. The appealing diet may be one that has not been fed recently. Sometimes cat owners trying a new commercial cat food observe this novelty effect and believe they have come across a more appealing food when in actuality it is the novelty of the new food, which will eventually fade away.

Eating Plants

Although eating grass and other plants seems to be normal for cats, if a cat munches on a favorite house plant it can become a serious problem to the owner. The function of grass eating is not understood; one perspective is that, as in grass eating by dogs (Chapter 16), grass that is consumed may provide some sort of chemical or physical way of expelling intestinal parasites. Given that in nature most felids carry some degree of intestinal parasite load, cats may be drawn by an evolved instinct to ingest the plant material on a regular basis. Alternatively, there may be stimuli from the gastrointestinal system that are interpreted as possibly signaling a heavy parasite load and that may then provoke an animal to seek out and consume grass.

Although the function of plant eating is not understood, the behavior of eating household plants can sometimes be prevented by providing a small garden of grass for the cat. Small feline gardens are even available commercially. When the grass garden is provided, one could go about using remote punishment to discourage cats from eating other house plants. This requires limiting the cat's access to plants except when the owner is nearby with some sort of remote punishment, such as a water pistol or ultrasonic noise maker. The use of upside-down carpet runners, upside-down contact paper, inverted mousetraps or sticky tape will require somewhat less vigilance by the owner. Although there is a tendency for cat owners to conclude that when a cat is eating grass its stomach is upset, and eating grass is a way of provoking regurgitation, this would appear not to be the basis for the behavior and most cats seem to be acting no differently before and after eating plants.

Chewing and Ingesting Inappropriate Substances: Pica

In the conventional medical sense *pica* refers to the abnormal behavior of consuming substances that are nutritionally inappropriate or even harmful. Dogs, for example, may ingest gravel, dirt, or children's plastic toys, sometimes causing a medical emergency. Cats, however, seem not to be afflicted with such severe ingestive problems with one prominent exception, that of wool chewing and ingestion.

Cats that typically chew and/or ingest parts of wool sweaters or terry cloth towels do not appear to be abnormal in other ways. There appears to be some drive or compulsion to chew and ingest wool and cloth objects with a similar texture. Despite repeated attempts with clinical cases, the behavior has not been closely related to a nutritional deficiency or other intestinal disorder, such as pancreatitis. One theory relates problems to early weaning of cats for those already predisposed to this pica; the idea is that wool chewing is related to nonnutritional sucking seen in prematurely weaned animals, but there is no empirical information to substantiate this hypothesis. The behavior is displayed primarily by Siamese and Burmese breeds and the behavior begins about the time of puberty.[2] Although wool seems to be preferred, cats may suck, chew or ingest chunks of material from stockings, sweaters, caps, towels and just about any type of cloth left where the cat has access to it.[2] Some cats can become such a problem that they cannot safely be maintained as indoor cats. Most cats seem to give up chewing within a year or two. For cats where this behavior persists, the problem seems to have many of the characteristics of compulsive and stereotypic behaviors and is covered in Chapter 26.

Anorexia

This problem, which refers to a loss or marked reduction of appetite, is seen by the owners as their cat going off food or eating relatively little compared with its typical feeding patterns. Anorexia can be life threatening and may require medical intervention in terms of supplying nutrients systemically if the behavior persists more than a few days. This is especially true in cats that are overweight because the weight loss can lead to hepatic lipidosis. One cause of anorexia can be just an alteration of the cat's appetite reflecting boredom with one type of food, or being presented with a new food for which the cat has a particular dislike. Cats may go off food because of the onset of an infectious disease.[3] Anorexia may also occur following development of some specific food aversions.

Typical History

Cat owners usually contact the clinician after more than 1 day of the cat showing little interest in food. One should distinguish between a cat with serious anorexia and a cat that was a voracious eater of a particularly palatable food and that now shows a more moderate appetite. Anorexia can be the first sign of almost any disease, including a febrile infectious disease or consumption of a poisonous substance. It is possible that treatment with certain drugs may suppress appetite and this needs to be explored in the history. The issue of appetite is confounded by the fact that pet food companies compete with each other to make cat foods particularly palatable. Thus, pet foods are often chosen on the basis of what the owner perceives the cat will be most anxious to consume. People have a remarkable tendency to want to nurture animals that is often expressed in finding the food they think the animal will particularly like.

Diagnosis

The major task in dealing with this problem behavior is to determine the cause of the anorexia from the standpoint of onset of acute sickness, specific food aversions, anosmia due to upper respiratory conditions, environmental conditions such as a hot environment, gastric disturbance due to accumulation of hairballs, ingestion of a poison, or change of diet. Infection-related anorexia is caused by the same endogenous pyrogens as those causing a fever and depression.[3] Therefore, one would expect to see an elevation in body temperature and perhaps signs of depression along with the anorexia (Chapter 7).

Anorexia due to an acquired food aversion may stem from certain foods being used to deliver medications that cause a degree of nausea or gastrointestinal illness. Research has shown that gastrointestinal illness or nausea is related to the food that accompanies the substance that produces the nausea even though the nausea may not occur for several hours after ingestion of the nausea-inducing substance. A food allergy is another cause of an acquired aversion.

Treatment Guidelines

Each of the following treatment approaches is related to the diagnosed cause of the loss of appetite.

Anorexia as part of sickness behavior

When it is clear that the anorexia is most likely due to the onset of a febrile response to an infectious disease or injury, attention is required in dealing with the illness or injury. After the illness is resolved, appetite usually returns. Unless the animal is particularly thin and the illness prolonged for several days, there may be no particular need to force-feed the cat while it is being treated for the illness.

Anorexia due to hairballs

Owners whose cats have a tendency to accumulate hairballs will be familiar with the depression of appetite that accompanies the buildup of a hairball. Some cat owners may not be familiar with this cause of anorexia. Usually appetite returns to normal within 12 hours after treatment of the hairball.

Anorexia due to anosmia

The anosmia that accompanies some types of upper respiratory diseases, even those that are nonfebrile, may be overcome by stimulating the taste receptors with techniques such as giving a food with fish flavors or warming the food in the microwave.

Food aversions

This type of food aversion, particularly with a food containing a poisonous substance, endotoxin, or a food that causes intestinal allergy and has made one temporarily ill with nausea and gastrointestinal upset, is common in people. In the laboratory, food aversions have been produced by lacing food with illness-inducing lithium chloride. The adaptive value of aversions to food is that the response protects wild animals from repeated ingestion of food substances that produce gastric distress and nausea. Food aversions have been seen in humans where a meal is given just after a chemotherapeutic drug used in cancer therapy.

The treatment of aversions due to an allergy would be to change the diet such that allergy-producing foods are avoided. One may have to devise a diet without the characteristics that were previously paired with the allergen. Over time, most aversions will weaken if the animal eats a diet that no longer induces gastrointestinal illness.

Obesity and Excessive Eating

This is where the owners' interest in nurturing their pet really comes into play. It is almost as if people want to be judged on how well they feed their cats, expecting that the cat will know they really love it if they are fed a highly favored food. In nature when an animal has access to a highly palatable food, it is adaptive to eat as much as possible while the food is available. This is true for a particularly large rodent or bird that a cat might capture in nature. The critical issue in weight control is whether caloric intake balances energy output. Frequently some cat owners will feed a highly palatable food in large quantities even though the cat does not expend the calories in moving about, playing, searching for food, or otherwise getting exercise.

Cat owners may suspect physical causes for their cat's obesity, such as a hormonal imbalance. In this regard, the possible influence of spaying or castration on obesity may come up. When it has been studied, ovarioectomy leads to an increase in body weight because estrogen has the effect of reducing appetite and reducing the efficiency with which animals extract calories from food.[4] Given the fact that female cats go through estrus cycles only part of the year, there is probably only a slight increase in body weight that may be attributed to gonadectomy. Removal of the testes generally does not promote the accumulation of excessive fat so much as the reduction of muscle mass leading to a replacement of muscle by fat.[4]

Typical History

Usually the issue of obesity is brought up by the attending veterinarian rather than an owner presenting a cat for obesity. However, when the cat owners decide that the animal's health is at risk, they may be willing to provide the details regarding their feeding regimen, the palatability of the food, and the frequency of feeding; and they may express an interest in following advice to reduce the cat's body weight.

Diagnosis

The main differential diagnosis with regard to pathophysiological causes is thyroid deficiency. Another consideration is that certain drugs may be contributing to an excessive appetite. The benzodiazepines, including diazepam, increase appetite,[5] and even have been used to stimulate appetite when animals are not eating sufficiently.

It is known that there is a genetic control of number of fat cells in an animal, as well as an influence of being overfed as infants, that may predispose some animals to be more obese than others. Generally the number of fat cells remains constant in the adult, and this may account for some of the differences between obese and normal individuals. Perhaps some cat breeders, in their concern to keep young kittens as healthy as possible, excessively supplement the mother's milk. This could cause hyperplasia of fat cells in the kittens and facilitate permanent obesity.

Treatment Guidelines

Aside from various pathophysiological factors or medical treatments that may contribute to obesity, the main cause of obesity in cats is that owners are offering their cats too much of a highly palatable food for the amount of exercise they get. It should be explained to clients that the physiological regulatory system of eating for urban cats is not refined enough to deal with modern urban living any more than it is with modern urban living in people. One has the choice of either maintaining a diet of highly palatable food and restricting the amount or perhaps substituting a less palatable food on a more liberal basis. As in other behavior problems, one of the best approaches might be to ask clients to experiment for a couple of weeks with a certain regimen before making a commitment to a lifestyle change in feeding their cat. One should counsel clients that love for a cat can be expressed in ways other than feeding and that after a new dietary regime is established, the cat will accept the routine.

A way to slow down the rate at which a cat consumes its food, as well as to increase its mental and physical exercise, is to use food-dispensing products. These products are commercially available, but owners can be creative in making their own. A plastic food container filled with dry food, with a hole cut into the lid, or a tennis ball with a hole cut into it and filled with dry food, are two options.

Predation

Cat owners, and the public at large, express a variety of feelings about the predatory behavior of cats. People love cats for their ability to keep the population of mice and rats at low levels on farms and other places where rodents may be a serious problem. However, in a suburban setting cats can have astounding effects on the population of songbirds and small mammals, such as squirrels and voles. And it is well-fed and cared-for cats that are the major threat. The hunting instinct is not triggered by hunger.[6,7] In several cities people are starting to organize to find ways to reduce cat predation especially on songbirds.

A cat and its hunting tendencies are not easily separated. When predation is a problem owners usually live with it, or they may attempt to manage the behavior by confining their cat or attaching a bell to the collar, hoping it will warn unsuspecting birds. In selecting and raising an urban cat from kittenhood, however, there are things one can do to reduce the likelihood of this problem. By the same token, action can be taken to enhance the pest control aspects for cats living on the farm.

Natural Predatory Behavior

The natural prey of cats is rats, voles, and mice, but songbirds are increasingly being taken. Prey animals often escape, especially if they are not taken by surprise. One estimate is that a cat makes about three attempts before it catches one mouse.[8] Generally a cat is more capable of catching small rodents that live in burrows than birds. With a rodent, a cat can watch the prey before pouncing on it and can time the attack. If a cat were to rush a mouse or rat as soon as it appeared at the entrance to its burrow, the rodent would simply run back into the burrow before the cat could nab it. The cat's strategy is to wait until the rodent strays away from its shelter. As a cat stalks, it also waits, slinking along a trail or ditch and then watching for the moment of opportunity. This waiting behavior can be counterproductive when applied to birds. The natural tendency of birds is to keep hopping while searching for food. When the bird hops along, the cat must also move and settle into its waiting mode. The bird may initiate this movement process several times and eventually fly away, usually without having seen the cat.

When rodents are plentiful the effect of feral cats on the rodent population can be very substantial. When the population of meadow voles surged in a northern California park, for example, feral cats ate approximately 88% of the entire population.[9] Around homes where vines are growing on fences, or where yards border on woods that provide food for rodents, cats prey on the rodent population and keep it within reasonable limits.

Cats are known to kill prey without immediately eating it, or they may kill more prey at one time than they can possibly consume. This behavior should be viewed from the standpoint of living in nature where, through multiple killings, a cat can store up a food supply. Most cat owners have seen cats play with their prey before eating it. Cats sometimes even delay delivering a killing bite as if to intentionally prolong their play with a half-live rodent. Prey is tossed into the air, batted around with the paws, rolled over, clasped, and kicked in the stomach with the hind claws. One explanation, without supporting evidence, is that this play is a release of pent-up energies associated with different aspects of predatory behavior.[8] Another possibility, also without evidence, is that injured rodents release a lactone related to the active ingredient of catnip, nepatolactone, that activates play behavior in much the same way as does catnip. By releasing a catniplike lactone, the rodent has some probability of escaping.

One of the fascinating aspects of feline maternal behavior is the manner in which mother cats introduce kittens to predatory behavior. Although some cats need no prior experience to prey on mice efficiently, others will not kill mice later unless taught by their mothers.[10,11] In general, cats exposed to mice as kittens gain in later predatory efficiency, but there is little carryover to preying on birds. Similarly, preying on birds does not improve a cat's skills with mice.

In nature the introduction of kittens to prey begins when the mother first brings dead prey to the kittens and eats it in front of them. Later the prey is presented to the kittens and the mother tries to provoke their interest in it without eating it herself, while not allowing the prey to escape. As a prelude to dispersion of the young, mothers continue to diminish their role, phasing the kittens into capturing prey on their own.

Selecting Cats to be Nonhunters

People who live in urban and suburban areas, who are determined to have their cats spend at least some time outside, and who want to select or acquire cats that are least likely to prey on songbirds or small mammals should consider the genetic aspects of predatory behavior. Selecting a kitten from a litter where the mother and sire are known to be nonhunters is the best way of reducing the probability that a kitten will become a hunter. If inquiries about siblings of previous litters reveal that few or none of them are known to be hunters, all the better. Regardless of the selection procedure, some cats do not become hunters even when the litter has been tutored by the mother to hunt. Other cats become hunters regardless of the fact that the mother did not hunt and the cats were not exposed to other cats who were hunters.

Regardless of whether one has a chance to get involved in the background of a kitten to be adopted, it is possible to discourage predation in a kitten or juvenile cat when predatory intention behavior is seen by surreptitiously disrupting the behavior with a remote punisher, such as with a water sprayer or ultrasonic noisemaker at these moments. These disrupters should be harmless but unpleasant enough to decrease this behavior.

Reducing Predation in Adult Cats

If an adult cat manifests predatory tendencies that are a problem to the owner, one solution is to manage the problem physically. It is becoming increasingly common and highly recommended to keep all cats indoors. Not only does this reduce disease transmission, but it certainly protects neighborhood songbirds. If keeping a cat indoors is not possible, cats can be outfitted with a bell, as mentioned earlier; this may alert birds being stalked and lower the probability of predation, but it does not eliminate it. The main threat of cats to the sustainability of songbird populations is predation on fledglings that spend a short period of time on the ground, and a bell will not help fledglings on the ground. The most it can do is increase the warning calls by parents of fledglings. Be aware that some cats learn how to move so as not to sound the bell. Owners of cats that are allowed outside should also be discouraged from maintaining bird feeders on their property. In many communities where outside cats are common, songbirds have no chance of reproducing, and the songbirds that are found have usually flown in from distant woods.

If the predatory problem is an indoor one, involving a cat pestering a caged bird or pet rodent, it may be possible to keep a cat away from specific areas where the potential prey is housed with remote punishment, such as a water sprayer (used by the owner without being seen by the cat) or barriers of upside-down plastic carpet runners, contact paper, or inverted mousetraps around the bird or hamster cage (Chapter 3).

References

1. Mugford RA. External influences on the feeding of carnivores. In: Kare MR, Maller O, eds. The Chemical Senses and Nutrition. New York: Academic Press, Inc., 1977.
2. Bradshaw JWS, Neville PF, Sawyer D. Factors affecting pica in the domestic cat. Applied Animal Behaviour Science 1997;52:373–379.
3. Hart BL. Biological basis of the behavior of sick animals. Neuroscience and Biobehavioral Reviews 1988:12L123–137.
4. Wade GN. Sex hormones, regulatory behaviors, and body weight. In: Rosenblatt JS, Hinde RA, Shaw E, Beer C, eds. Advances in the Study of Behavior. Vol. 6. New York: Academic Press, Inc., 1976:201–279.
5. Mereu GP, Fratta W, Chessa P, Gessa GL. Voraciousness induced in cats by benzodiazepines. Psychopharmacology 1976;47:101–103.

6. Adamec RE. The interaction of hunger and preying in the domestic cat (*Felis catus*): An adaptive hierarchy. Behavioral Biology 1976;18:263–272.

7. Churcher PB, Lawton JH. Beware of well-fed felines. Natural History 1989;7:40–48.

8. Leyhausen P. Cat Behavior. New York: Garland STPM Press, 1979.

9. Pearson OP. Carnivore-mouse predation: An example of its intensity and bioenergetics. Journal of Mammalogy 1964;45:177–188.

10. Caro TM. The effects of experience on the predatory patterns of cats. Behavioral and Neural Biology 1980;29:1–28.

11. ———. Effects of the mother, object play, and adult experience on predation in cats. Behavioral and Neural Biology 1980;29:29–51.

Chapter 25
Problems with Sexual and Maternal Behavior of Cats

More than any other area, cat owners look to veterinarians and other professionals for behavioral advice regarding reproductive behavior. Sexual behavior in particular is closely aligned with medicine and physiology. It is an area that many people feel embarrassed about, but expect professionals to be competent in discussing. The problems in this area, relating to deficiencies in sexual responsiveness in breeding cats and problems from inappropriate or objectionable sexual behavior, require the clinician to differentiate normal from abnormal behavior.

The topic of maternal behavior brings up another set of problems. Of all domestic animals, cats are probably the most capable of going through parturition and raising of their young without human care or intervention. In the classic example, a mother cat that has secretly gone through parturition in some obscure location reveals a litter of perfectly healthy kittens to the human family members after the kittens have been born. This romanticized view of feline motherhood has given way to the more formalized cattery operation or the family breeder where a mother cat may give birth to her litter of kittens in the midst of an overly concerned human audience. Problems with maternal behavior manifest themselves primarily as either lack of proper attention to the kittens, resulting in inadequate care and nutrition of the kittens, or infanticide with cannibalism of the kittens.

This chapter deals first with normal feline sexual behavior and then with some of the problems with breeding animals and with objectionable behavior of nonbreeding cats. The topic of maternal behavior is taken up next, starting with a discussion of normal maternal behavior and followed by the problems with maternal behavior.

Normal Sexual Behavior

Cats are nocturnal, which means that much of their general activity takes place at night, including interactions with the opposite sex. Most cat owners, therefore, are less familiar with the sexual behavior of cats than dog owners are of dogs because dogs are much easier to observe. Many veterinarians have been called at late hours by anxious feline owners wondering why their gonadally intact female cat is acting as though she were in pain.

When a female cat is in estrus her behavior is very distinct, including heightened activity and nervousness. Her mating call apparently attracts male cats, and sex attractants in her urine stimulate visiting male cats to stay around. Unfamiliar male cats may appear on the doorstep of an amorous female and emit courtship cries, unequivocally communicating their interest in meeting the female. In the presence of a male cat, or even if she can only hear or smell him, the female is likely to assume the receptive posture, consisting of elevation of the pelvic region, deviation of the tail to one side or the other, and treading or stepping of the back legs. As the male cat investigates and starts to mount the female these responses usually become more intense.

Female cats differ from females of other domestic species in that this receptive behavior is sometimes displayed to the pet owner. The pelvic elevation, tail deviation, and treading of females in estrus can often be induced by human handlers stroking the back of the female cat and touching the perineal region (Fig. 25-1). The response may be intensified by grasping the skin over the back of the neck while stroking the perineal region with the other hand.

If a male is comfortable with the surroundings, he will then approach the female, typically engage first in nose-to-nose and then genital investigation. The latter often evokes a flehmen response called a *gape,* in the male. He then proceeds to take a neck grip on the female with his teeth. The male usually engages in treading or stepping of the back legs after he mounts. His initial mount is usually fairly high on the female's back, but he generally slides backward over the female as he continues leg stepping until he is aligned for intromission. Leg treading by the female also aids in bringing about genital contact. The male then begins pelvic thrusting, and copulatory intromission is followed by a deep pelvic thrust. The male remains motionless for a few seconds after intromission, and during this time a degree of excitement seems to build up within the female as her eyes dilate. Soon after ejaculation she begins to pull away from the male, typically emits a loud cry, and turns as if to hit at the male as he springs back. She then begins licking her genitalia and goes into the after-reaction, which consists of rolling and rubbing on the floor. These stages in mating are shown in Figure 25-2.

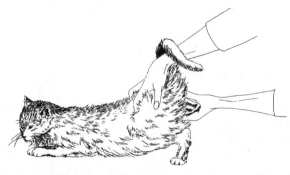

Figure 25-1   The receptive posture of female cats in estrus can often be elicited by the owners. In some instances this is a test for receptivity before males are brought to females for breeding.

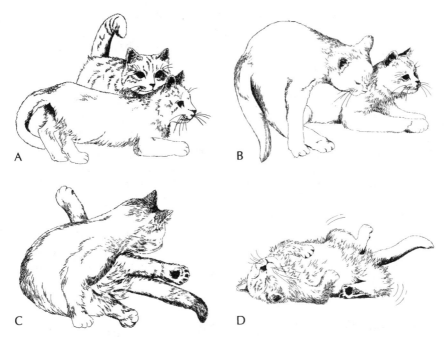

Figure 25-2   Stages of mating: A, male approaches a female while the female displays the receptive posture; B, male mounts female and engages in pelvic thrusting, eventually achieving intromission and ejaculation; C, after male dismounts, female cleans genitalia; D, at the end of the mating sequence, female briefly engages in rolling and rubbing, referred to as an *after-reaction*.

The male, meanwhile, engages in licking of his penis. This behavior is probably more than just surface hygiene. Cats seem to be afflicted with few sexually transmitted diseases, and one of the reasons probably is due to the fact that the transmission of genital diseases is broken by the male physically cleansing the penis and then applying antibacterial saliva.[1,2]

Because the female cat is a reflex ovulator, the duration and number of estrous periods during the breeding season is affected by the frequency of mating. When she is mated, estrus lasts for only 4–6 days, but if she is not mated, estrus may last for as long as 10 days, and subsequent estrous periods may occur at intervals of 2 or 3 weeks. Ovulation can be induced by probing the vagina of a female cat with a smooth blunt instrument such as a metal or glass rod. Several insertions of about 10 seconds duration and 5 minutes apart for 2 successive days will usually induce ovulation.[3] Often females will display the copulatory after-reactions to these insertions. Hence, in this way repeated or prolonged estrous periods can be avoided if ovarihysterectomy or breeding is not desired.

Problems with Sexual Behavior

Male cats may fail to copulate with a receptive female because of lack of interest in females or discomfort with an unfamiliar breeding environment. Inability to perform could also reflect physical interference with the copulatory process even with a highly motivated male. Objectionable sexual behavior usually takes the form of mounting of other cats.

Lack of Apparent Motivation

When cat owners have decided they have a male worthy of carrying on the family genes, they may find to their disappointment that he lacks the sexual prowess equal to the task. A few precautions may save the owners some dismay. If a specific area is reserved for breeding, the male cat may eventually come to anticipate copulation when he is placed in that area. For each mating occasion, the male should be given time to acclimate to the area, and after a few minutes a receptive female placed with him. The male should be allowed to mate with the female several times in succession if both sexes are motivated. During the initial sessions, the male may wait 30 minutes to several hours before copulating. However, usually after a few weeks of frequent presentations of a receptive female, he will copulate within 15 minutes or less.

Apparent Inability to Sexually Perform

A hair ring sometimes develops around the glans penis, preventing intromission and, hence, successful mating.[4] One clue that this problem exists is a male that continually thrusts but does not intromit. The glans penis of the male cat is covered with epithelial papillae which project backward, and the papillae apparently collect hairs. The hairs may come from the preputial sheath or, perhaps with frequent mating, from the fur of the female when the erect penis is rubbed over the back and perineum of the female. The hair ring is sometimes removed by the males themselves. One can also remove the ring by gently sliding it over the penis. Animals are able to mate immediately after removal of the hair ring, and the rings do not appear to be painful.

A male's lack of interest in mating could theoretically be due to abnormally low levels of testosterone. One way to evaluate male cats in this regard would be to analyze the blood testosterone level and compare it to a normal range. However, it would be necessary to submit several blood samples taken throughout the day because blood testosterone concentrations fluctuate. Evidence available indicates that less than half of the usual level of testosterone can maintain normal copulatory activity in male cats. Thus, testosterone levels would have to be quite depressed to account for a male's lack of sexual interest in females.

One area where testosterone levels may be important is in regulating sexual behavior during seasonal fluctuations. For males, the lowest period of sexual activity is in the fall. One would not expect this to be an important factor in breeding, because females usually are not in estrus at this time. However, a seasonal fluctuation should not be automatically disregarded in a consideration of an otherwise unexplained decline in the sexual prowess of a breeding male.

A male cat may fail to perform effectively if a painful or fear-eliciting event happened during the mating sequence. Any stimulus that caused a cat to be fearful should be identified and removed from the breeding area, or the breeding should be moved to another area. If these options are not feasible, the owners should desensitize and countercondition the cat to the stimulus. Antianxiety medications should not be used, because there is the potential for sperm abnormalities to occur. If the level of anxiety in the cat is so elevated, the owners should be counseled that this behavior is not desirable to pass on to the progeny. The personality of kittens in a litter can often be related to the personality of the tomcat, even without any parental care by the male.[5]

Problems with Breeding Females

In order to breed females, it is crucial to pinpoint the time of estrus carefully. If owners carefully observe the queen's behavior or listen to tomcats in the neighborhood, they will usually find it easy to know when the time has arrived. Problems with females fall into two categories: difficulties with estrus detection in which the female is overdue for coming into estrus but shows no behavioral signs, and rejection of a male's sexual advances even though the female shows other signs of sexual receptivity.

Females that the owners desire to breed do not usually live with sexually active males, and the owners are thus faced with the problem of determining when the queen is in estrus. Unlike the dog, the female cat does not have noticeable vulva swelling or vaginal bleeding as an indication of impending estrus. Of course, the sexual attractants emitted by females can attract wandering tomcats to the house, providing a clear signal. Estrus may be expressed by sexual vocalizations and rubbing and rolling on the floor. With many female cats the behavioral signs associated with sexual receptivity are a useful indication of estrus. These signs may be evident when the female hears or smells a tomcat. Petting on the back will often cause the female to crouch and elevate the pelvis (Fig. 25-1). Although rubbing the perineal region while holding on to the skin over the dorsum of the neck (as the male cat would do) frequently evokes treading of the back legs and deviation of the tail to one side, such responses cannot be evoked from all females in full estrus. Therefore, it would be a mistake to rely on this behavioral response as the sole indicator of estrus. One may have to place the female in the vicinity of a sexually active male to observe behavioral signs of estrus.

A complaint regarding breeding females is that a queen that appears to be in full estrus will not accept the male. Gently restraining the reluctant female could be tried in these cases. Even though some male cats are reluctant to mate with a restrained female, an experienced and regularly active stud will often breed a female restrained by the breeder. If the restraining does not work, one might resort to leaving a male and female together for several hours and hope for the best. The drawback with just putting animals together is that one cannot be sure if mating has occurred. If the female remains in estrus for a week or more after this type of mating, she presumably has not ovulated. Some females may reject one particular male but accept others. If it were thought that the female is responding differentially to different males, it would be advisable to try the female with a different stud male. The breeding of cats is fraught with individual idiosyncrasies and special sensitivities. From the standpoint of our management of this aspect of a cat's life, persistence and patience are invaluable.

As with males, painful or fear-eliciting stimuli may also affect female sexual performance. Alleviating the pain, removal of the stimulus, or moving the breeding area away from the stimulus should all be attempted. If these options are not feasible, systematic desensitization and counterconditioning should be done. Antianxiety medications should not be used because the safety of treating pregnant or nursing animals generally has not been examined, and there is a potential for teratogenic effects. Also as discussed previously, if the level of anxiety is so great, the owners should be counseled against breeding that cat.

Objectionable Mounting of Other Cats or Objects

On occasion castrated males may persistently mount other males in the household or females that are spayed. A cat may mount and even perform thrusting upon inanimate objects, such as stuffed animals or towels. One approach is behavior modification based on the principle that a cat will not mount other cats if the other cats do not tolerate it. Remote punishment with a water sprayer (see Chapter 3) might prove effective if the cat being mounted is sprayed each time it allows mounting, and if the water spraying is done so that the cats do not know who is delivering the punishment. The owner must take care not to frighten the cat being mounted. When no one is around to deliver remote punishment, the cats should not be allowed together until the problem is solved.

Normal Maternal Behavior

In nature basic necessities must be provided to neonates by the mother. Mothers with inadequate mothering behavior leave few or no offspring, and hence poor mothering is rarely seen in nature. On the domestic scene when maternal care, such as nursing the kittens, has not been adequate, we step in and take over; the result is a survival of kittens whose mothers were possibly lacking in the genetic programming of maternal behavior. Thus, our intervention may help perpetuate the genes for poor mothering. The result is individual variability in the behavioral patterns that were previously under natural selection.[6] This variability in maternal behavior among cats is especially evident to managers of catteries. Although many cats are perfectly normal attentive mothers, some never seem interested in their own kittens, even after several litters. Normal maternal behavior is not only necessary for survival of kittens, but the experiences the kitten receives as a result of maternal attention and interaction with littermates have a critical influence on its behavior and health as it grows into adulthood.

Behavior Before and During Parturition

As the time of parturition nears, pregnant females become less active, and licking of their mammary and genital areas increases. Keep in mind that the anogenital and ventral abdominal areas are the first surfaces outside the sterile uterine environment with which the neonate mouth comes in contact. Newborn kittens with a vulnerable intestinal tract seem to be saved from an overdose of bacteria in their initial suckling attempts by the licking of the mammary area and teats by the mother cat. Not only does she physically cleanse with her tongue, but she applies antibacterial saliva as well.[2]

Shortly before parturition some females may seek out a dark, dry, and relatively undisturbed area where they will deliver their young. Other cats that are strongly attached to their owners may not choose a location isolated from them. In fact, some cats become quite emotional during parturition if the owners are not nearby. Still other cats may become irritable or aggressive toward other cats or people as the time of parturition nears.

The four stages of labor are contraction, delivery of the fetus, delivery of the placenta, and the interval between deliveries. The interval between deliveries includes initial maternal care and leads into the immediate postparturient care of the young. Uterine contractions begin in the first stage with a good deal of straining. Cats usually lie down during this stage of labor, although they may frequently sit up to change positions. Contractions of the uterine and abdominal muscles become more intense in the second stage, and the fetus moves rather rapidly through the birth canal. The female often breaks the fetal membranes with her teeth when the head or buttocks of the fetus appear at the vulva. She may actually pull the fetus through the birth canal by tugging on the membranes. Her typical posture is lateral recumbency with her head bent to the hindquarters through her back legs. After the newborn has passed through the birth canal, the mother rapidly consumes the fetal membranes and begins licking the newborn vigorously, which usually stimulates the first respiratory movements.

During placental delivery in the third stage, the mother continues to lick and groom the newborn. The placenta is usually eaten by the mother as it is passed. While the mother eats the placenta, she generally bites off the umbilical cord. The pulling and stretching involved in eating the placenta and umbilical cord seem to cause vessel constriction of the cord. Occasionally, movement of the newborn and the mother causes breakage of the cord. At other times the umbilical cord does not get broken shortly after birth, and it may be necessary for a person to intervene, cut the cord and tie it off. Between deliveries the mother not only continues to lick and groom the newborn kittens and her own genital region, but she also cleans the bedding that has been soiled with amniotic fluids.

There is a wide range of normal variation in the duration of stages in kitten birth. The stage of contraction ranges from 12 seconds to more than 1 hour, and the stage of delivery from 30 minutes to 1 hour.[7] Only minor differences have been reported in parturient behavior between primiparous and multiparous females. Experienced mothers are less disturbed by physiological changes during birth and appear to respond more readily to the neonates in licking, grooming, and retrieving. Immediately after the birth of the last kitten, a female lies almost continuously with her young for 12 hours or more. Newborn kittens usually begin to suckle within an hour or two after delivery of the last fetus. The mother cat remains almost constantly with her litter for about the first 2 days and leaves the nest only for very short periods to move about and feed. She takes breaks away from the nest more frequently after these first 2 days. Later, the amount of time the mother spends nursing the young relates to the size of the litter. A mother may spend 70% of her time nursing if she has a litter of several kittens, but with only one or two kittens, it may be considerably less. Group rearing of kittens by more than one lactating queen is observed in groups of feral cats.[8]

Nursing

For the first 3 weeks, the mother initiates essentially all nursing sessions. While hovering over the litter or lying near them, she licks the kittens and arouses them. She typically lies with her body arched around the litter with her nipples exposed. With time the newborn become very adept at finding nipples and responding to the mother's solicitous behavior. Many kittens are able to take specific nipple positions with some regularity just 2 or 3 days after birth. Others do not seem to prefer a particular nipple location. From about the third week of life, the eyes and ears of kittens function well, they are able to leave the nest, and they recognize and interact with the mother outside the nest. The young now initiate most nursing episodes, which can take place inside or outside the nest.

From about the fifth week of life until weaning, the kittens initiate all nursing. As time progresses the mother begins evading the nursing attempts of the young. For example, she may lie with her mammary region against the floor or climb up on objects so that the young cannot reach her. Weaning occurs near the end of this phase with the mother becoming less available to the young. At the same time, the young are becoming more capable of taking adult food. Mothers of wild feline species typically provision the young near the end of this phase with rodents brought back to the nest. She will first bring killed rodents back to the nest. Then she will bring live prey, but prevent the prey from leaving the nest area, thus allowing the kittens ample opportunity to learn to catch the prey.

Grooming the Newborn

The mother cat licks the newborn rather extensively through the first 3 weeks. Grooming with the tongue is effective in controlling fleas,[9] and in nature this frequent grooming aids in removing nest-borne ectoparasites such as fleas that have hatched from flea pupae. Infections such as conjunctivitis may be eliminated by the mother's licking of these areas and application of antibacterial saliva. Grooming the anogenital region also evokes elimination, and the urine and fecal material are consumed by the mother, thereby keeping the nest clean. As the young begin leaving the nest area, the anogenital licking subsides, and the young deposit feces and urine away from the nest in another part of the room or along the side of the nest box. The mother continues to keep the nest area clean.

Retrieving Behavior

The classical sign of interaction between a mother and her young is the sight of a mother carrying a kitten by the nape of the neck. The reflexlike immobility posture that the young assume when being carried by the nape of the neck may sometimes be temporarily induced in adult cats. In fact, minor procedures such as giving subcutaneous injections and taking rectal temperatures may be performed on cats restrained in this fashion.

Mother cats retrieve young when they hear their vocalizations, particularly when the sound reaches a high intensity; kittens that are marooned from the nest and emit stress vocalizations are readily retrieved. The tendency for a mother cat to shift her litter from one spot to another in response to environmental disturbances is well known. This tendency to move a litter is strongest between 25 and 35 days after birth.[7]

Adoption of Strange Kittens

The ease with which some mother cats lavish care upon strange kittens is quite surprising. When two or more females in a house or cattery have given birth to kittens around the same time, one is likely to find the mothers stealing kittens back and forth or harassing each other for the other's kittens. This behavior may result in a type of communal nursery with all the kittens piled together, while mothers take turns caring for the kittens. At other times the mothers jointly lie with the kittens. Feral cats have been observed to raise their kittens communally.

Although this behavior of willingness to provide resources to kittens of another female may seem to be maladaptive, it should be noted that strange kittens were never present in the natal nest of ancestral lactating cats; thus, natural selection did not act to produce a rejection of other kittens.

Problems with Maternal Behavior

Maternal reactions that create problems fall at the emotional extremes, ranging from ignoring the kittens and allowing them to die, to killing and eating newborn kittens. This is the place to emphasize that the tendency of cat owners to intervene and help mothers with inadequate maternal behavior should be balanced against the knowledge that aiding the survival of young from mothers that provide inadequate care removes the selection pressures against poor mothering in the feline population. The result is increasing the extent to which poor mothering behavior is perpetuated in the offspring of poor mothers, who then live to reproduce at almost the same rate as the offspring of exemplary mothers.

The rather incomprehensible occurrences of maternal neglect or cannibalism can be extremely upsetting for clients. The clinician's role is to cast all aspects of maternal behavior in a biological perspective. Cats cannot be blamed for being poor mothers any more than they can be blamed for being poor hunters or for not being outgoing and friendly. A main concept to get across is that maternal behavior is at least as much a reflection of genetic predisposition as it is learning or experience. Although some cat mothers improve with experience, cat owners should be discouraged from feeling that they are likely to be able to teach their cats to be good mothers.

Maternal Neglect

If a mother does not remove the fetal membranes and dry the kittens, or she does not keep them close to her, the kittens may die of hypothermia. In large litters tangled umbilical cords may occur as the kittens arrive quickly and the mother does not clean off the fetal membranes. Hypothermia occurs if kittens are allowed to leave the nest and the mother fails to retrieve them. Once in a while a kitten gets dropped outside the nest because it held onto a nipple when the mother left the nest. Mothers may attend to a kitten in the nest and not notice one that is lying alone on the cold floor. Hypothermia also occurs when the mother does not stay with the litter. Stranded kittens or kittens that a mother has abandoned can be gently warmed and presented to the mother again. Sometimes such kittens may be accepted by the mother and recover completely. Others are rejected by the mother even after being repeatedly presented to her.

The following are recommendations for the management of catteries. The mother should be in an individual parturition box at least 3 days before she is due so she can adapt to the new surroundings. The queening box should be stable so that it will not be knocked over by the mother, and the sides high enough to prevent kittens from falling out. At the time of parturition mothers should be checked to see that they are cleaning the kittens and that the kittens are suckling soon after birth. Mothers that have presented problems in the past should be watched closely.

Infanticide and Cannibalism

A mother cat that is reported to have killed one or more kittens in a litter may appear normal and attentive to the remaining kittens. Circumstances that have been reported to be related to the occurrence of infanticide and cannibalism are having a litter larger than usual, going through a second pregnancy of the season, and the presence of kittens that are ill or deformed. Previous experience in being a mother does not appear to be related to cannibalism.

Perhaps the most accurate explanation of cannibalism is that the ability to kill newborn and eat them is a genetically programmed behavior that would appear to have an adaptive role on some occasions in nature. If a kitten is sick and likely to die from disease, the mother, by killing and eating it, keeps the nest from becoming contaminated by pathogens from the sick kitten. By reacting to what could be an early sign of disease, the mother may be protecting the other kittens by promptly removing a sick kitten before it is incubating billions of potential pathogens.[1] Rather than just depositing the dead kitten outside where it could attract scavengers, the mother removes the evidence by consuming it. And at the same time she gains some additional nutrition, which means she will need to be gone from the nest one less time to replenish her nutritional resources for lactation. The fact that a mother's cannibalism must be triggered by the very first sign of illness in a kitten means that a noninfectious disturbance of the kitten, or other type of ambiguous signal in the domestic environment, such as strong novel odor, noise or vibration, might also trigger cannibalism.

Infanticide and cannibalism may also occur if a mother detects a congenital deformity. In this instance it is not the risk of a pathogen that may affect the rest of the litter. Rather, the behavior represents selection for a behavior that removes a newborn that is unlikely to reproduce later in life (thus of no genetic benefit to the mother). Maternal cannibalism of the deformed kitten conserves otherwise wasted resources for the remaining normal kittens.

A type of infanticide committed by males occurs in some wild felids and a few primate species. Males that have fought with another male and taken over territory in which there is a resident female and her litter may indiscriminately kill the kittens. Removing the newborn causes females to come into estrus again soon. The male can then breed her and sire the next round of offspring. Domestic tomcats have been reported to commit this type of infanticide. Thus, there is some reason to keep strange tomcats away from lactating female cats. One would expect a resident tomcat that has sired the kittens to be quite safe around kittens, and, indeed, this is what some breeders have found.

References

1. Hart BL. Behavioral adaptations to pathogens and parasites: Five strategies. Neuroscience and Biobehavioral Reviews 1990;14:273–294.
2. Hart BL, Powell KL. Antibacterial properties of saliva: Role of maternal periparturient grooming and in licking wounds. Physiology and Behavior 1990;48:383–386.
3. Diakow C. Effects of genital desensitization on mating behavior and ovulation in the female cat. Physiology and Behavior 1971;7:47–54.
4. Hart BL, Peterson DM. Penile hair rings in male cats may prevent mating. Laboratory and Animal Science 1970;21:422.
5. Reisner IR, Houpt KA, Erb HN, Quimby FW. Friendliness to humans and defensive aggression in cats: The influence of handling and paternity. Physiology and Behavior 1994;55:1119–1124.
6. Price EO. Behavioral aspects of animal domestication. The Quarterly Review of Biology 1984;59:1–32.
7. Schneirla TC, Rosenblatt JS, Tobach E. Maternal behavior in the cat. In: Rheingold, HL, ed. Maternal Behavior in Mammals. New York, John Wiley & Sons, Inc., 1963: 122–168.
8. Macdonald DW, Apps PJ, Carr GM, Kerby G. Social dynamics, nursing coalitions and infanticide among farm cats, *Felis catus*. Advances in Ethology 1987;28:1–64, Supplement to Ethology.
9. Eckstein RA, Hart BL. Grooming and control of fleas in cats. Applied Animal Behaviour Science 2000;68:141–150.

Chapter 26
Repetitive, Compulsive, and Stereotypic Behaviors

Almost all the behavior problems addressed in the preceding chapters on cats deal with behaviors that can usually be considered normal or adaptive from the cat's standpoint. This chapter, however, deals with compulsive and stereotypic behavioral patterns that appear abnormal with no adaptive or functional value in nature for the ancestral cat or the modern cat living under feral conditions. This does not mean these behavioral patterns do not have a link to a normal behavior; indeed some behaviors discussed here will be linked to a normal adaptive behavior, but in which the manifestation is abnormal.

In the chapter on compulsive and stereotypic behavior in dogs, behavioral patterns discussed were excessive tail chasing, repetitive snapping at imaginary flies, chasing light flashes or shadows, flank sucking and excessive licking of the carpus or tarsus. Not unexpectedly, given differences in innate behavioral predispositions, the compulsive and stereotypic behavioral patterns of cats differ markedly from those of dogs. The ones that are of primary concern are excessive grooming or biting off the hair, resulting in areas of the skin that are devoid of hair cover, and wool chewing or wool ingestion. Both abnormal behaviors seem to be related to an aberrant form of a normal behavior. Thus, excessive grooming is an exaggeration of normal grooming. Wool chewing and ingestion seems similar to chewing and eating grass, at least in form. Cats may also display other repetitive behavioral patterns that could fall into this category or would eventually be diagnosed as attention seeking. As with dogs, common to the behavioral problems discussed in this chapter is that they show a high degree of constancy from one occasion to the next, both within the same cat and between cats.

Most readers are familiar with the syndrome of obsession-compulsive disorder (OCD) in humans, and sometimes parallels are drawn between repetitive stereotypic behaviors in cats and dogs with those of humans with OCD. In human patients, compulsive behaviors appear to prevent or reduce anxiety or stress coming from an internal emotion referred to as an obsession, rather than being attributed to an environmental source, such as that induced by crowding, isolation, or boredom. In humans an obsession with ideas, thoughts, impulses, or images may produce stress or anxiety, and it is believed that the compulsive performance of a repetitive act in some way relieves this stress or anxiety. The connection between the obsession and the compulsive behavior has led to the term *obsessive-compulsive disorder*. As mentioned, human OCD patients usually do not seem to be suffering from environmental stressful situations analogous to captive environments of zoo animals or farm animals, and which can be related to the performance of stereotypic behaviors.

Because the term *OCD* implies a verbal report on the part of the patient about obsessions with ideas, thoughts, impulses, or images, one is not in a position to say whether such mental activity occurs in cats or any other animal. However, the term *compulsion* seems to apply because cats, like similarly affected dogs, seem to be driven to perform the repetitive behaviors independent of any identifiable external stimulus. The stereotypic behaviors such as pacing, swaying, and mouthing frequently seen in farm and zoo animals kept in confinement appear to be different from those seen in pet cats and dogs. In farm and zoo animals, the stereotypic behaviors can often be attributed to environmental stress, crowding, or isolation. The environmental extremes of farm and zoo animals seem not to apply to cats. Cats engaging in wool chewing or excessive licking appear to be normal and not particularly stressed in day-to-day living. When the behaviors are prevented with special collars, the affected cats do not perform an alternative stereotypic behavior.

Wool Chewing and Wool Ingestion

Wool chewing and wool ingestion are common behaviors in some cats. One can even find pictures of cats engaging in this behavior in some of the popular cat books. In the conventional medical sense the ingestion of a substance that is nutritionally inappropriate is referred to as *pica*. Clearly the most common pica in cats is chewing or consuming wool or other fabrics. Wool is the preferred material, although cotton and even synthetic fabrics are chewed by some cats. Because the behavior is somewhat compulsive, wool ingestion would appear to be a syndrome different from other types of pica, such as ingestion of wood chips, sand, or litter material. Grass chewing and eating, though sometimes referred to as pica, would appear to be normal with a possible parasite control function (Chapter 24), although wool chewing or eating could be an aberrant form of grass eating.

Cats that engage in wool chewing do not appear to be abnormal in other ways. There has been some tendency to explore whether there was an attractive element or substance to the articles being chewed that might explain the attraction. As of yet no physiological explanation has been presented despite repeated attempts to relate the behavior to a nutritional deficiency, intestinal disorder, or pancreatitis. Some feel that early weaning of cats may predispose them to this problem, but there is no empirical information to substantiate this hypothesis.

Typical History

This behavior is particularly prominent in cats of the Siamese and Burmese breeds, but it may also be shown on occasion by cats of other breeds.[1] The behavior seems to have an onset about the time of puberty. Some cats may go through a transient phase of chewing and ingesting wool; others continue to engage in chewing and eating wool into adulthood, sometimes to the point where the owners complain of destruction of valuable sweaters or socks. Some cats seem to go from chewing and ingesting wool to showing the same behavior toward other substrates, whereas others may engage in chewing other substrates from the beginning. The behavior can be so severe that the cat cannot be maintained as an indoor cat.

Diagnosis

The diagnosis of this behavior problem is straightforward with few competing alternative diagnoses. One possibility is to examine the onset or concurrent presence of stressful events that may have led to the behavior.

Treatment Guidelines

Sometimes the behavior can be controlled by restricting the cat's access to target woolen or other objects. In more severe cases, some form of behavior modification can be employed involving staged trials. A target object that the cat is likely to chew is left accessible to the cat and then booby-trapped with electronically activated sirens or some sort of startling stimulus to produce an aversion to the object (Chapter 3). All other possible woolen targets for chewing should be made unavailable. If successive exposures indicate that the cat has acquired an aversion to the object that is booby-trapped, then other similar objects can also be booby-trapped and the process carried out until it is likely that the cat has lost its attraction to chewing these objects as well.

This type of remote punishment is going to be most successful if the cat's motivation in engaging in the behavior is reduced. Providing the cat with consistent, regular periods of interaction with the owner, such as play with a ball on string may be useful in providing some structured interaction to counteract a rather boring lifestyle. Similarly one might also provide the cat with a perch or resting place near a window so the cat can observe action outside the house. In the event that the behavior is an aberrant form of eating grass, in the absence of access to grass, a grass "garden" should be provided. Food-dispensing toys, including homemade ones made out of tennis balls with holes cut into them and filled with dry kibble, increase the amount of time that a cat spends eating and may reduce the problem.

In some instances a pharmacological approach might be implemented in addition to behavior modification. If the behavior responds to a conventional serotonergic drug, such as fluoxetine or clomipramine, one should consider treatment for at least 16 weeks, followed by phasing the cat off the medication.

Excessive Grooming (*Psychogenic Alopecia*)

The term *psychogenic alopecia* refers to the diagnosis used by dermatologists for the syndrome in cats presented with extensive hair loss from excessive grooming, or where other forms of dermatitis, including flea hypersensitivity and other ectoparasite infestations, were ruled out.[2] The excessive grooming may take the form of excessive licking of the hair to the point where the hair is worn off or from biting off of hairs in the infected area. Some dermatologists express the perspective that most would-be cases of psychogenic alopecia can be found to have a medical cause related to dermatitis or ectoparasite allergy. A thorough medical workup is required before arriving at this diagnosis.

Whether the problem stems from a cat's "overreaction" to a relatively minor dermatological or allergic stimulus, or simply an aberrant behavior, an understanding of this problem is facilitated by a discussion of normal grooming in cats. For one, cats are probably easily triggered to grooming. The grooming, for which cats are famous, enables them to maintain a sleek pelage. With the exception of long-haired cats, grooming is frequent enough that one rarely sees problems with excessive shedding of fur. Cats can accumulate hair in the stomach in the form of hairballs, which occasionally cause some gastrointestinal discomfort, or even obstruction, and must be treated. Oral grooming, which accounts for an estimated 8% of nonsleeping or nonresting time, is characterized by the cat drawing the conified papillae of the tongue over the surface of the pelage repeatedly in multiple bouts of licking. Scratch grooming, delivered in single bouts, is directed to one region at a time and occupies a very small proportion of waking time. Oral grooming in cats appears to be governed primarily by programmed grooming, in which bouts of grooming are periodically activated by a central grooming control center, rather than peripheral stimulation.[3] One of the important functions of grooming in cats is removal of ectoparasites, including fleas, and when cats are exposed to fleas, the grooming clock appears to be accelerated and there is an increase in the rate of grooming bouts.[4] A possible model to explain the occurrence of excessive grooming in cats is an abnormal activation of the grooming control center such that oral grooming on some areas is markedly increased. The hairs are also bitten off with the teeth, resulting in broken hairs.

Typical History

This problem is often presented to veterinarians when owners notice areas of the pelage from which the hair coat is denuded. In contrast to excessive licking in dogs, which is directed toward the carpus and sometimes the tarsus, affected areas may be anywhere on the body that the cat can easily reach and usually involve a fairly large area. No breed predispositions are noted, and both genders seem to be afflicted equally with this syndrome.

The behavior is usually presented as a *dermatological* problem when there is a careful examination for fleas in the event that the excessive licking is a reflection of a flea allergy or hypersensitivity. The problem is considered to be a *behavioral* problem when, after exhaustive medical evaluation, there is no other explanation. Licking can generally be controlled with the use of a conical Elizabethan-like collar, which allows the hair to grow out. Not infrequently when the collar is removed, the excessive grooming starts again, with the possibility of removal of hair from the same or other parts of the body. Because the collar used to limit grooming undoubtedly causes some stress for the cat, the return to excessive grooming following removal of the collar may, in part, reflect the stressful effects of the collar.

Diagnosis

After a dermatological problem has been ruled out, one can turn to behavioral explanations for the excessive grooming. Although unlikely, enough history should be explored to rule out that there is any attention-seeking aspect to the behavior by noting whether the behavior primarily occurs in the presence of the owners. If the excessive grooming primarily occurs when the owners are absent, stress from separation from the owner should be considered.

It is important for the clinician to evaluate carefully the circumstances regarding when the excessive grooming seemed to have first started, although this may not be known because it takes some time for damage to the pelage to be noticed. The history should explore the current environment for any signs of conflict, confinement or boredom. Because cats take to a solitary lifestyle more easily than dogs, boredom is less likely to be a cause of abnormal, excessive licking than in dogs. Any measures that the owners have taken to stop the behavior should be evaluated and indications explored as to whether the owner's attempts at dealing with the problem have helped or exacerbated the problem.

Treatment Guidelines

Any evident environmental source of stress, boredom, or conflict should be resolved. Although the use of a restraint collar may prevent excessive grooming, there is a need to implement measures that may resolve the problem so that such collars are not necessary. Regular playful interaction between the cat caregiver and the cat—in the form of pulling a sock tied to a string, teaching the cat tricks, or other creative types of interaction—may be useful. Providing one or more perches for the cat to follow the goings-on in the street outside the house may be helpful. It is not unheard of for cat owners to provide a television program with images designed for cats, but whether this actually reduces boredom remains to be tested.

The use of serotonergic drugs such as fluoxetine or clomipramine to reduce anxiety and eliminate the excessive grooming has been tested with varied success. The drug regimen that can be tried is the administration of a serotonergic drug for at least 4 months. Drug treatment will be most successful if combined with one or more of the above-mentioned behavior modification measures. After 4 months of drug treatment, the resolution of the problem could be evaluated by gradual withdrawal of drug treatment.

References

1. Bradshaw JWS, Neville PF, Sawyer D. Factors affecting pica in the domestic cat. Applied Animal Behaviour Science 1997;52:373–379.
2. Sawyer LS, Meon-Fanelli AA, Dodman NH. Psychogenic alopecia in cats: 11 cases (1993–1996). Journal of the American Veterinary Medical Association 1999;214:71–74.

3. Eckstein RA, Hart BL. The organization and control of grooming in cats. Applied Animal Behaviour Science 2000;68:131–140.
4. ———. Grooming and control of fleas in cats. Applied Animal Behaviour Science 2000;68:141–150.

Chapter 27
Selecting and Raising Kittens

Although many people enjoy both dogs and cats as companion animals, cats and dogs fill different household and owner-personality niches. The size of cats makes them more suitable for small living spaces. For people with busy schedules and long hours at work, the fact that cats will use a litter box for elimination, as opposed to the necessity of being taken on a walk 2–3 times a day, can be very important. These differences contribute to the increasing popularity of cats in urban settings where regular access to the outdoors is not available. In addition, cats can usually deal with being left alone better than dogs as a reflection of the evolved solitary lifestyle of their wild ancestors. Thus, cats are much less likely than dogs to experience separation anxiety than dogs upon being left alone by a working household. Finally, cats do not appear to challenge human members of the family for dominance as do dogs, and hence aggressive behavior is farther down the list of complaints of cat owners than in dog owners where aggression toward human family members is the most frequent complaint.

Most cats live in multicat households.[1] The adoption of multiple cats may reflect a person's love of cats or it could reflect the mistaken feeling that a single cat, left home alone much of the time, will be lonely; therefore, cat owners may feel obligated to find a companion. As many cat owners will testify, the addition of a new cat often makes matters worse for the resident cat. The resident cat may reject the stranger, or the cats may tolerate each other. Worse yet, the resident cat may start urine marking when a new cat is brought into the house because of the extra agitation and emotional upset it creates (Chapter 21).

One thing becoming increasingly clear, however, is that cats are much more flexible in social interactions than one would predict from their African ancestors. Thus, some cats get along famously with feline housemates and can form recognizable social bonds and hierarchies.[2] This flexibility in social system structure may represent the absence of selection against sociality as well as human selection for a modest degree of sociality

Age and Source of Adoption

As a rule people are much less concerned about breed identification of a prospective cat than they would be in adopting a dog. If one wants a cat of a particular breed, one should go to a family breeder or cattery where loving attention and care

are given to the kittens. Breeders and catteries are also an excellent source for adoption of cats of mixed breed, loosely referred to as *domestic shorthairs or domestic longhairs*. At a breeder or cattery, one should look into behavioral predispositions of the dam and the sire and whether the kittens are all handled and socialized to people. If a cat is left alone with the mother and littermates, it may be very difficult to socialize to people later. Animal shelters usually have large numbers of kittens available for adoption and, in many instances, volunteer shelter personnel have devoted considerable hours to socializing these cats, making them good pets for adoption.

Behavioral Characteristics of Cat Breeds

What breed of cat is best with children? What would be the most appropriate breed for a single person who wants minimal interaction with a cat? These are the kinds of questions to ask anyone recommending a cat. As with dogs, one must be wary of trusting the tradebooks that deal with particular breeds; either they mention very little about behavior that can be counted on, or they point out only the desirable behavioral patterns of the breeds in question.

The information on the more common breeds presented here is from an informal survey of cat show judges who had a wealth of experience with various breeds.[3,4] Collectively, the judges emphasized that there are major individual differences in behavior between cats of the same breed, and that generalizations about a breed are not going to hold for all cats of that breed. Domestic shorthairs and domestic longhairs are more common than dogs of mixed breed, but are not included in the breed behavior profile.

Siamese

This most popular of all breeds originated in what is now Thailand and is reported to be the most outgoing with strangers and demanding of affection and attention. Although Siamese do not display the one-person cat behavior that we associate with more fearful cats, they become strongly attached to their owners and recognize their owner's voice at a distance. Siamese cats extensively vocalize in a style that many people refer to as "talking." They easily vary the pitch of their meows, especially if this gets a reaction from the owners. The vocalizations are objectionable to some people, especially in small apartments or when females come into estrus. Loving to be held, snuggled, and carried about, the Siamese can be a good choice for gentle children.

Burmese

Like their close Siamese relatives, the Burmese are reported to be demanding of affection. They are considered good family pets, if the family members want a cat that is affectionate, easygoing, and playful. Compared with the Siamese, they vocalize less and are less outgoing to strangers, but are not as withdrawn as some other breeds. This breed is considered suitable for a family with gentle children.

Persian

This breed, originating from what is now known as Iran, has a beautiful long fur coat that attracts many people. This beauty requires more upkeep, however, in combing and brushing. Behaviorally, these cats are reported to be somewhat reserved, inactive, and do not seek affection as do the Siamese. Seemingly not desiring close contact they are more comfortable with being petted as they lie on the floor. Persians have a dense and long hair coat and the aversion they seem to have to being held may reflect their tendency to get too warm on a person's lap. Persians are also not very active compared to other breeds and they may be the safest breed if one wants to avoid a song bird predator.

Himalayan

This breed has the heavy, short, well-rounded body and long fur of a Persian and the coloring of a Siamese, and its behavior is apparently intermediate between the two breeds. The Himalayan is not as outgoing to strangers as the Siamese but is not as reserved as the Persian. Like the Persian, a Himalayan may become too warm with close human contact and thus may not appreciate extensive cuddling.

Abyssinian

This breed is the most feral looking of the popular breeds and is reportedly usually more shy and fearful of strangers. The Abyssinian may be too nervous to make a good cat for children. Apparently it does not like snuggling as a lap cat, but enjoys being petted from a distance.

Manx

People are attracted to this breed by its overall roundness: a rounded head, arched back, round rump, and lack of a tail. The behavior of the Manx seems to be more variable than in other breeds. Some are apparently withdrawn and wary of strangers and others quite playful.

Russian Blue

Members of this breed are reportedly likely to be shy and withdrawn with a tendency to avoid strangers or visitors to the home. The dense, plush fur coat feels like a short-coated beaver. An unusual feature is the hair coat; trace a design in the coat with your finger and it remains.

Rex

People that are allergic to cats are often able to tolerate the Rex, which has no undercoat. Like the Russian Blue, members of this breed may also be withdrawn and shy.

Gender Considerations and Effects of Neutering

If a cat has a behavior problem that becomes intolerable to the owner, it is not going to be much of a companion. One of the most important behavioral problems in cats for which veterinary consultation is sought is urine spraying. In fact, because of the seriousness of the behavioral problem, the animal may have to be given up if therapeutic measures are not successful or the owner is unwilling to pay for medication needed to control the behavior (Chapter 21). Thus, the adoption process should take into account the likelihood that the cat will become a problem urine marker as an adult.

It is abundantly clear that females are much less likely to become problem urine markers or engage in fighting than neutered males. Therefore, by selecting a female the likelihood of having a cat that engages in urine marking and fighting can be minimized. The degree of difference between neutered males and females in a tendency to be problem urine markers is at least 2 to 1 and possibly as great as 5 to 1 (Chapter 21).

There is no information to suggest that breed differences, littermate composition, or early experiences are related to the occurrence of urine marking. Neutering as early as 1 or 2 months of age, as increasingly practiced at animal shelters, is not associated with adverse medical or behavioral conditions.[5,6] In males, castration somewhat later, but before puberty, seems to have about the same effectiveness in preventing urine marking as an adult castration of tomcats has in elimination of a urine marking problem (Chapter 21). In either case one can expect abut 10% of males to be problem urine markers.

Influence of Early Experience

In the neonatal period, a kitten is relatively nonresponsive to the rest of the world, but it is susceptible to tactile, olfactory, and thermal stimuli. Some handling appears to actually have effects that would be considered desirable in the sense that a brief period of being picked up and handled on a daily basis for a few minutes seems to activate or accelerate normal development. Under controlled conditions, Siamese kittens that are handled for as little as 10 minutes a day starting just after birth, are reported to have eyes open a day or so sooner than nonhandled kittens, and they develop the characteristic color pattern slightly earlier. Handled kittens emerge from the nest about 3 days sooner and, in general, are more active.[7] Beyond the neonatal period, handling kittens for several hours per week may increase their boldness and tendency to approach people.[8,9]

Although handling kittens that are with the mothers may have positive developmental effects, long-term social isolation from the mother can be detrimental. Among the studies revealing the detrimental effects of very early weaning is one showing that kittens separated from their mothers at about 2 weeks of age, even if left together with littermates, are likely to be more suspicious and cautious than those weaned at the usual time of 6–8 weeks.[10] These adverse effects of early weaning seem not to occur if kittens are left with the mothers until 4 weeks of age. This indicates that for separation from the mother to produce adverse behavioral effects it must occur at a very early age.

Although it has not been studied, there is reason to wonder if the wool chewing displayed by some cats of the Siamese and Burmese breeds might sometimes reflect the separation stress of early weaning—especially if these breeds are particularly sensitive to this separation process. Some breeders have reported that they are able to reduce this tendency in their line of cats by allowing the kittens to suckle the mother for longer than the normal weaning time. Because wool chewing or wool ingestion is a serious problem for some cats, especially of the Siamese and Burmese breed, it may be worth keeping this possibility in mind.

While with the mother and littermates, kittens go through an early socialization process that is particularly important with regard to developing suitable social interactions with people and other pets in the adoptive family. As a general rule 6–8 weeks of age would appear to be the best time to adopt a cat to enhance these effects. This gives the new owners ample time to facilitate socialization to people in the new home. If kittens are exposed to dogs early in life, they will often continue to be friendly to dogs, at least to the dogs the cat knows. In fact, about the only circumstance in which one sees a cat that is a "buddy" to the family dog is when the cat has been raised as a kitten with the dog.

Those cats who seem to do best in social interactions with other cats, and are the most tolerant of living in a household with other cats, are also those that have been exposed to other adult cats when growing up and that continue to live in a household with several cats. A cat that is adopted into a home with no other dogs or cats and is then exposed to dogs or other cats only as an adult, frequently reacts in an aggressive or withdrawn manner.

Fear of strange people can often be traced back to a lack of exposing the kitten to strangers, especially in a rewarding fashion. As the cat gets older and shows some timidity around people, forcing the cat to be held or handled by other people often will exacerbate the problem. This is one of those problem behaviors where one can take advantage of the ease with which cats may be socialized at an early age and before normal adultlike fear responses develop. When the cat shows some degree of fear or timidity around other people, the cat should not be forced on them but rather allowed to habituate to people gradually and given food treats for approaching and interacting with the visitors.

Avoiding Problem Behaviors

House Soiling

Undoubtedly what helps endear cats to people is the ease with which they can be "house-trained." Just add box and litter and the cat is house-trained. However, keep in mind that house soiling is the most frequent problem for which professional help is sought by cat owners. For adult cats this topic is handled in Chapter 21. There are some important principles to keep in mind in dealing with kittens that are expected to use a litter box. One is that they may have been accustomed to a certain type of litter or litter box in the previous home, cattery, or shelter, and if the cat was regularly using this litter box, it is best to try to duplicate that in the new home. In fact, as is explained later in this chapter, one should bring home some of the soiled litter of the kittens being adopted to act as a "starter" for the litter box in the new home.

Aside from this early experience, some types of litter are preferred by cats over others; the fine, clumping litter seems to be favored by most cats although it is not invariably the favorite.[11] Thus, if a kitten is not using a litter box regularly, one should offer the kitten its choice of two or three types of litter to see the one to which it is most attracted. Remember that cats do not necessarily want to use a litter box used by other cats—not a bad strategy for cats in nature. When introducing a kitten into a household where there is one or more other resident cats, it is important to bring in at least one other litter box.

Any stimulus that is frightening or creates an emotional reaction associated with a litter box may cause cats to use alternative toilet areas. As with cats in nature, a frightening experience in the toilet area could spell danger in the future and would naturally lead to choosing a safer area. If a puppy or child were to grab a kitten while it is using the new litter box this might be all that is needed for the cat to change litter habits to a corner of the carpet in the living room.

In nature a toilet area that has mild residual odors of urine and feces attracts use of this area, a behavior that helps keeps other areas in the territory clean. However, an area that is too soiled has the potential to be a land mine of intestinal parasites; the cat may choose a place just alongside the soiled area or start a new toilet area. With this background it is obvious that attention to litter box hygiene is important in reducing the likelihood of inappropriate elimination. The litter box should be cleaned of all waste material at least on a daily basis; twice a day is the best practice. If the litter box itself becomes visibly soiled with feces it is necessary to wash the box. Washing the box once a week is advisable. Because residual urine and fecal odors indicate a toilet area, it is important that at the first sign that a cat has chosen an alternative toilet area, one should immediately clean the area with an enzymatic cleaner. If possible one could also cover the area (with plastic sheeting) to make it unavailable or employ deterrents such as reverse sticky tape while doing all that is possible to make the litter box or boxes attractive.

Cats that are expected to spend some time outdoors present a somewhat different set of concerns. Cats can be encouraged to use one or two specific toilet spots outside by digging a shallow hole at least the size of a large litter box and adding an inch or two of sand. To further indicate that this is a toilet area one could add some fecal- or urine-tainted old litter material to begin the orientation. After it is being used, this area can then be cleaned and scooped out just as one would a litter box.

Management procedures to avoid house soiling problems should take into account the triggers of urine marking, especially agonistic interactions with other cats inside or outside the house. The onset of spraying is often related to unfriendly or agonistic interactions with other cats.[12] This can occur with the introduction of new cats into the household. If a cat seems to be having unfriendly interactions with other cats through a window or door, it is advisable to block this access so that it will not lead to in-house urine marking in the future. For the same reason, one should not let agonistic interactions between cats of the same household continue on a chronic basis within the house, but should make arrangements so that the cats each have their own primary domains of living area. Food and water availability should not be concentrated in one area nor should litter boxes all be placed in one area. It should be easy for the cats to withdraw from each other and live in separate areas. Later they can be gradually allowed more visual and physical contact.

Furniture Scratching

Scratching environmental objects is a natural behavior for wild or feral cats and is usually directed toward one or more prominent trees within the territory. By scratching, trees cats create scruffed-up visual marks which are overlaid with chemical marks from the feet. With free-ranging cats, such territorial marks are presumably noticed by feline intruders cruising through. At the same time as marking their territory, cats condition the claws of the front feet by removing the outer cuticle to expose a new sharp claw beneath.

Because scratching is a natural behavior, cats are going to attempt to scratch on some objects in whatever environments they find themselves. They are likely to seek substrates that are prominent, are vertical, and have the most suitable textures for scratching. Unfortunately this often ends up being furniture or drapes. After a cat starts to scratch an area, such as a corner of a couch, the scent glands in the feet allow a chemical mark to be deposited, and the cat is drawn back to that area to freshen the scent. This freshening up maintains an adequate visual marker—as on trees in nature—and adds a fresh olfactory marker that allows would-be intruders to know that the territory is occupied.

It is important to get a kitten started on an appropriate scratching object as soon as possible. If the kitten being adopted has been using a scratching post in the previous home, one should request also adopting the old scratching post and offering to pay for a replacement. This win-win offer allows the kitten to have a familiar scratching post in its new home so that at least one item in the new home will smell familiar. Furthermore, they are likely to continue scratching on this object rather than the couch. Irrespective of this ideal, most cats should be supplied with a scratching post or cardboard scratcher obtained at a pet store. The standard post should be turned on its side so that it is easy for the kitten to have access to it and later placed right side up. The corrugated cardboard scratchers, placed horizontally on the floor, have wide appeal among cats. In the area of free option for felines, one might even offer a cat the choice of suitable scratching objects in different locations to see which is preferred.

As soon as a kitten shows any tendency to scratch areas other than the acceptable area, one should thoroughly wash the scratched area with a strong detergent to remove oily foot-gland secretions, and if possible, the new target should be covered to make it temporarily unavailable. One could also use upside-down sticky tape to repel the cat from the previous target. The intended scratching area should immediately be made as appealing and accessible as possible. This may even mean testing different covering materials on the scratching post, offering a cardboard scratcher, and providing more than one scratching location in the house. The new scratching post or cardboard scratcher should be placed near the problem scratching area and later gradually moved to the side.

Biting or Scratching People

Biting or scratching people often reflects a rough style of play. Some cats may have experienced rough play sessions with a human family member where the kittens were encouraged or allowed to scratch or bite. Objectionable biting and scratching in older cats might be reduced through avoiding rough play with kittens. When biting or scratching does occur, discourage this behavior with the use of a water sprayer rather than directly hitting or pushing away the kitten; direct contact with the kitten may tempt it to bite or scratch playfully all the more. Keep in mind that biting or scratching are part of normal play and cannot be totally avoided. An acceptable outlet for such play is to fashion a string with a cloth tied to it and structure play sessions where the hands and feet of human family members are not used in play.

Predation

Many cat owners and environmentalists are concerned about the predation on birds by cats. The best solution is to keep cats inside always. For indoor-outdoor cats the best recommendation is to adopt a kitten from a litter in which the mother was a nonhunter. If the mother is known to stalk and kill songbirds and the kitten has been around that mother for a considerable period, the kitten is likely to have learned bird predatory behavior from the mother. There is a genetic component to the predatory behavior and, even if the kitten is adopted before it had any experience with the mother's hunting, it may still take up hunting birds. Previous research has shown that approximately half of cats that have never experienced predatory behavior by the mother will go on to develop predatory behavior.[13]

Conclusions

In addition to addressing the advantages of cats for certain households and human family life-styles, this chapter discusses sources of kittens that are important to consider from the standpoint of the behavior of the adult cat. Of primary importance are favorable social interactions with people in the natal family. The best time for adoption of a kitten is 6–8 weeks of age because this is a period when the cat can be easily socialized to people in the new home. In adopting a kitten that has established litter box and scratching routines, it is important to give consideration to using the same kind of litter material in the new home and the same scratching post.

Although breed selection is generally less a concern in adopting cats than it is in dogs, some prospective kitten owners will be interested in looking into the behavioral characteristics of various breeds. If one decides to get a purebred cat, it is usually necessary to go to a breeder or cattery. A primary concern in adopting a kitten from a cattery is whether there was adequate socialization through handling and playful interaction with the kitten by people prior to adoption. If such favorable social interaction is not the rule for that cattery, and one still wants to adopt a cat from the location, pushing the adoption age to 6 weeks or so may allow more adequate human socialization in the new home.

There are specific behavioral problems with adult cats that can be reduced in likelihood with attention to details either in the selection process or in raising kittens. A major concern is that of urine marking. Females are much less likely to become problem urine markers than neutered males. Kittens that are adopted into multicat households are more likely to take up urine marking, or evoke it in a resident cat, than kittens adopted into a home with no other cats. The safest bet for a cat that does not urine mark is a female in a single-cat household. Close attention to litter box hygiene helps prevent both inappropriate elimination as well as urine marking. Rough playful interaction with a kitten, where it is encouraged to scratch and bite, should be discouraged. Furniture scratching can wreak havoc with a new home, and here it is important to see that the cat has at least one acceptable and appealing scratching area. At the same time one should be vigilant for any sign of scratching damage to household furniture and take measures to prevent the behavior.

References

1. American Veterinary Medical Association. U.S. Pet Ownership and Demographics Sourcebook. Schaumburg, Ill: American Veterinary Medical Association, 1997.
2. Macdonald DW, Apps PJ, Carr GM, Kerby G. Social dynamics, nursing coalitions and infanticide among farm cats, *Felis catus*. Advances in Ethology 1987;28:1–64, Supplement to Ethology.
3. Hart BL. Breed-specific behavior. Feline Practice 1979;9(6):10–13.
4. ———. Prescribing cats. Feline Practice 1980;10(1):8–12.
5. Stubbs WP, Bloomberg MS, Scruggs SL, Shille VM, Lane TJ. Effects of prepubertal gonadectomy on physical and behavioral development in cats. Journal of the American Veterinary Medical Association 1996;209:1864–1872.
6. Spain CV, Scarlett JM, Houpt KA. Long-term risks and benefits of early-age gonadectomy in cats. Journal of the American Veterinary Medical Association 2004;224:372–386.
7. Meier GW. Infantile handling and development in Siamese kittens. Journal of Comparative Physiology and Psychology 1961;54:284–286.
8. Lowe SE, Bradshaw JWS. Ontogeny of individuality in the domestic cat in the home environment. Animal Behaviour 2001;61:231–237.
9. McCune S. The impact of paternity and early socialization on the development of cats' behavior to people and novel objects. Applied Animal Behaviour Science 1995;45:109–124.
10. Seitz P.F.D. Infantile experience and adult behavior in animal subjects. II Age of separation from the mother and adult behavior in the cat. Psychosomatic Medicine 1959;21:353–378.
11. Borchelt PL. Cat elimination behavior problems. Veterinary Clinical North American Small Animal Practice 1991;21:257–264.

12. Pryor PA, Hart BL, Bain MJ, Cliff KD. Causes of urine marking in cats and effects of environmental management on frequency of marking. Journal of the American Veterinary Medical Association 2001;219:1709–1713.
13. Caro TM. Effects of the mother, object play, and adult experience on predation in cats. Behavioral and Neural Biology 1980;29:29–51.

Section IV

Human-Companion Animal Interactions

The two chapters in this section are intended to help the clinician understand the role of the dog and cat in the lives of people and how this impacts the clinician's interaction with clients. Topics covered in Chapter 28 include health-related benefits of pets, dealing with disturbed clients, and community support of relationships with pets. In Chapter 29 the phenomenon of pet loss, and anticipation of the loss of a pet, is discussed along with suggestions for helping in these difficult times. Because of the relatively short life span of pet dogs and cats, pet loss emerges as a frequent and important consideration.

As most animal health care providers know, each animal is an individual, with specific unique habits and mannerisms. In fact, the intriguing and curious predictability of their special personalities, combined with some surprises, are what draw people to a particular animal. Knowing the animal well enough to recognize its unique qualities draws us closer and grabs our emotions. Skillful clinicians recognize these aspects of human-animal interactions in every client they deal with and express this acknowledgment to their clients. Although the particular traits of each animal are somewhat unique, our feelings for our animals, as we perhaps dote on them, may have similarities to those of other people as they are doting on their animals and for which they know the special behaviors and habits. The strong bonds of people with their companion animals serve as bridges for social interactions with other people. This is evident even for dog owners at a dog park, who may feel they share more with people there than with those they may meet at a cocktail party.

Veterinarians see clients who on average are willing to provide preventive and medical care and are more likely to retain the animal for its natural healthy lifetime. Veterinary clients invest time and money in looking after their animals, and they benefit from the veterinary guidance for enhancing the relationship with their animal. The committed clients take the steps they can to optimize and sustain a positive relationship with the animal. They are more likely than nonclients to know something about animal behavior and to be realistic in their expectations of the animal. Such clients are usually open to suggestions for avoiding or resolving problem behavior. These investments in a positive relationship position clients to enjoy the potential benefits of interacting with an animal, because living with unsolved behavior problems disrupts the quality of the relationship and can prevent clients from enjoying the pleasurable benefits of interacting with companion animals.

One might say that people can be themselves the most with their companion animals—playful, free, and nurturing. The childlike sweetness and simple needs of a pet are uncomplicated by content and lead to the well-known perspective that pets are not judgmental, never talk back, and are always welcoming. No wonder that in many cases the pet becomes part of a cherished emotional connection. Deep feelings within caregivers can arise, often unanticipated by the client. For some clients, especially those without close human companions, this becomes their most intimate relationship—comprised of joy and a sequence of dependable daily pleasures.

Clients with such beloved animals are likely to be the most conscientious in following instructions and willing to pay for a full range of health care services, including behavior therapy. Unlike the children of pet owners, the pets do not become independent, but are in a permanent dependent state when receiving medical care or assistance. Thus, for veterinarians, the strong emotions of people for their nonspeaking animals are inevitably a prominent force that arises in practice. Chapters 28 and 29 address the nature of the emotional bond, and how the bond may influence the approach of the clinician in dealing with clients and the implications of loss of a companion animal.

Chapter 28

Role of the Dog and Cat in Families

People often remember when they first adopted their companion animal and enjoy talking about how the relationship began; if the animal was injured or rescued, that in particular will be prominent. An animal may be the centerpiece of the client's daily routine, which includes nurturing the animal and drawing the person's attention outward. Inevitably, the animal stimulates interactions with other people and conversations about animals.

The relationship the person had with the animal is unique, but the person's aroused feelings can be understood by others who have had similar experiences. The clinician who accurately assesses the significance of the animal to the family is better prepared to make some estimates of the likely commitment of the family to solve behavior problems. This chapter presents the results of scientific studies on the role and impact of pets on their owners and the human family and society in general.

The Psychosocial and Health-Related Benefits of Animals

The beneficial effects of pets are perhaps most evident in providing companionship and preventing or alleviating depression. Among college women living alone, those with companion animals report being less lonely.[1] Similarly, among elderly women living alone, those with pets report less depression and more interest in planning for the future.[2] This comfort provided by companion animals is the most universally noticed benefit of sharing lives with them.

Protection from depression and loneliness are most reliably measured with people who are especially vulnerable to depression and to isolation.[3] Pets calm people with Alzheimer's disease such that their caregiving relatives report that they engage in fewer aggressive outbursts.[4] Companion animals can somewhat compensate for limited human social companionship, and this has been especially evident among bereaved elderly people who have lost a spouse. Those with companion animals are less likely to be depressed, especially if they are very attached to the animal.[5] Companion animals are protective against depression for people with AIDS, especially for those with few friends.[6]

Having a pet cannot cure cancer, resolve a cardiovascular disorder, or normalize the mental activities of someone with Alzheimer's disease, but pets can contribute to a better outcome. For example, pet owners have better average indicators of cardiovascular health, such as cholesterol and triglyceride levels, than nonowners.[7] Research that is now classical in the annals of health benefits of pets is the demonstration in two epidemiological studies of an enhanced likelihood of survival from heart attack for people with canine companionship.[8,9] The effect is of the same order as the well-known contribution of social support to recovery from heart attack.

Not only do animals themselves provide comfort, they also provide a medium for social contact among human companions. A pet, especially a dog, can become a hub for relationships with friends and family as a person moves through major landmarks in life, including residential moves, going away to school, marriage, and divorce. A dog or cat stimulates positive social approaches and conversations from other people apart from the immediate circle of family and friends. This social lubrication has been quantitatively documented; people walking their dogs in the park receive more social approaches and greetings than those without dogs, including even those with young children.[10] An assistance dog working in the service of someone in a wheelchair normalizes the social interactions with passersby.[11] Similarly a hearing dog normalizes the responses of people that interact with them in a public setting.[12]

Aside from companionship, social facilitation, and prevention of loneliness, there are other benefits. Inadequate exercise is a problem of almost epidemic proportion for people in modern society. The tremendous enjoyment that dogs express for going on walks motivates people to increase their amount of walking and regularly getting outside, meeting other neighbors and friends in the process.[13] Dogs motivate some people to take on an altruistic hobby—that of visiting long-term care centers for the elderly and disabled.

Not only dogs but a variety of animals inspire and motivate their human companions to provide social support to those in nursing homes where the visitors share this animal with the residents. The profound social movement of volunteers providing animal-assisted activities for residents of hospitals and residential nursing facilities is fueled by the joy of sharing companion animals.

These various benefits are best experienced in highly compatible human-animal relationships. Severe behavior problems can disrupt the relationship and upset the person to such an extent that these benefits do not occur. As with any relationship, some challenges in the animal's behavior are to be expected. Even people with well-trained hearing dogs reported some behavior problems in half of the cases.[14] This was a challenge not anticipated by people awaiting placement of a hearing dog and is estimated to involve about half of the dogs placed with hearing-impaired people. Clearly, increasing use of dogs in the service of people is going to be accompanied by a lack of realistic knowledge that animals present behavioral challenges that need to be addressed as one goes along. This is necessary to maintain and nurture the high quality of the relationship.

The Human-Animal Bond in Selecting and Raising a Dog or Cat

Ideally, a client would consult with the veterinarian prior to acquiring the animal to gain some assistance in thinking through how the proposed animal will mesh with the client's life-style, what will be required in caring for the animal, and whether the proposed animal is a good fit in this particular family setting. In the ideal situation, the family is off to a good start and makes the initial appointment to have the animal checked over and perhaps get a schedule for immunizations. Regardless of the state of the family's relationship with the animal at the first office visit, some clinicians schedule a longer initial appointment when a new animal is acquired and provide the client an educational introduction to the anticipated life stages of the animal, including the typical lifespan. This is especially helpful for clients with large dogs with a short life expectancy. Such meetings with a new client are an opportunity to demonstrate the tone of respect that is most desired by the client. Preparing the client with information concerning the species and breed behaviors, listening carefully to the client's concerns, and referring to the animal by name are behaviors of the veterinarian that the client notices and values most.[15] Although clients seem to take for granted that the veterinarian will provide excellent medical care to the animal, they scrutinize the way they are treated, valuing being treated with respect as the most essential of traits. Getting off to a good beginning, a veterinarian can strongly advocate a puppy class for dogs and even "kitty kindergarten" for cats, as well as permanent microchip identification of the animal, actions that reduce the likelihood of later relinquishment or loss of the animal.

Unfortunately, when acquiring their animals, many people still make their decisions without knowing that some challenges are inevitable. Bringing home a dog that is likely to be too aggressive around young children, or a cat that is probably not going to be as affectionate as desired by the client, are examples. Thus, right from the beginning, the veterinarian's first contact with the animal may be one where already the client is asking for help in improving the animal's behavior. Even though the misbehavior appears within a day or two of adopting the animal and the relationship quickly has become problematic, usually the family has become attached to the animal and hopes to resolve the problem. They may feel distressed from being concerned as to whether the problem can be resolved. The fresh anticipation of enjoying the new animal already is jeopardized by the immediate appearance of problems.

A person's past experience and family tradition with animals inevitably shape emotional feelings about the species, breed, appearance, and behaviors of a prospective companion animal. Thus, a person's previous experiences create an expectation and some knowledge of what to expect in living with this animal. Layered upon this perspective are societal changes still in progress; older people who grew up surrounded by farm animals and outdoor dogs today may reside in small apartments that they find inadequate for dogs.

Someone looking for an active companion who will join in jogging is likely to be happiest with a medium or large dog, whereas someone interested in a sedate or cuddly cat may plan mostly to spend time at home with the animal. Although the number of dogs in the United States is stable or declining, the increasing number of cats reflects the smaller family size, the increased time many people spend away from home, and a generally more complex life-style. Either a cat or dog can provide inestimable comfort, companionship, and entertainment while also being a welcoming presence in the home. Clients who think in advance about their particular situation in the context of their home prior to acquiring companion animals, are more likely to be content in their evolving relationships with the animals.

With regard to dogs in general, they are interactive, and to a varying extent, they require considerable interaction throughout the day. Enjoying walks, greeting their owners, being affectionate, and seeming intelligent and expressive, dogs are remarkably consistent, and these are the traits that we find so endearing. That said, breeds show a remarkable range in physical and behavioral attributes. People differ in their perceptions about what comprises the ideal dog. Not surprisingly, the idealized behavioral traits judged as most important in a dog almost perfectly matched the behavior of dogs owned by those responding to the questions.[16]

The consistent increase in the popularity of cats as companion animals reflects the changing demographics and growing urbanization in the United States. Shifting to smaller family households and smaller living quarters, such as condominiums, fewer people can easily accommodate the daily requirements and provide the social interaction that most dogs need. Many people cannot consistently walk a dog daily, nor can they easily make satisfactory arrangements for the dogs when they leave town. Cats are less demanding of attention. They can be more self-sufficient. Clients can leave the cat alone for a 10-hour day and not fret that the cat's social needs are being compromised. Even being gone for an overnight can be dealt with more easily than with a dog. In short, it is possible for clients to enjoy cats with a clear conscience and without feeling seriously encumbered by the responsibilities of providing the time-intensive care often needed by a dog.

A further advantage of cats as pets is that they are suitable for someone who is bedridden or weakened by poor health. They provide warm comfort and acceptance without requiring frequent interactions, playing, and walks. The client is free to enjoy the animal with relatively minimal requirements to provide care.

As mentioned, the profound benefits of relationships with companion animals can be eroded or even obliterated if behavior problems intrude. By now many studies of people who adopt and relinquish companion animals reveal some simple steps toward success in relationships with companion animals. Selecting an animal that is likely to be manageable and fit the family's life-style is the first step. Being aware of the basic responsibilities and some guidelines of pet ownership at the beginning prepares the family. Promoting an understanding of behavior is a part of a full-service animal health practice, just as is providing identification by means of microchips; managing reproduction; and providing veterinary care, nutritious food, and adequate shelter. Being a good canine or feline neighbor is increasingly important as objectionable barking, roaming, and aggression in dogs have become profiled as a social issue—as has predation on birds by cats.

Coping with Disturbed Clients

A real problem for veterinarians and their staffs are the difficult clients. Some clients facing financial straits, believing veterinarians may offer services out of their love for animals in general, may seek or expect free or low-cost veterinary care. Clients who are extremely disturbed may make verbal or physical threats against the veterinary team, or even threaten suicide. As part of the general preparation of the veterinary team for crisis management, veterinarians need an explicit plan and strategy for dealing with difficult, disturbed, or violent individuals. Although violent occurrences are rare, their tragic potential merits careful thought. The veterinary group should be alert to problems that develop and have knowledge of appropriate interventions and ready access to emergency services. Phone numbers for police, the poison control center, an emergency ambulance, suicide centers, and emergency rooms should be available. Establishing a network with mental health professionals in the community makes help accessible when it is required.

Less dangerous to the veterinary team, but still challenging, are clients who have such strong emotional ties to their animals that their attachment may impede resolution of some medical problems. These clients may experience anxiety or depression when their animals require veterinary care. Active listening in a calm, relaxing setting with clear communication can facilitate interactions with these clients. Speaking slowly with simple words and writing down instructions can be helpful. Maintaining eye contact while listening to the client's experiences with the animal can facilitate management of clients with special needs. Among people that are most likely to have such strong attachments are the elderly, clients living alone with an animal, clients with disabilities and with assistance animals, and clients with a recent loss of a family member.[17]

From the moment a client enters the office, offering a comforting and soothing environment at the clinic can reduce a person's anxiety, especially among those who are already concerned about a pet's medical problems. Soft lighting, attractive artwork, beautiful scenes or views, and comfortable furniture make it easier to start off on a positive note with relaxed communication.

A universal finding is that clients of all types want to be treated with respect. From the standpoint of the family veterinarian, ways of expressing such respect are listening carefully and knowing the animal's name and breed traits.[15] Apparently, clients take for granted that the veterinarian will provide excellent veterinary care, so they may tend to focus on whether the veterinarian pays full attention to their concerns. A safe assumption is that it is hard to exaggerate the importance of the animal to the person. In one widely cited study, clients consistently rated the importance of their animals higher than their veterinarians rated the importance of the animal to them.[18] Biomedical advances for humans have been paralleled by enhanced veterinary care, as represented in the wide range of specialties. At the same time, veterinary clients themselves have come to expect being treated with respect and compassion.

Today's veterinarians realize they are dealing with families. Successful veterinarians build lifelong relationships with families and their animals, addressing their specific needs. For families with children, pets are special friends and confidants that provide experience in nurturing.[19] Child-friendly practices provide a play area with toys and include the children in examinations and discussions of the animal's behavior.

Caring clinicians can anticipate their clients' needs and help them avoid problems by facilitating or providing information about puppy and dog obedience classes. Veterinarians can enhance harmonious relationships regarding animals among the various constituencies of the community by providing leadership in conflict resolution. An increasing practice among veterinarians is to sponsor puppy socialization classes. This practice not only helps recruit loyal clients but conveys an ambience of respect and caring. As respected members of the community with integrity, veterinarians can assume an informed middle-road position in seeking to solve problems.

To the extent possible, successful veterinarians provide personalized care and understanding as they address the special needs of their clients. Physical disabilities, grief, hospitalization, allergies, immunocompromised status, and caring for an assistance animal are a few of the particular circumstances that affect needs of veterinary clients.[17] Veterinarians who can respond appropriately to the particular needs of their clients inspire great loyalty and respect.

Some clinicians manage to develop a niche practice that attracts a particular category of pets. A veterinarian who has special expertise with cats, for example, will find that the word spreads among those pet owners; that part of the practice may expand because the clients with these species are very confident that their pets will get optimal care. It is also probably more incumbent on a veterinarian in a species specialty to become more knowledgeable about behavior and behavior problems than the generalist.

Community Support of Compatible Relationships with Pets

The local community sets a context that affects the convenience of pet keeping. Having available housing where pets are permitted and ready access is provided to dog exercise areas and pet kenneling simplifies the responsibilities and complications that pets impose on a family. For an individual wanting to keep a pet, these amenities comprise a supportive environment that increases the likelihood of responsible pet ownership.

Some companion animals, especially dogs, assume specialized roles as service dogs to assist with various disabilities. Other clients prepare their animals to participate in animal-assisted activities or therapy. Effective practitioners attend to particular needs of clients whose dogs perform special roles in addition to serving as companions. Even so, the community as a whole faces inevitable challenges and conflicts related to animals. The rural, urban, and suburban backgrounds of residents lead to contrasting expectations on how dogs and cats should live. People who live alone, or who are elderly or with disabilities, may have particular requirements for assistance with their animals. Retirement facilities and those offering assisted care, as well as landlords allowing pets in rental properties, will consider appropriate policies that limit property damage by pets and their intrusions on other residents. Interventions may be required for individuals who are suicide prone and for whom pets offer life-saving benefits.

Uses of space for dog parks and policies regarding feral cats are topics that can polarize communities. Fortunately, the issues are being addressed at the community level. Unwelcome natural disasters precipitously demand attention and care for animals and also involve dealing with the strong emotions of the animals' caregivers. Each of these many topics has been a focus of scientific study, and a variety of information resources is available.[20] Issues involving animals that cannot be ignored, such as the development of an off-leash dog park, invariably are thrust upon communities. Veterinarians are the best-positioned individuals to provide leadership and assist in bringing together the various community constituencies to seek solutions. Veterinarians are viewed with respect and their breadth of knowledge and experience uniquely prepares them for assisting in this kind of community problem solving.

Recognizing the crucial role of animals, cities, states, and the nation offer some legal protection for people with disabilities to keep animals, especially when they reside in assisted housing. A broader appreciation in society for the psychosocial value of relationships with pets has led to a greater support for animals and willingness to offer some accommodations for pet keeping. Veterinarians can provide informed leadership within the workplace and the broader community, paving the way for enhanced relationships with animals.

References

1. Zasloff RL, Kidd AH. Loneliness and pet ownership among single women. Psychological Reports 1994;75:747–752.
2. Goldmeier J. 1986. Pets or people: Another research note. Gerontologist 1986;26:203–206.
3. Hart LA. Psychosocial benefits of annual companionship. In: Fine A, ed. Handbook of Animal Assisted Therapy. New York: Academic Press, 1999:59–78.
4. Fritz, CL, Farver TB, Kass PH, Hart LA. Association with companion animals and the expression of noncognitive symptoms in Alzheimer's patients. Journal of Nervous and Mental Disease 1995;183:359–363.
5. Garrity TF, Stallones L, Marx MB, Johnson TP. Pet ownership and attachment as supportive factors in the health of the elderly. Anthrozoös 1989;3:35–44
6. Siegel JM, Angulo FJ, Detels R, Wesch, J, Mullen A. AIDS diagnosis and depression in the Multicenter AIDS Cohort Study, the ameliorating impact of pet ownership. AIDS Care 1999;11:157–170.
7. Anderson W, Reid P, Jennings GL. Pet ownership and risk factors for cardiovascular disease. Medical Journal of Australia 1992;157:298–301.
8. Friedmann E, Katcher AH, Lynch JJ, Thomas SA. 1980. Animal companions and one-year survival of patients after discharge from a coronary unit. Public Health Reports 1980;95:307–312.
9. Friedmann E, Thomas SA. Pet ownership. Social support, and one-year survival after acute myocardial infarction in the Cardiac Arrhythmia Suppression Trial (CAST). American Journal of Cardiology 1995;76:1213–1217.
10. Messent P. Correlates and effects of pet ownership. In: Anderson RK, Hart BL, Hart LA, eds. The Pet Connection: Its Influence on Our Health and Quality of Life, Minneapolis, Minnesota: Center to Study Human-Animal Relationships and Environments, University of Minnesota, 1984:331–340.
11. Eddy J, Hart LA, Boltz RP. The effects of service dogs on social acknowledgments of people in wheelchairs. Journal of Psychology 1988;122:39–45.
12. Hart LA, Zasloff RL, Benfatto AM. The socializing role of hearing dogs. Applied Animal Behaviour Science 1996;47:7–15.

13. Serpell J. Beneficial effects on pet ownership on some aspects of human health and behavior. Journal of the Royal Society of Medicine 1991;84:717–720.

14. Hart LA, Zasloff RL, Benfatto AM. The pleasures and problems of hearing dog ownership. Psychological Reports 1995;77:969–970.

15. Case DB. Survey of expectations among clients of three small animal clinics. Journal of the American Veterinary Medical Association 1988;192:498–502.

16. Serpell J. The personality of the dog and its influence on the pet-owner bond. In: Katcher AH, Beck AM, eds. New Perspectives on Our lives with Companion Animals. Philadelphia: University of Pennsylvania Press, 1983:57–63.

17. AVMA Committee on the Human-Annual Bond. AVMA guidelines for responding to clients with special needs. Journal of the American Veterinary Medical Association 1995;206:961–976.

18. Catanzaro TE. A survey on the question of how well veterinarians are prepared to predict their client's human-animal bond. Journal of the American Veterinary Medical Association 1988;192:1707–1711.

19. Melson GF, Schwarz RL, Beck AM. Importance of companion animals in children's lives—Implications for veterinary practice. Journal of the American Veterinary Medical Association 1997;211:1512–1518.

20. http:www.vetmed.ucdavis.edu/AnimalAlternatives/main.htm.

Chapter 29
Dealing with Loss of the Companion Animal

Having a good beginning in the relationship with the client and the companion animal paves the way for the veterinarian to offer support at the end of the animal's life. By preparing clients in advance to deal with animals that are dying, veterinarians can alleviate some of the inevitable distress experienced by clients and the veterinary staff. Clients who are fully conscious of the shorter life span of their animals from the time of acquisition may be somewhat less shocked by a dog's death at the age of 10 years, or a cat's at 15 years. As specific preparation for dealing with the death of animals, veterinarians can polish their skills for helping clients by reading up on methods for dealing with this issue.[1] To prepare clients, clinicians can talk about the expected life cycle of the particular breed and give clients some preparation for pregrief therapy.

Caring for an Aging Pet

A prelude to the loss of a pet is often a period of physical and mental decline. Caring for an aging pet can be very stressful. A clinician can offer some guidelines to make life more comfortable and reduce stress for both the pet and the caregiver. When a pet has special requirements for care, the human caregiver can benefit by learning efficient and labor-saving methods of assuring comfort for the pet.[2] Arthritis is one of the most common ailments of aging animals; specialized diets or food supplements might delay or ameliorate discomfort while promoting optimal health. Accommodations such as padded ramps and beds, nonslip floors, and elevated bowls facilitate the animal's mobility and functioning. Visual and auditory impairments are also common in aging animals. A consistent environment with frequent verbal communication helps animals with visual decrements. Animals that are hard of hearing are assisted by hand signals, clapping, or stamping on the floor to get the animal's attention. House soiling can particularly challenge the caregiver's patience. This problem can be managed with reduced effort by using diapers, floor or bed liners, barriers to protect certain rooms, and easy access to the outdoors.

Emotional Impact of Loss of a Companion Animal

In any clinical practice, the client's loss of a companion animal poses a challenge that is stressful to both clients and their practitioners. The loss is most devastating in long-term relationships where the person has enjoyed a myriad of daily routines with the animal over many years. Often the clinician has been part of this satisfying relationship, and effects of the loss radiate through the clinic as well.

Effects of Pet Loss on Veterinary Hospital Staff

Veterinarians as a group are closely attached to animals, both their own pets and those in their practice. Inevitably, involvement in animal death inflicts pain and stress on the veterinary staff. In a study of veterinarians in England, half reported they had felt guilty after euthanizing a pet; virtually all remembered the death of a pet of their own and 22% reported that the death of one of their own pets had led to long-term emotional effects.[3] Euthanasia encounters of veterinarians inevitably resonate with their previous experiences, and they represent the most time-consuming and emotionally wearing clinical exchanges in which veterinarians are routinely involved.[4] Not surprisingly, veterinarians may feel a need, as a way of coping, to separate themselves emotionally from routinely dealing in death. Given their own extensive involvement in such experiences, veterinarians may not always perceive that some clients are extremely emotionally involved with their animals.

In dealing with animals nearing the end of their lives it is important to recognize and express the unique qualities of each animal. Veterinarians and their staff, in the course of working for years with a particular family and animal, have learned a great deal about the nature of the relationship between a client and their animal. They can prepare the veterinary staff for offering the appropriate care for the particular situation. In general, those individuals who seek out regular veterinary care for their animals truly value their relationship with their animals and can be presumed to be among the more closely attached individuals. They are a group who are most closely bonded and attached to their animals. Information about the extent to which an animal is a member of the family, and how upset a family would be if something happened to the animal, has revealed that veterinarians and their staff may underestimate these aspects of attachment.[5]

For a protracted illness, especially one leading to death, the veterinarian is faced with weighing the extent of the animal's discomfort, illness, and care required with the commitment and ability of the client's family to provide the daily assistance that the animal may require. For an animal with a disabling illness, knowing convenient methods to provide comfort and palliative care to the animal allows the client to carry on and also know that the animal continues to enjoy life to the extent possible. As with aging pets, clients frequently require education in methods for providing the animal with a good quality of life, comfort, nutrition, and supportive care. A goal is that the animal's end of life and death occur with full respect and honoring of the animal to help the client avoid regret and guilt, while also doing well by the animal.

Preparing the Client for Loss of the Companion Animal

Nothing can prepare a person for the unexpected sudden death or disappearance of an animal. The shock reverberates within the person, sometimes for an extended period of time, and the person may not be able to accept such a piercing loss. This loss is exemplified in the following quotation from a bereaved client. "Loss leads us to have new identities. We are not the same person we were before the loss. Because my babe Phoebe died unexpectedly in November, I find even colors seem different to me. We buried her under our red dogwood, which was then brown sticks, of course, but is now gloriously deep pink. It's never been so beautiful. And I feel it as Phoebe emerging" (Ann, personal communication, April 2003). Clearly, the attending veterinarian is also impacted by this disrupted relationship. Although the loss cannot be ameliorated, the veterinarian can offer supportive understanding of the magnified effect of this particular circumstance as the person slowly evolves toward some acceptance.

In some situations that involve a highly vulnerable person, the likelihood of extreme grief can be anticipated and some preparations made in advance.[6] Veterinarians know their clients and often have identified extremely emotional ones early, usually prior to a crisis. Difficult grief is more likely for anyone who has especially strong emotional ties to an animal, including those who have suffered recent human losses, live alone, are unemployed, and/or have little social support. Grief is also more likely for those who feel guilty about causing the death of the animal, who have rescued the animal, who have experiences with the same disease as the animal, or who consider the animal a last link with another person who is deceased.

Children or elderly persons may be especially affected by a loss. Clients with physical disabilities, including those with assistance animals and those with particular medical needs, require special consideration. Understanding and anticipating the special needs for support of these individuals can buffer the stressful process of the animal's death. Clinicians are advised to provide a quiet place for upset clients, personally advise clients on sensitive matters involving an animal's death, and develop a specific protocol for euthanasia of companion animals. Veterinarians should be prepared for occasions when clients may become inappropriately angry, aggressive, or suicidal, with an unanticipated aspect of loss or impending loss of a beloved pet.

Conducting Euthanasia with Respect for the Animal and Client

Deciding where and when to perform the euthanasia, or otherwise accommodating clients, is a first step that can increase the comfort for the client and animal even before the event. A study in Ontario, Canada, indicated that virtually all clinics scheduled euthanasia at quiet times during the day or evening and most offered to perform euthanasia at clients' homes.[7] For many clinicians, performing euthanasia is the most difficult aspect of their practice. If some principles are followed, this process may proceed more comfortably for the clinician, the client, and the patient. In fact, the more authoritative, relaxed, and calm the clinician is, the better things will go for the client. As implied, complete respect for the animal, the client, and the animal's body is an essential hallmark of the occasion of euthanasia. It is worthwhile to think methodically about and develop a euthanasia protocol that establishes a basic foundation for effective practice in this challenging area.[6] The practitioner then can fine-tune the basic protocol to fit particular needs of the presenting situation. Some items to consider include promptly selecting a special time and place, making arrangement for the animal's remains, and explaining the procedure simply. One should discuss the animal's reactions beforehand and offer time for the client with the animal prior to euthanasia. Sending a sympathy card is clearly in order as is handling the billing in a sensitive fashion.[8]

When euthanasia of an animal is performed, members of the family are in a state where they scrutinize and bring their full emotional sensitivity to the entire proceeding. What might appear to others to be a minute aspect of the occasion can become a riveting memory for the person. For example, if the animal is not carried in a comfortable way, or the animal's body is not treated with full respect and presented in an attractive manner, the person may focus grief and anger on that aspect. Occasions of euthanasia are significant family ceremonies that require the thoughtful preparation of the veterinary staff. Some features of a euthanasia generalize across many situations, such as sedating the animal prior to the euthanasia. Some clients prefer conducting a euthanasia in a special location where they and the animal are comfortable, such as their living room or backyard.

When dealing with grieving clients, veterinarians are advised to meet with the client in a quiet area, leaning forward attentively with eye contact, and speaking slowly and clearly with the client. If information needs to be given, such as the names of pet cemeteries or memorial sites, this should be written down because clients are distracted and find it difficult to remember.[9]

The Experience of the Clients During Euthanasia of a Companion Animal

The memory of the day an animal is euthanized pierces the person's reality and the details persist as visual images that intrude or can continue to be recalled. The client may repeatedly review the process of deciding on the euthanasia, questioning whether it was the right decision. The experience of another bereaved client, Barbara, offers some insights. "She was taken to the pet cemetery for her last resting place. She was lying on her pillow, tucked in with her blankets, a couple little angels, St. Francis statue, some favorite toys, tee-shirts, and sweater." The daily routine of life is changed forever. "I can still see her, telling me it's time to take a nap. When we got up, she would run to the kitchen and sit by the cabinet to wait for her pill. She wouldn't start to eat her dinner till I got her vitamin pill . . . how she'd grab a toy and run and wait for me to chase her. After 17 years, part of my life is gone. It will never be the same.

"He said everything had been done for her medically and love. Her precious little body had just 'given out,' regardless of how much I loved her and she loved me and she had the very best life anyone could have . . . but many times I feel there must have been something else that I could have done" (Barbara, personal communication, October 10, 2001).

For some clients, being in the room is helpful in finding closure. Veterinarians may have concerns about including the client, fearing the reactions of the animal or client and the increased emotion of the occasion. Increasingly, though, clients insist on choosing the details of the occasion, sometimes preferring that the euthanasia be conducted elsewhere than the clinic, and expecting to be present. Those who do not may later suffer regret. "I only wish I could have stayed in the room with her till the very last. Although she was not alone and someone she really liked was with her, she trusted me and I should have been with her." (Barbara, personal communication, 2002).

Stages of Grief and Emotional Healing

It is now well established that a caregiver of a companion animal that has died goes through the complex process of grief that is seen in people grieving the loss of a loved one. Grief in general from loss of a loved one is characterized as proceeding through five stages, including denial, anger, bargaining, depression, and acceptance.[9] A general pattern of initial disbelief, followed by anguish and upset, may resolve over time to acceptance. The time course and array of painful feelings are unique for each person. Veterinarians can draw from the theoretical framework and practical suggestions offered by authors in pet loss and grief resolution.[1] The qualities of grieving can cover a spectrum of manifestations, such as physical crying or nausea, intellectual denial or confusion, emotional sadness or anger, social withdrawal, and spiritual bargaining. When dealing with a grieving client, veterinarians are advised to assume a role as educator, support person facilitator, and resource and referral guide.

A particularly destructive aspect of electing euthanasia for companion animals is that caregivers often then are burdened with extraordinary feelings of guilt stemming from their responsibility for the animal's death. Among callers to a pet loss support hotline, 41% expressed feelings of guilt, and 4% had pondered suicide.[10] Another study found about half of participants felt guilty about their decision to euthanize their pet, and 16% said they felt like a murderer.[7]

The veterinary staff can provide essential emotional support before and after a euthanasia by listening sensitively and accepting the grief as clients express it. Providing time to discuss the euthanasia and aftercare options assists clients in mentally preparing.

The Magnitude and Extent of Grief Following Animal Loss

The veterinary profession over the past decade has embraced the significance to clients of losing their animals, providing grief support and referrals to pet loss support groups or hotlines. Many veterinarians send cards or flowers to clients following the death of an animal and check in with clients who live alone during the initial weeks following the loss. What might be surprising to many is the duration of grieving. In a study of people who had called pet loss support hotlines, it is clear that grief may be extremely prolonged. For some people, the extreme grief never really resolves and the person may feel that life will never be the same. Many people may take a year of holidays and experiences without the animal before they fully understand and accept that their companion is really gone. For bereaved clients it is not unreasonable to send a card of remembrance of the animal 1 year after the death, to acknowledge the special qualities and honor the memory of that animal. Veterinarians themselves are deeply attached to their animals and may grieve for many years following the death of a special animal. Veterinarians commonly express having feelings of deep attachment to animals themselves. By realizing that clients may have similar feelings, they can more easily understand their clients' distress.

As has been found in studies of grieving for human family members, people have various methods for coping, and the patterns of grieving differ with the individual. Upon losing the unconditional love, companionship, and daily routines with their animal, some people are absolutely devastated and may feel they have lost a life line. Individuals suffering prolonged grief benefit from support of friends and may rely on comfort and guidance from the veterinarian. They may need to express their grief in a particular way by memorializing the animal in a ceremony or with some other remembrance. Pet loss support groups and hotlines provide essential support for some persons.

The proliferation of virtual cemeteries on websites is a clear testimony to the widespread need of many people to express their grief and acknowledge the special and unique traits of their beloved animals. They offer a low- or no-cost and convenient way to recognize and memorialize their animal while retaining their personal privacy. Many of these websites address the concept of animals in heaven, attesting to the compelling wish for the relationship to be continued and to be reunited with the animal. Perusing some of these sites reveals a window on the emotions people feel at such times. Viewing some of these brings home a reality that many people grieve deeply at the time of such a loss.

Turning to Barbara once again, one can see that each client seeks an appropriate source of comfort. "Not a day goes by without some tears. There are very few people that understand my feelings. Everyone has families, and because I'm alone, there is no one to really talk to. What has really helped is keeping journals. Since the day I lost her, I've written eight volumes with thoughts, remembrances, poems, prayers . . .. I feel so guilty because I did what had to be done. I feel like I really let her down, but there was nothing else medically or otherwise that could be done. Will I ever get over this feeling? Are there other people that feel this way? There are times I feel that she is near and I can almost touch her, then know it's not possible."

References

1. Lagoni L, Butler C, Hetts S. 1994. The Human-Animal Bond and Grief. Philadelphia: W.B. Saunders Co.

2. Hart LA, Dorairaj K, Camacho S, Hart BL. Nurturing older dogs: Attitudes and experiences of caregivers. Journal of the American Veterinary Medical Association 2001; 37:307–310.

3. Fogle B, Abrahamson D. Pet loss: A survey of the attitudes and feelings of practicing veterinarians. Anthrozoös 1990;3:143–150.

4. Sanders CR. Killing with kindness: Veterinary euthanasia and the social construction of personhood. Sociological Forum 1995;10:195–214.

5. Catanzaro TE. A survey on the question of how well veterinarians are prepared to predict their client's human-animal bond. Journal of the American Veterinary Medical Association 1988;192:1707–1711.

6. Hart LA, Hart BL, Mader B. Humane euthanasia and companion animal death: Caring for the animal, the client, and the veterinarian. Journal of the American Veterinary Medical Association 1990;197:1292–1299.

7. Adams CL, Bonnett BN, Meek AH. Predictors of owner response to companion animal death in 177 clients from 14 practices in Ontario. Journal of the American Veterinary Medical Association 2000;217:1303–1309.

8. AVMA Committee on the Human-Animal Bond. AVMA guides for responding to clients with special needs. Journal of the American Veterinary Medical Association 1995;206:961–976.

9. Kubler-Ross E. On Death and Dying. New York: Collier Books/Macmillan, 1969.

10. Mader B, Hart LA. Establishing a model pet loss support hotline. Journal of the American Veterinary Medical Association 1992;200:270–274.

Index

DATE DUE

OCT 2 1 2010			
SEP 0 4 2019			
GAYLORD			PRINTED IN U.S.A.